Cardiac Pathology

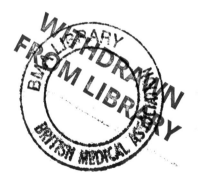

S. Kim Suvarna

Editor

Cardiac Pathology

A Guide to Current Practice

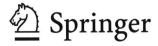 Springer

Editor
S. Kim Suvarna, MB, BS, BSc, FRCP, FRCPath
Histopathology
Sheffield Teaching Hospitals
Sheffield
UK

ISBN 978-1-4471-2406-1   ISBN 978-1-4471-2407-8   (eBook)
DOI 10.1007/978-1-4471-2407-8
Springer Dordrecht Heidelberg New York London

Library of Congress Control Number: 2012943693

Printed on acid-free paper

Springer is part of Springer Science+Business Media (www.springer.com)

Preface

Having a personal passion for education and a strong interest in cardiac pathology, it was an honour to be asked to edit and help produce *Cardiac Pathology: A Guide to Current Practice*. Reflecting upon current and previous trainees reminded me that more than just pathology is required for a good understanding of cardiac pathology. With this consideration in mind, the chapters include cardiac embryology, therapeutics, modern imaging techniques and cardiac electrophysiology. It is hoped that better understanding of these areas, alongside the cardiac pathology, will allow an enhanced ability when considering surgical cardiac pathology specimens and routine/specialised autopsy workload.

Cardiac Pathology: A Guide to Current Practice aims to support the daily work of those active in this field of medicine. I hope it is clear and easy to use whether one is a pathology trainee, senior practitioner or a non-pathologist working within the wider cardiac medical/surgical arenas.

This book owes much to the work and support of others. Firstly, the chapter authors deserve credit for their hard work and enthusiasm. Secretarial support and diligence with the revisions and editing process has been provided by Seonaid Ashby. Connie Walsh and the Springer staff have to be thanked for editorial guidance and incredible patience! I am grateful for the new elegant line drawings created by Jeremy Chui and Adam Parsons. Finally, as the book came towards completion, I found myself aware of my gratitude for the general encouragement towards things academic from my parents many years ago, and currently to Grace, Miranda and Elara for allowing me the time to indulge myself in this project.

January 2012 , Sheffield   S. Kim Suvarna

Contents

Contributors

Abdallah Al-Mohammad, M.D., FRCP(Edin), FRCP(Lond) Department of Cardiology, Northern General Hospital, Sheffield Teaching Hospitals NHS Foundation Trust, Sheffield, UK

Michael T. Ashworth, M.D., FRCPath Department of Histopathology, Great Ormond Street Hospital for Children, London, UK

Ulrik Baandrup, M.D., Ph.D. Department of Pathology, Center for Clinical Research, Vendsyssel Hospital, Aalborg University, Hjoerring, Denmark

Peter W. G. Brown, MBChB, FRCS(Ed), FRCR Department of Diagnostic Imaging, Sheffield Teaching Hospitals NHS Foundation Trust, Sheffield, UK

Susan J. Davies, MBBS, FRCPath Department of Histopathology, Papworth Hospital, Papworth Everard, Cambridge, UK

Siân Hughes, MBBS, M.Sc., Ph.D., FRCPath Department of Histopathology, University College Hospital London, London, UK

Peter R. Jackson, Ph.D., FRCP, FFPM(Dis) Department of Pharmacology and Therapeutics, Royal Hallamshire Hospital, Sheffield, UK

Department of Clinical Medicine, Sheffield Teaching Hospitals NHS Foundation Trust, Sheffield, UK

Katarzyna Michaud, M.D. Department of Community Medicine and Public Health, University Hospital of Lausanne, University Center of Legal Medicine of Lausanne and Geneva, Lausanne, Switzerland

Paul D. Morris, BMedSci(Hons), MBChB(Hons), MRCP(Edin) Department of Cardiology, Sheffield Teaching Hospitals NHS Foundation Trust, Sheffield, UK

Desley A. H. Neil, BMedSc, MBBS, Ph.D., FRCPath Department of Cellular Pathology, Level − 1, Queen Elizabeth Hospital Birmingham, Edgbaston, Birmingham, UK

Department of Histopathology, Queen Elizabeth Hospital Birmingham, Birmingham, UK

Doris M. Rassl, MBBS, FRCPath Department of Histopathology, Papworth Hospital, Papworth Everard, Cambridge, UK

Jonathan Sahu, MBChB, MRCP, FACC Department of Cardiology, Sheffield Teaching Hospitals NHS Foundation Trust, Sheffield, UK

S. Kim Suvarna, MBBS, B.Sc., FRCP, FRCPath Department of Histopathology, Northern General Hospital, Sheffield Teaching Hospitals NHS Foundation Trust, Sheffield, UK

S. Kim Suvarna

Abstract

Any understanding of cardiac disease requires a clear appreciation of normality at the macroscopic and microscopic level, and it is therefore reasonable to commence the book with this understanding. This chapter is therefore solely devoted to normal adult heart. The sections include the gross architecture of the heart, dealing with the external and internal tissues and their arrangements. Each chamber is individually considered in terms of the anatomical landmarks, in a manner/sequence akin to blood passing through the heart in sequential format. The histological features of the myocardium, as assessed by routine and special histological stains, are considered alongside each other. In addition, internal related structures are also reviewed, both at the light microscopy and ultrastructural level. Specialized tissues, such as the cardiac conduction system and the cardiac valves, are individually considered. There is specific mention of the cardiac vasculature.

Keywords

Heart • Anatomy • Histology • Ultrastructure • Valve • Conduction system • Ventricle • Atrium • Normal • Adult

Introduction

The heart is a complex, folded, and hollow muscular structure situated just to the left side of the mid-low sternum when viewed from the front, being enclosed by the pericardial sac and joined to the great vessels [1]. The surface/external landmarks of the cardiac tissues, viewed from the same direction, are the right and left parasternal second intercostal spaces down to the right sixth costal cartilage with the apex of the heart being in the fifth left intercostal space midclavicular line.

To appreciate any cardiac disorder, one must understand normality. This simple statement is deceptive since the heart is an organ which has a complex three-dimensional architecture

with mechanical and motile functionality. It is made mostly of muscle, but the tissue varies in format across the chambers, with a dynamic microscopic layout and an elegant electrophysiological function. Other non-muscular tissues are also present within the heart.

In this chapter, the normal heart is considered purely from the macroscopic and histological perspective, along with attention to specialized cardiac tissues and structures. It should be appreciated that many of the images have been derived following standard autopsy examinations [2], and this often involves separating the midventricular tissues in transverse section through to the apex. Other views in this chapter and elsewhere in the book show cardiac tissues with the ventricles intact.

It is recognized that there is no single, or perfect, method to consider and assess cardiac tissue. Indeed, all examination should be guided by the clinical query to be considered by the pathologist or other medical practitioner. However, the cardiac sample examination and evaluation require a clear

S.K. Suvarna, MBBS, B.Sc., FRCP, FRCPath
Department of Histopathology, Northern General Hospital,
Sheffield Teaching Hospitals NHS Foundation Trust,
Sheffield S5 7AU, UK
e-mail: s.k.suvarna@sheffield.ac.uk

S.K. Suvarna (ed.), *Cardiac Pathology*,
DOI 10.1007/978-1-4471-2407-8_1, © Springer-Verlag London 2013

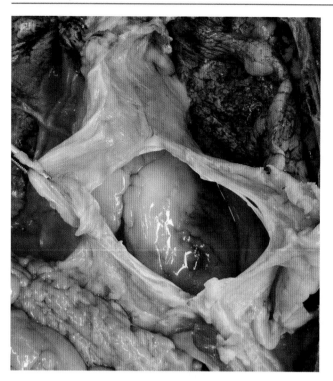

Fig. 1.1 The pericardium has been opened anteriorly revealing the enclosed heart and local fatty soft tissues of the mediastinum. The lungs are seen on either side

understanding of relevant clinical data – which often include a variety of tests (see sections on Chaps. 2 and 3).

Pericardium

The pericardium is a serous cavity/ saclike structure (Fig. 1.1), with slight distensibility, encasing the heart and large vascular connections. It measures about 1 mm in thickness and has a well-defined dense fibrous wall with collagenized tissue. A variable amount of fat lies immediately adjacent. There is normally only a scanty amount of clear (serous) fluid within the pericardial sac, generally less than 0.5 ml. This freely allows for thoracic and heart movement.

The pericardial sac (containing the heart) is in direct continuity with the adjacent mediastinal soft tissue structures of the esophagus, thymus, and the lungs on either side. The inferior aspect of the pericardial sac is bounded by the diaphragm with the superior aspect, comprising the great vessel tributaries and soft tissues, running up to the thoracic inlet.

Histologically, the pericardium, and the surface of the heart, is lined by a monolayer of mesothelial cells (Fig. 1.2). The wall of the pericardial tissues comprises dense fibrous connective tissue with some adjacent fatty connective tissue.

There is a blood and lymphatic vascular network present with scanty nerve fibers.

External Cardiac Morphology

The external (epicardial) surface has a smooth aspect with some fat usually being evident (Fig. 1.3). There may be minor fibrous thickening on the anterior epicardial wall of the right ventricle where the heart "rubs" against the pericardium/chest wall. A moderate and variable amount of fat is usually seen alongside the blood vessels and in the grooves between chambers. There is a small blood and lymphatic vascular network present, and a few lymphoid cells are often to be found.

The heart is generally about the size of one's fist in health, growing from childhood through to adult status – but it may be considerably enlarged if diseased. The weight of a normal heart may be assessed *only* if empty of blood and detached from adjacent tissue. There exist tables to compare cardiac weight against body mass, which may assist analysis – with predicted weights and a population range [3, 4]. Alternatively, one may make a basic calculation against the body mass, with expected values of 0.45% and 0.4% for males and females, respectively [5]. However, the standardized charts and calculation derivations might be argued to be dated and thereby not reflective of current diets and exercise habits. Thus, some caution always needs to be exercised when considering any cardiac weight. Indeed, there is some evidence to suggest that a higher figure (possibly 0.51% of body mass) might be more appropriate [6, 7].

In simple terms, there are four chambers with great vein and artery connections. The two atrial and two ventricle compartments are separated at the level of the coronary sulcus and central fibrous body with septation into right and left halves by the interatrial and interventricular tissues. While often displayed in planar two-dimensional view, it should be appreciated that, when the individual is standing, the anatomy points the heart partially downward and to the left side of the body. Thus, when standing upright, the base of the heart is mainly the right atrium and right ventricle.

The chambers are best considered in sequential format, and convention has it that all analysis follows "the flow of the blood" [1, 2, 8].

Right Atrium and Tricuspid Valve

Externally, this vaguely round chamber is noted to have an external slightly triangular appendage (auricle) (Fig. 1.4). Histologically, the epicardium (outer cardiac layer) has a thin layer of fibrous tissue. The outer surface of the heart is bounded by a monolayer of mesothelial cells – akin to the pericardium (see Fig. 1.2). As noted, there is variable fat, accentuated adjacent to the coronary vessels.

Fig. 1.2 Histology of the pericardium demonstrates mesothelium on either side, reflecting the pericardial and pleural aspects. There are scattered vascular channels and some fibrous and fatty connective tissues. The high magnification (*low right inset*) shows detail from the regular monolayer of mesothelial cells (hematoxylin and eosin)

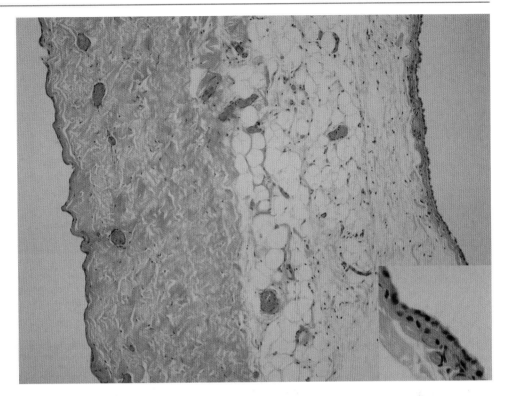

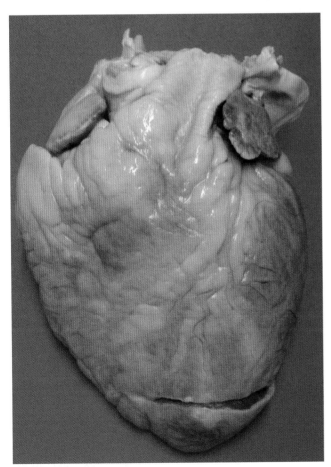

Fig. 1.3 The heart is seen from the anterior aspect with two auricles at the top. The ventricular chambers are seen with coronary vessels coursing across the surface

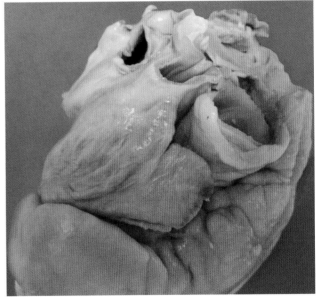

Fig. 1.4 The heart specimen is seen from the upper right aspect, allowing inspection of the right atrial appendage in detail. The appendage has a roughly triangular structure

The right atrium derives venous blood flow from the superior and inferior venae cavae, the coronary sinus, and other minor cardiac veins. The venae cavae enter the posterior and basal aspect of the right atrial chamber. There is also cardiac venous blood inflow from the coronary sinus, covered in part by a flap of tissue (Eustachian valve). This sinus receives blood from the great cardiac vein, but there are small anterior cardiac veins draining the anterior wall of the right atrium.

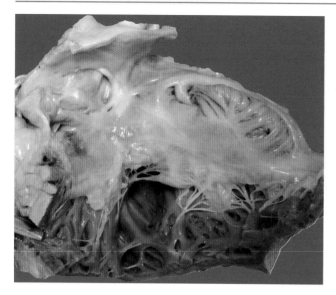

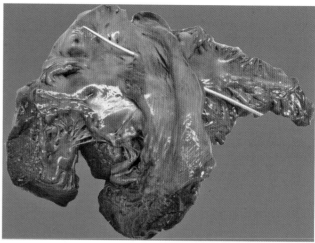

Fig. 1.6 This autopsy specimen shows left atrial tissue displayed from the posterior aspect with a probe passing between from the right atrium through the septum into the left atrium; being a probe patent foramen ovale

Fig. 1.5 The right atrium has been opened, from the posterior aspect with a cut between the superior and inferior venae cavae and with a further cut running alongside the atrial and ventricular septum. Focally there is the trabeculated appendage/auricular architecture. There are smooth endothelial surfaces elsewhere (venous inlet, vestibule) and the tricuspid valve at the base. The tricuspid valve chordae are noted to run from edge of the valve to the papillary muscle tissues of the ventricle

The chamber internally (Fig. 1.5) consists of three parts. There is a smooth-walled posterior part (venous inlet), joining the superior and inferior venae cavae, also deriving blood from the coronary sinus. On the anterior aspect and fully involving the appendage are parallel (trabeculated) muscle bands. The auricular appendage itself consists of the triangular projection running anteriorly across the upper anterior cardiac tissues. There is a groove externally (sulcus terminalis) that divides the venous and trabeculated zones with a ridge (crista terminalis). The other part of the chamber is the smooth-surfaced vestibule, (at the base of the chamber) being the support tissue for the tricuspid valve and the outflow for this chamber.

The interatrial septum shows an oval residuum from closed-off (gestational/ante-natal) blood flow (foramen ovale). In about 15–20% of the population, there is probe patency of a part of the septal tissues (Fig. 1.6). This is a normal variation and without functional deficit. The coronary sinus/Eustachian valves are noted posterior-laterally in the right atrium.

Blood flows from the right atrium across the atrioventricular orifice/tricuspid valve (see Fig. 1.5). This usually has a circumference of 10–12 cm entering into the posterior aspect of the right ventricle. The tricuspid valve has a thin pliable trileaflet structure (less than 1-mm thickness), anchored onto the myocardial wall tissues and by chordae tendinae onto the right vestibular wall. The right side of the atrioventricular orifice is part of the fibrous skeleton of the heart.

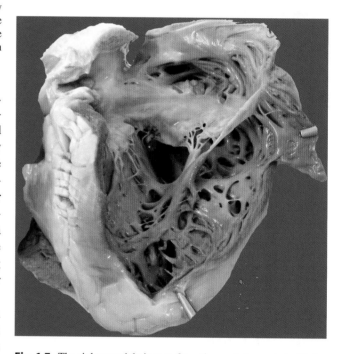

Fig. 1.7 The right ventricle is seen from the posterior aspect with the atrium above. The coarse trabeculations are noted, and the chordae/papillary muscles are also evident. The inlet is seen immediately below the tricuspid valve. The ventricular trabeculated part is clearly demarcated, and the blood passes toward the outlet/conus

Right Ventricle and Pulmonary Valve

The second chamber is the right ventricle (Fig. 1.7). This makes up the anterior and inferior part of the heart (when one is standing erect) and has a vaguely ovoid/crescentic architecture on transverse section (Fig. 1.8) with some features suggesting an inverted cone shape. There is a variable fat

Fig. 1.8 A transversely sliced view of right and left ventricle tissues. The variably trabecular architecture can be fully appreciated in this view along with comparative detail of the two ventricular wall thicknesses. This view of the cardiac tissues (standard in autopsy examinations) allows the cross section of the chamber diameters to be defined. The coronary arteries are seen running through the epicardial fat peripherally

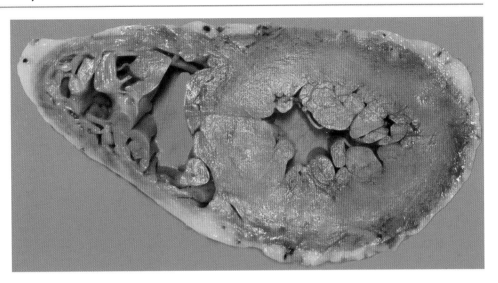

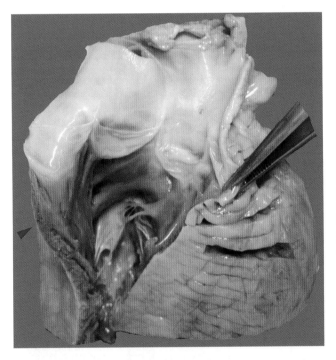

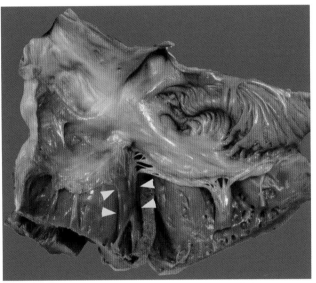

Fig. 1.10 The right ventricle and right atrial tissues have been opened to allow definition of the septomarginal band of myocardial parenchyma (*arrowed*) as it runs from the high septal tissue toward the right ventricle trabeculations and papillary muscles

Fig. 1.9 The right ventricle outflow tract has been opened anteriorly allowing inspection of the pulmonary valve, smooth aspect conus tissue, and proximal pulmonary artery. Measurement of the right ventricle outflow tract at this point is recommended (*arrow*) as this thickness is easy to define and repeat – particularly as no trabeculations are present

(adipocytic) component clearly seen by the naked eye. Internally, there are three evident parts: inflow, trabecular, and outflow components (see Fig. 1.7).

There are coarse trabeculations across the chamber evenly, apart from the outflow tract (conus) that is relatively smooth walled (Fig. 1.9). The right ventricle is normally thinner than the left (see Fig. 1.8). The normal and variable amount of fat present in the free wall of the chamber should not be confused with the fat/fibrous tissue replacement of arrhythmogenic

(right ventricular) cardiomyopathy. Given that the wall varies markedly in thickness around the circumference and has variable fat content, it may be pragmatic to assess right ventricle wall thickness in the outflow tract approximately 10 mm below the pulmonary valve – being an area easy to regularly identify and measure (see Fig. 1.9). It also has less peripheral fat along with a smooth surface allowing for easy assessment. The outflow tract measures 3–4 mm normally.

There are three papillary muscles running from the walls of the ventricle that insert into the free margins and ventricular surfaces of the tricuspid valve by fibrous cords (chordae tendinae).

The septomarginal trabeculum (Fig. 1.10) is a notable band of muscle crossing the cavity of the right ventricle from the septum to the anterior papillary muscle, importantly carrying part of the atrioventricular bundle of conducting tissue. This ensures that the papillary muscles have already contracted (tensioning the chordae tendinae) as ventricular contraction commences. This permits efficient closure of the tricuspid valve.

At the apex of the outflow tract is the pulmonary valve (see Fig. 1.9). This valve has three roughly equal, semilunar leaflets joined minimally to each other at the wall. The ring circumference is generally 5.5–7.5 cm, and the valve function permits unidirectional deoxygenated blood to flow into the pulmonary artery and thence into the lungs. The pulmonary artery is discussed later.

Left Atrium and Mitral Valve

Oxygenated blood returns from the lungs to the left atrium through the four pulmonary veins. These enter high/posteriorly into the chamber. For the chamber itself, there are no specific landmarks externally – apart from the oblong (rather "dog-ear") appendage (Fig. 1.11). Otherwise, it has a rounded architecture.

Internally, the left atrium has a predominantly smooth endocardial surface, but the left side appendage is trabeculated. The only other landmark is the closed fossa ovalis, which may be easily seen on the interatrial septal aspect, being the closed formen ovale (see above). The chamber (Fig. 1.12) can also be divided into the three parts, analogous to the right side (venous inlet or posterior, appendicular, and vestibular: supporting the adjacent valve). After atrial contraction, blood passes across the left atrioventricular orifice/mitral valve (ring circumference = generally 8–10 cm) into the left ventricle. Contrasting with the right atrium, there are only two mitral (bicuspid) valve leaflets present. These also have a similar structure and attachments to the tricuspid valve, with papillary muscle anchors. The anterior cusp/leaflet is longer in circumference and/or larger than the posterior, with the valve opening having a slightly curved architecture when viewed from above [2].

Left Ventricle and Aortic Valve

The final chamber is the left ventricle on the left side of the heart (see Fig. 1.3). There is scanty fat present, although this is normally only distributed on the epicardial aspect of the heart mostly alongside vascular channels (Figs. 1.3 and 1.13). This chamber "as the blood flows" is longer than the right and has a rounded cross section with an inverted

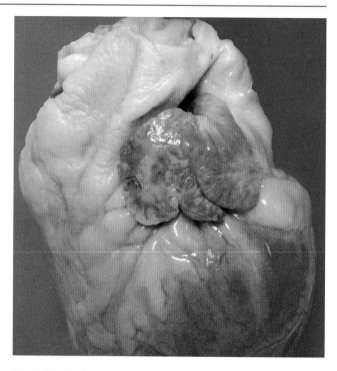

Fig. 1.11 The left atrium is seen from the cardiac specimen from the upper left aspect. The appendage has a somewhat square architecture

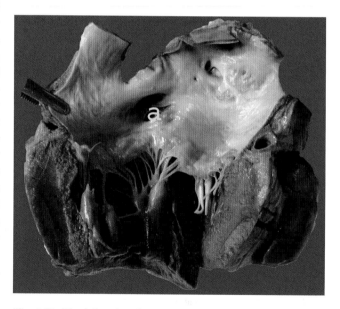

Fig. 1.12 The left atrium has been opened by cuts interlinking the pulmonary veins and with a further cut running alongside the atrial and ventricular septum. The two leaflets of the mitral valve are seen with adjacent chordae and papillary muscles. The auricle (*a*) can be inspected directly. The left atrium is largely smooth surfaced. The great cardiac vein is arrowed

cone architecture. The chamber has trabeculations throughout, apart from the very apical part of the outflow tract. The trabeculations are finer than the right side, but are most marked toward the apex. There are two large papillary

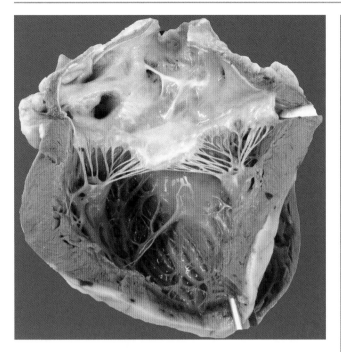

Fig. 1.13 The left ventricle has been opened from the back to demonstrate the atrial and ventricular chambers. As with the right side, there is the inlet, ventricular trabeculated, and outlet components evident. The trabeculations are slightly finer than those on the right side

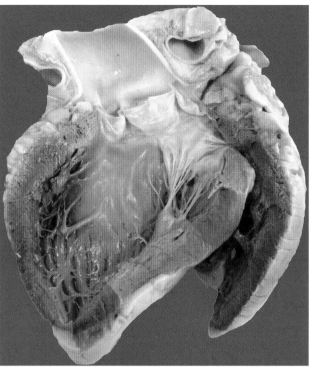

Fig. 1.15 The left ventricle outflow tract has been opened by running a cut up the anterior wall of the left ventricle, alongside the left anterior descending artery, and then turning between the left main stem artery and left auricle across the aortic valve. The inner aspect of the outflow tract can be appreciated along with the left ventricle wall thickness. This is a good point to measure ventricular wall thickness as it is easy to define and standardize. The proximal aortic tissues can also now be examined for arterial disease and the coronary ostia are also seen

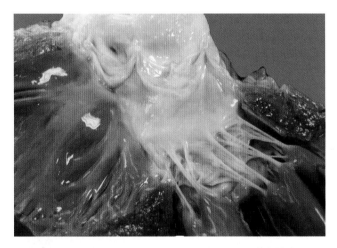

Fig. 1.14 The mitral valve is seen in detail, folded toward the side, from the ventricular aspect. Firstly, its close alignment to the aortic valve tissues can be appreciated. Secondly, it should be noted that the chordal tissues insert not only at the edge of the valve but also at other positions along the valve undersurface

muscles, attached via chordae tendinae to the mitral valve. The chordae insert into the free margins and ventricular surfaces of the valve (Fig. 1.14).

Within the chamber (Fig. 1.15) there is the usual inlet, trabecular, and outflow ventricular compartment subdivision. The aortic outflow tract/vestibule is a thin muscle and, in part, is largely fibrous. The left ventricle outflow tract passes behind the right ventricle outflow tract, approximately in perpendicular fashion, to finish at the aortic valve. The aortic valve ring has an average circumference of 5.5–8.5 cm. It is centrally positioned within the fibrous body/skeleton of the heart. It is sometimes described as wedged, centrally within a triangle, between the pulmonary valve (anterior) and the atrioventricular valves (posteriorly) when viewed from above, if one imagines the atria removed.

The muscular wall of the left ventricle is thick (see Figs. 1.8 and 1.15), on average between 14 and 20 mm in the outflow tract (albeit varying from childhood to adulthood). The same limitations of wall thickness assessment exist for this chamber. Indeed, it has been said that if you give the same heart to ten pathologists you will get *at least* ten different thickness assessments! This clearly is an unsatisfactory solution, given the pivotal role this chamber has for systemic circulation realities. It is thus recommended that measurements are taken 10 mm below the outflow tract anteriorly as a simple standard position – unless the case involves asymmetric hypertrophy or a local mass lesion.

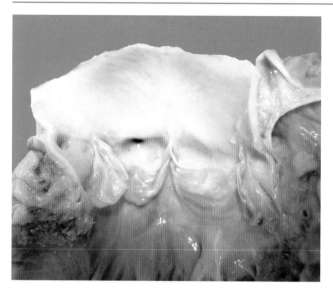

Fig. 1.16 The opened aortic outflow tract has the right and left coronary artery ostia in the right and left coronary sinus positions. The posterior sinus has no coronary artery ostium

It should be noted that those involved in heavy sports training may have a considerably greater left ventricle muscle mass than average members of the population. It should also be noted that some similar hypertrophy is seen at the end of normal pregnancy. Both of these physiological situations will return to the average ventricular mass after the end of training or in the postnatal period, respectively. Contrastingly, as one passes to old age, some general mild/cardiac tissue mass reduction may occur.

One of the most important components of the left ventricle is the septum, being the wall between the two ventricles. This is normally of relatively uniform thickness. However, it is thinner at the top, with apex of the septum comprising a slender band of fibrous tissue (membranous septum) that can be transilluminated if desired. This structure is in communication with the tricuspid valve ring through which passes the His bundle (see conducting system below). This membranous portion is developed from the same tissue that forms the valves and develops separately to the muscular part of the septum.

Blood leaving the left ventricle is at high pressure as it passes across the three semilunar valve leaflets of the aortic valve. The aortic valve (Fig. 1.16) structure is similar to the right-side pulmonary counterpart. However, immediately above the aortic valve, two (left, right) of the three valve sinuses have the orifices of the left main stem and the right coronary artery. The third (posterior) sinus has no coronary artery orifice (see Fig. 1.16). Occasionally, the small conus artery has origin adjacent to the right coronary artery, appearing as a separate small vessel. This should not be confused with a coronary anomaly.

Aorta and Pulmonary Artery

These are large muscular and elastic arteries, similar to each other in caliber and architecture (see Figs. 1.9 and 1.16). The wall of the aorta is thicker as it has to cope with a higher blood pressure. Macroscopically, the normal lumen aspect shows a bland and smooth endothelial-lined surface.

The basic histological structure (Fig. 1.17) is that of an inner thin loose fibrous connective tissue intima, surfaced by a bland monolayer of endothelial cells. Enclosed centrally is the media which comprises the bulk of the artery wall. There is an inner elastic lamina between intima and media. The outer layer of the vessel is vascularized fibrous connective tissue and fibroadipose parenchyma. There is an outer elastic lamina at the interface of the media and adventitia. Small arteriolar and capillary blood vessels (vasa vasorum) penetrate the wall of these large arteries (as common with all such vessels) to supply the vessel wall tissues. Even in young apparently very fit individuals, there is often a minimal amount of nonspecific/intimal focal fibrous thickening histologically - rarely amounting to more than 5% stenosis, although larger amounts may develop with increasing age.

The Histology and Ultrastructure of the Myocardial Wall

The majority of the heart is muscle, but there also is a fibrous tissue framework, a rich vascular network with some innervation. The muscle cells are different to smooth and skeletal muscle tissues, although many similarities exist. While the tissues are similar across the whole organ, the chambers and the walls of each of the four chambers are histologically distinct. The cardiac myocytes [9, 10] in the left ventricle and septum are somewhat brick-like and are closely applied to one another, with little other tissue (Figs. 1.18 and 1.19). Those in the right ventricle have a variable amount of admixed adipocytes (Fig. 1.20). With regard to the fatty tissue component of the right ventricle, it should be noted that this varies between the sexes and also increases with age [11]. Myocytes of the atria are often more slender and supported in a fibrous and variably fatty stroma.

The cardiac myocytes (see Fig. 1.18), generally of the order of 125×30 μm (length and width), have central nuclei and abundant cytoplasm – the latter element mainly containing eosinophilic myofibers [9]. There is usually a single nucleus, although this may not always be present in the plane of section. A small number of cardiac myocytes may have more than one nucleus. The striated quality of the

Fig. 1.17 Histological examination of the aortic and pulmonary arterial tissue shows a thicker aortic wall, reflecting the greater pulse pressures, with otherwise similar content and structure. Note that the intima is very thin, being almost impossible to define. The bulk of the wall comprises the muscular media and elastic tissue. The outer fibrous adventitia is seen peripherally (Elastic van Gieson)

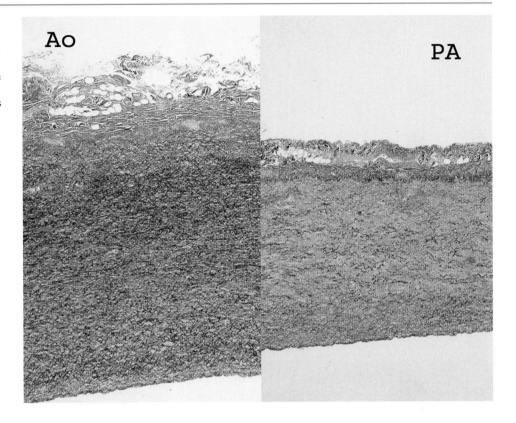

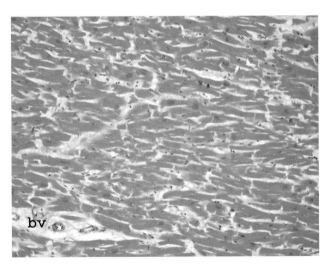

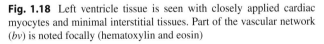

Fig. 1.18 Left ventricle tissue is seen with closely applied cardiac myocytes and minimal interstitial tissues. Part of the vascular network (*bv*) is noted focally (hematoxylin and eosin)

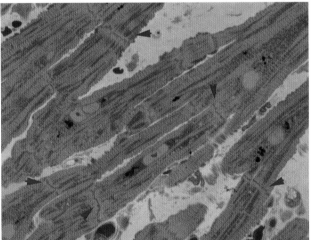

Fig. 1.19 Resin-embedded thin section of cardiac myocytes demonstrating the banded muscular structure. Intercalated discs can be seen at the longitudinal ends of the myocytes (*arrowed*) (*toluidine blue*)

muscle can be appreciated with phosphotungstic acid hematoxylin, Masson's trichrome, or toluidine blue (resin thin section) histochemistry (see Fig. 1.19), but is less defined than skeletal muscle. The cells may often exhibit focal lipochrome accumulation, often immediately adjacent to the nucleus. The nucleus itself often varies in shape and size, being enlarged and roughly square in hypertrophic states.

The terminal junctions of the myocytes have dense eosinophilic bands (intercalated discs) (see Fig. 1.19). These are sites of cell-cell adhesion and electrical communication, the latter effectively allowing the heart to act electrically and functionally akin to a syncitial mass.

The ultrastructure of the heart largely recapitulates that seen at light microscopy. The cardiac myocytes classically

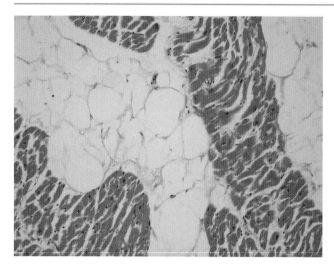

Fig. 1.20 High magnification of the right ventricle shows cardiac myocytes with significant amounts of mature adipose connective tissue interspersed. It should be noted that there is no significant fibrous tissue associated (hematoxylin and eosin)

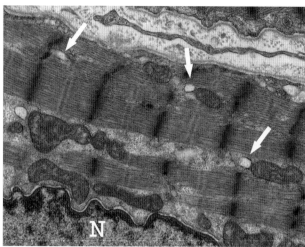

Fig. 1.22 Electron microscopy of a cardiac myocyte showing nucleus (*N*) and banded muscular tissue immediately adjacent. Small tubular/cisternal spaces are noted, representing sarcoplasmic reticulum (*arrowed*). Scattered mitochondria are also evident

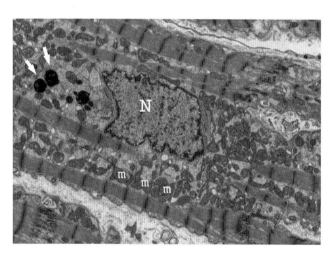

Fig. 1.21 Ultrastructural view of a cardiac myocyte showing a central nucleus (*N*) with associated lipofuchsin (*arrowed*) along with the banded muscular tissue. Abundant mitochondria (*m*) are evident

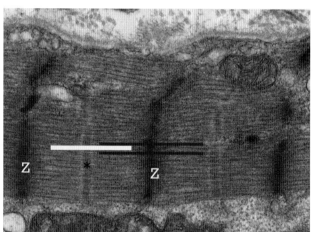

Fig. 1.23 Electron microscopy high-magnification detail of the banded myofilament architecture. There are well defined Z bands. The M band (and lighter H zones) is marked by the asterisk (*). Overlaid in schematic form are representations of the thin actin and related protein filaments (*black*) and thick myosin/related protein filaments (*white*). The contraction of cardiac myocytes is accomplished by the ratcheting of the proteins to allow greater/lesser interdigitation and thereby cardiac myocyte shortening and later relaxation

are seen as having a block-like architecture with a well-defined nucleus and myofibrils (Figs. 1.21 and 1.22). Electron microscopy also allows detailed inspection of the banded myofibril structure. These bands reflect the different protein filaments, which vary in architecture according to whether the tissue fixation occurs when there is relaxation or contraction. The portion of tissue between the two consecutive Z lines is called a sarcomere. There are two main types of interdigitating filaments (Fig. 1.23), being designated thick and thin. The thin actin filaments overlap variably the thick myosin filaments. During contraction, a ratcheting of the filaments occurs, and the two Z lines are drawn closer together, resulting in cellular contraction.

The higher magnification also allows inspection of the cytosolic/ non-myofibril compartment. There are usually abundant mitochondria, glycogen stores, and lipid droplets (see Fig. 1.21). There is some smooth and rough endoplasmic reticulum as would be expected. These parallel the standard features seen in other tissues. Special attention to the mitochondria, with their relatively uniform folded membranous architecture, is recommended, in order to exclude mitochondrial myopathy.

Fig. 1.24 Three-dimensional reconstruction of cardiac muscle cells in the region of an intercalated disc, a junctional complex between neighboring cells. The interdigitating transverse parts of the intercalated disc form a fascia adherens, with numerous desmosomes; gap junctions are found in the longitudinal parts of the disc. The organization of the transverse (*T*) tubules and the sarcoplasmic reticulum is also shown (This figure was published in Borley et al. [9], page 140, copyright Elsevier 2009)

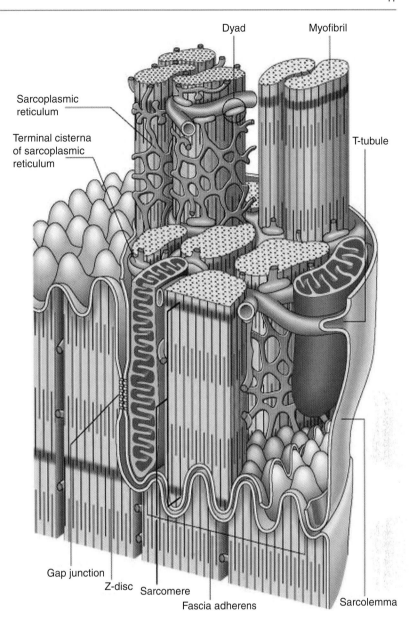

At the longitudinal poles of the cells are the intercalated discs. These are best appreciated in schematic form (Fig. 1.24) initially, but clearly have a complex folded structure (Fig. 1.25). These are the junctions binding cells to one another and also permit the cell-cell depolarization wave to propagate rapidly. The intercalated discs have several types of junction. Firstly, there are fascia adherens (linking different cells in line with myofibrillar apparatus and cell skeleton elements). Then there are the gap junctions [12, 13]. These are sometimes known as nexi and contain the connexins/gating domains which allow cell-cell depolarization. After childhood, the intercalated discs are only found at the ends of the long axis of the cells. There are also undifferentiated regions usually present between the desmosome/myofibrillar insertion sites of the intercalated discs (see Fig. 1.25).

Contraction follows the cell membrane (sarcolemma) depolarization wave being swept inward along the invaginated membrane elements. These are called the T-tubule system, allowing deep cellular depolarization in uniform fashion. The T-tubules pass directly toward the Z-bands of the myofibers, but interact with the sarcoplasmic reticulum closely, at regions called dyads. The sarcoplasmic reticulum (see Fig. 1.24) is a complicated folded cistern-like network, layered around the bundles of myofibrils that serve to store calcium. At depolarization, the sarcoplasmic reticulum activation allows calcium to be liberated resulting in myocyte contraction. The filament contraction involves adenosine triphosphate (ATP) lysis, increasing the interdigitation, thereby shortening the cell. Relaxation is dependent on new ATP production – thus, being energy dependent.

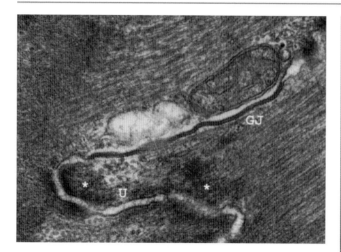

Fig. 1.25 Part of an intercalated disc is seen with a gap junction (*GJ*) being defined as a thin dense structure running between two adjacent myocytes. There are some "undifferentiated" cell membrane (*U*) and insertion points of the muscular apparatus of each cell (*)

Of note, within the atrial tissues, there are dense membrane-bound granules, containing atrial natriuretic factor, that are responsible for diuresis following atrial distension. These granules are found close to the nucleus/Golgi apparatus.

The interstitial tissues comprise a small amount of fibrous (collagenized) connective tissue and a vascular network of blood and lymphatic vessels. Scattered mast cells are occasionally seen in the background, but no other significant inflammatory cell population (beyond that seen in the circulatory compartment) should be present. Fibroblastic elements may be seen in the interstitial compartment, and their nuclei can occasionally be confused with lymphocytes at light microscopy. The interstitial tissues are best appreciated with Masson's trichrome histochemistry, and the tissues may be investigated for inflammatory components and the vasculature by means of immunohistochemistry. The use of trichrome stains is of particular value in the right ventricle, serving to exclude the enhanced fibrous tissue of an arrhythmogenic cardiomyopathic status.

The interstitium ultrastructurally contains collagen and elastic tissues together with adhesive fibronectin molecules. In addition, there is some proteoglycans and loose amorphous matrix. The collagen (principally types 1 and 3) is required to maintain cell: cell alignment and structural integrity during contraction and relaxation. The collagens connect individual myocytes together with linkage to capillaries and the adjacent interstitial tissues. Fibronectin links the cardiac myocyte with local extracellular matrix.

Coronary Blood Vessels

The cardiac vasculature is divided principally into outer arteries and veins with some lymphatics. The coronary arteries run from the root of the aorta over the heart, progressively

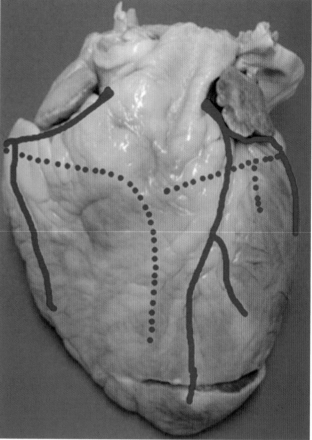

Fig. 1.26 The anterior surface of the heart is displayed with a diagrammatic representation of the main coronary artery branches. The *dotted lines* represent coronary tissues on the posterior aspect of the heart

subdividing on the epicardial surface (Fig. 1.26), and only later pass inward to supply the myocardial tissues. They have a smooth intimal/lumen aspect and muscular walls measuring less than 1-mm thickness. They are normally accompanied by the venous circulation and have fatty connective tissue adjacent (Fig. 1.27).

The right coronary artery arises from the right aortic sinus just above the aortic valve leaflet, passing in a groove (sulcus) between the appendage of the right atrium and upper part of the right ventricle. It turns inferiorly and round onto the posterior-inferior aspect of the heart. In its midsection, it gives rise to the acute marginal artery (passing perpendicularly down along the lateral wall of the ventricle). The right coronary artery continues and terminates at the top of the posterior interventricular septum, merging with the terminal part of the circumflex artery. At this point the combined vessel runs down along the midline of the heart posteriorly as the posterior interventricular descending artery.

The left coronary artery arises from the left aortic sinus, likewise just above the valve, as the left main stem. This artery runs downward and forward between the pulmonary trunk and left auricle where it divides (after about

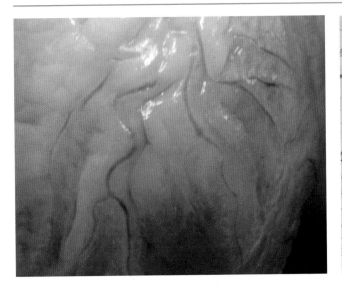

Fig. 1.27 The epicardial surface of the heart shows both coronary veins as well as coronary arteries running alongside each other within the fatty tissue parenchyma

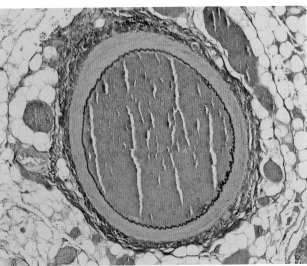

Fig. 1.28 A coronary artery is seen in cross section with well-defined elastic laminae and muscular walled structure. The peripheral fibrous adventitial tissue is seen. There is no significant thickening of the intimal layer (Elastic van Gieson)

5–15 mm) into the left anterior descending and circumflex arteries.

The circumflex artery curves left around the atrioventricular sulcus toward the left side passing round the back of the heart. The circumflex vessel can end, either merging with the right coronary artery, as above; or may terminate as a set of obtuse marginal artery branches (usually one, but up to three are seen occasionally). The obtuse marginal artery (or group of arteries) runs along the lateral and posterior wall of the left ventricle.

The left anterior descending artery runs anteriorly over the anterior septal tissues (between the ventricles) with penetrating branches running directly downward penetrating into the septal tissues. There is also often a variable caliber diagonal artery starting in the midsection of the left anterior descending artery running obliquely left and downward across the left ventricular tissue.

In most people (about 65% population), the right coronary system is larger, referred to as dominant. Aside from the main arteries described above, there are also small radicular arteries evident that are quite variable, but still part of normality. The coronary arteries anastomose poorly and can be considered as end-arteries. Since the arteries' blood supply is from the aortic root, it should be noted that the bulk of coronary blood flow occurs during diastole – which also blends with the reality that blood flow is better through relaxing phase ventricular tissue.

The arteries have a similar histology to the aorta (Fig. 1.28), with thin intimal tissues surfaced by endothelium. The medial smooth muscular/medial tissues have an internal and external elastic lamina on the inner/outer aspect. The adventitia is likewise bland vascularized fibrous tissue.

The arteries described progressively subdivide, become progressively smaller, and eventually connect into a rich capillary network. The capillaries drain into venules and thence veins, broadly following the pathways of the coronary arterial system. The main venous system comprises the great cardiac vein, running in the posterior/left-sided atrioventricular groove with drainage from the anterior, lateral, and posterior aspects of the left ventricle. The small cardiac vein (draining the right side of the heart and right atrial tissue) joins close to the great vein termination point at the coronary sinus. It should also not be forgotten that there is a moderate network of lymphatic vessels within all the tissues of the heart. These lymphatic vessels have a monolayer of endothelium and have a simple basement membrane as the outer layer.

The Valves

There are two types of valve. The atrioventricular (tricuspid and mitral) valves separate the atrial and ventricular chambers, preventing reflux of blood into the atria upon ventricular systole (see Figs. 1.5 and 1.12). The semilunar (pulmonary and aortic) valves, situated at the ventricular outflow, prevent reflux of blood back into the ventricles after ventricular systole ends (see Figs. 1.9 and 1.16). Their anatomy is described above alongside that of the chambers.

Histologically, the atrioventricular valves (Fig. 1.29) have several parts best visualized by connective tissue stains. The central part (zona fibrosa) is the strength of the valve, composed of a plate of dense collagenous matrix. The fibrosa, accounting for the valve structural function,

Fig. 1.29 Composite diagram of the tricuspid valve showing the ventricular wall attachment and the valve arching across the center and top of the image toward the left side. Chordae (*c*) are noted running from the under surface of the valve tissue. The high-magnification cross section of one of the chordae is noted in the bottom left corner (*h*). High magnification (*inset low right*) of the valve tissues shows a variably collagenized framework with thin endothelial surfaces and some elastic parenchyma with the ventricular suraface marked (**) (Elastic van Gieson)

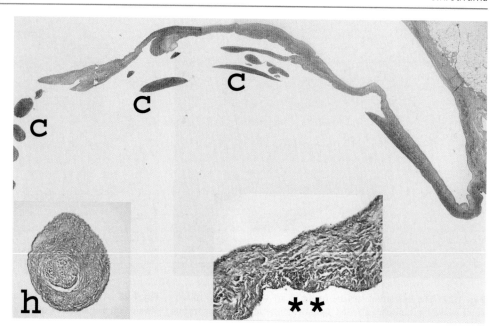

is tied in with the annulus (wall interface) of the valve tissue, being composed largely of collagen. There are very sparse nerve fibers and lymphatics present. The ventricular aspect tissue (ventricularis) lies immediately below the monolayer endothelium and has a loose structure with elastic. Within this there are also the fibrous anchor points of the chordal tissues. The chordae tendinae are similar to tendons with parallel collagen fibers running along the long axis of the fiber. They enmesh with the adjacent papillary muscles (see Fig. 1.29). The atrial aspect (atrialis and spongiosa) is composed of loose connective tissue with minor elastic tissue. The amount of loose spongy connective tissue (mainly proteoglycans with some collagen and elastic fibrous tissue) varies along the length of the valve cusp with scanty fibroblast-like cells being present. There is normally no blood vessel component present within the valve.

The semilunar valves (Fig. 1.30) also show similar layers, being covered with endothelial cells. Proceeding from the ventricle to the artery outflow, there are ventricularis, spongiosa, fibrosa, and arterialis compartments, respectively. The fibrosa again shows dense collagen with some elastic tissues. There may be occasional fibroblasts, but there is no significant vasculature. The fibrosa blends with the adjacent annulus/wall tissues. The ventricularis contains elastic tissue with some collagen. The spongiosa is only partially present toward the outer rim of the valve. The ventricularis layer is focally thickened on the semilunar valves producing nodular bulges (noduli Arantii). The atrialis layer has some loose collagen and elastic tissue.

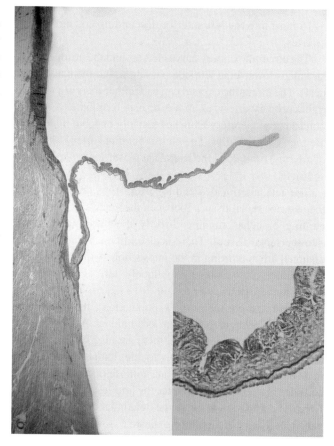

Fig. 1.30 The pulmonary valve tissues are seen here with the outflow tract of the right ventricle and proximal pulmonary artery root running along the left-hand border. A high-magnification *inset* of the valve tissues is seen allowing appreciation of the valve substructure (Elastic van Gieson)

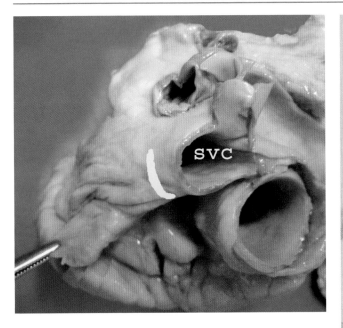

Fig. 1.31 The right atrium is seen from above, with some tension applied to the auricular appendage. At the root of the superior vena cava is a representation of the sinoatrial node (*yellow*). This cannot be specifically identified from the external or internal aspect, and histological sampling of the tissues is required to completely block this area if it is to be considered

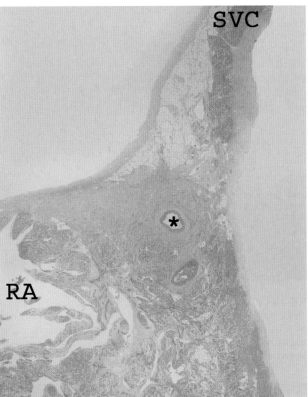

Fig. 1.32 The sinoatrial node tissue is seen immediately adjacent to the sinoatrial artery (*). The right atrial and superior vena cava tissues are seen adjacent (hematoxylin and eosin)

Conduction System

All cardiac myocytes have pacemaker (spontaneous rhythmic arterialis depolarization) potential, but coordinated organ contraction is managed by the cardiac conduction system. As none of the components of the cardiac conduction are visible by the naked eye, it is necessary to block the tissue around the appropriate landmarks and section diligently through the tissues, often with multiple levels, in order to identify all the appropriate structures histologically (see Chap. 5). Fixation of tissues prior to section (i.e., not sampled fresh in the mortuary) is often an advantage for providing orientated blocks of the conduction system parenchyma.

The sinoatrial node (SAN) tissue acts as the pacemaker for the heart. It is positioned at the apex of the crista terminalis at the top of the right atrium (Fig. 1.31). Depolarization from this area of tissue spreads in a wavelike fashion across the atrial muscle toward the atrioventricular node. The node itself is a banana-shaped structure lying immediately in the subepicardial tissues at the junction between the superior vena cava and right atrium. Its position can be predicted to an extent by identifying the sinoatrial artery. Histologically, the SAN comprises a meshwork of irregularly orientated and rather slender myocytes (Figs. 1.32 and 1.33) within a poorly

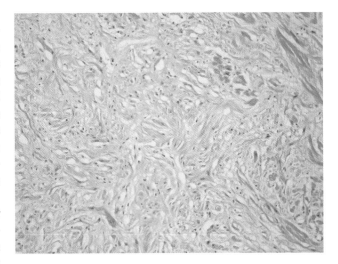

Fig. 1.33 High magnification of the nodal tissue shows a somewhat haphazard myocyte arrangement set within fibrous stroma (hematoxylin and eosin)

defined, connective tissue matrix. Another clue to the location of this tissue is the local sympathetic and parasympathetic autonomic nerve tissue.

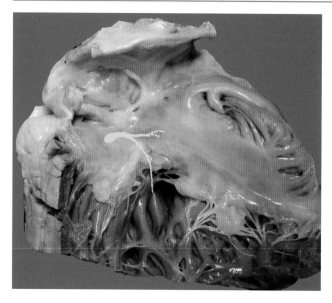

Fig. 1.34 Right atrial tissues are seen with a schematic representation of the atrioventricular node and the proximal pathways for the bundle branch tissues. Given the absence of clear anatomical landmarks of the nodal tissue, one needs to block this entire area when considering nodal and bundle histology

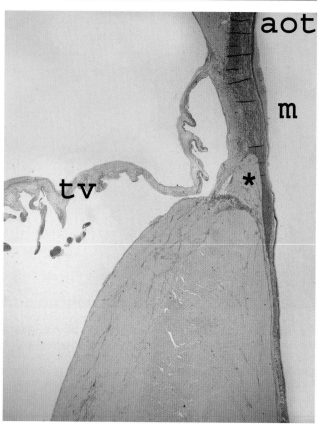

Fig. 1.36 Membranous septal tissue (*m*) with local aortic outflow tract (*aot*), tricuspid valve (*tv*) and high ventricular septal tissues in the plane of section. The base of the His bundle is noted (*), and there is clear fibrous tissue separation of the atrial and ventricular component requiring electrical depolarization to pass along the bundle of His for ventricular excitation (Elastic van Gieson)

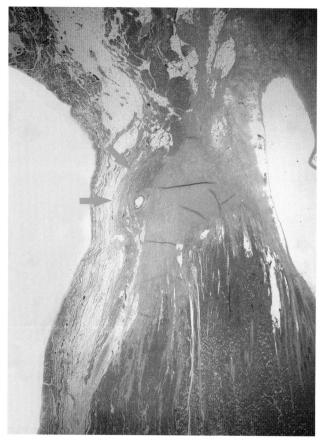

Fig. 1.35 Histological view of the atrioventricular node sitting immediately adjacent to the central fibrous body and part of the membranous septal tissues. The nodal tissue is *arrowed* and is seen as a well-defined group of cardiac myocytes with similar morphology to that of the sinoatrial node (hematoxylin and eosin)

Atrial depolarization is not transmitted directly to the ventricle as the central fibrous body and fat act as an insulator, with a two-stage contraction of the heart thereby being possible. The atrioventricular nodal tissues are also supplied by both sympathetic and parasympathetic nerve parenchyma.

The atrioventricular node (AVN) (Figs. 1.34 and 1.35) is found at the base of the right atrium at the apex of the triangle of Koch in the subendocardial tissue. It lies below the tendon of Todero (running from the superior limb of the Eustachian valve/coronary sinus toward the membranous septum, and above the annulus of the tricuspid valve). It also has a rather haphazard histological myocyte architecture within a fibrous stroma. The node tissue tapers to enter the membranous septum and then runs as a slender tract of muscle (His bundle) fiber through this fibrous boundary zone (Fig. 1.36). Occasional adipocytes can be seen, but there should be no other tissue present in the bundle.

The base of the His bundle splits into two bundle branches to supply the right and left ventricles. The bundles (Fig. 1.37) are conceptualized electrically as well-defined tracts, but the

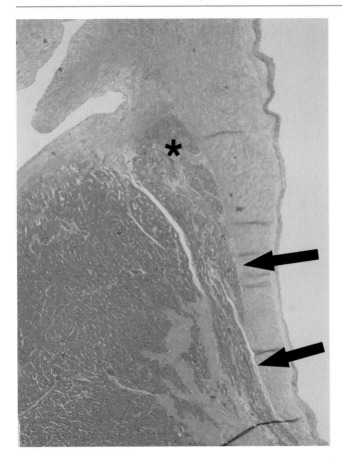

Fig. 1.37 The base of the membranous septum has the bottom part of the His bundle displayed (*) and part of the left bundle branch group radiating downward and into the endocardial tissue adjacent (*arrow*) (hematoxylin and eosin)

reality is that they run in small fascicles and in a mesh-like array across the ventricular subendocardial parenchyma distally. These conducting cells appear paler than standard cardiac myocytes and often have a slender disposition. These specialized bundle branch muscle cells also pass in the subendocardial tissues along the septomarginal trabeculum (see Fig. 1.10), described above.

Acknowledgments Grateful thanks are expressed to Mr. B. Wagner, Senior Electron Microscopist, Sheffield Teaching Hospitals, for his expertise and photography of ultrastuctural histology.

References

1. Anderson RH, Becker AE. Normal cardiac anatomy. In: Anderson RH, Becker AE, Roberts WB, editors. The cardiovascular system. Part A: general considerations and congenital malformations. Edinburgh: Churchill Livingstone; 1993. p. 3–26.
2. Suvarna SK. National guidelines for adult autopsy cardiac dissection: are they achievable? Histopathology. 2008;97–112:53.
3. Kitson DW, Scholz DG, Hagen PT, Ilstrup DM, Edwards WD. Age-related changes in normal human heart during the first ten decades of life. Part II. Maturity: a quantitative anatomical study of 765 specimens from subjects 20–99 years old. Mayo Clin Proc. 1988; 63:137–46.
4. Sheppard M, Davies MJ. Cardiac examination and normal cardiac anatomy. In: Practical cardiovascular pathology. London: Arnold; 1998. p. 1–16. 103–8.
5. Silver MM, Silver MD. Examination of the heart and cardiovascular specimens in surgical pathology. In: Silver MD, Gotlieb AI, Schoen FJ, editors. Cardiovascular pathology. 3rd ed. New York: Churchill Livingstone; 2001. p. 1–29.
6. Lucas SL. Derivation of new reference tables for human heart weights in light of increasing body mass index. J Clin Pathol. 2011;64:279–80.
7. Gaitskell K, Perera R, Soilleux EJ. Derivation of new reference tables for human heart weights in light of increasing body mass index. J Clin Pathol. 2011;64:358–62.
8. Becker AE, Anderson RH. Cardiac adaptation and its sequelae. In: Cardiac pathology. An integrated text and color atlas. Edinburgh: Churchill Livingstone; 1982. p. 1.2–8.
9. Borley NR, Collins P, Crossman AR, Gatzoulis MA, Healy J, Johson D, Mahadevan V, Newell RML, Wigley CB. Smooth muscle and the cardiovascular and lymphatic systems. In: Standring S, Borley NR, Collins P, Crossman AR, Gatzoulis MA, Healy J, Johson D, Mahadevan V, Newell RML, Wigley CB, editors. Gray's Anatomy. The anatomical basis of clinical practice. 40th ed. Spain: Churchill Livingstone Elsevier; 2008. p. 127–43.
10. Veinot JP, Ghadially FN, Walley VM. Light microscopy and ultrastructural of the blood vessels and heart. In: Silver MD, Gotlieb AI, Schoen FJ, editors. Cardiovascular pathology. 3rd ed. New York: Churchill Livingstone; 2001. p. 30–53.
11. Tansey DK, Aly Z, Sheppard MN. Fat in the right ventricle of the normal heart. Histopathology. 2005;46:98–104.
12. Yeager M. Structure of gap junction intercellular channels. Gen Struct Biol. 1998;121:231–54.
13. Severs MJ, Coppen SR, Dupont E, Yeh HI, Co YS, Matsushita T. Gap junction alterations in human cardiac disease. Cardiac Res. 2004;62:368–77.

Cardiac Electrophysiology

Paul D. Morris and Jonathan Sahu

Abstract

This chapter provides a review of cardiac myocyte electrophysiology, including the molecular mechanisms and tissue adaptations underlying the generation, propagation and control of electrical impulses in the heart. There is a brief review of key clinical subject areas such as the ECG and implantable pacemaker therapies. The pathological mechanisms behind arrhythmia are covered, along with a brief description of the catheter-based electrophysiological studies and therapies, which can be used to diagnose and treat cardiac rhythm disturbances.

Keywords

Ion channels • Electrophysiology • Pacemaker • Electrocardiogram • Autonomic nervous system • Action potential • Ablation • Arrhythmia • Automaticity

Introduction

In order to serve its primary function of pumping blood, the heart depends upon a continually cycling sequence of complex electrophysiological processes. These processes rely on specialized molecular, cellular, and anatomical adaptations which generate and propagate electrical impulses through the heart in an organized fashion, ultimately resulting in coordinated myocardial contraction. The key components in this sequence involve

- *A resting electrochemical gradient* across the myocyte cell membrane

- *Automaticity* which allows certain myocytes to spontaneously discharge electrical depolarization impulses and act as cardiac pacemakers
- *Gap junctions* between cells which convey these impulses to adjacent cells
- *Specialized conduction tissues* which rapidly propagate the electrical impulses across the myocardium in an organized fashion
- *Excitation–contraction coupling* which links electrical stimulation to myofibril conformational changes and cellular contraction
- *Repolarization* which returns the myocyte membrane to the resting state before the process restarts

This process commences in utero and cycles continually until death. A derangement at any level can result in inefficiency and reduced cardiac performance, whether this is due to arrhythmia or uncoordinated cardiac contraction.

This chapter will focus on the normal electrophysiological and cell contraction processes listed above to provide a basic knowledge of cardiac electrophysiology from the molecular level up to the tissue adaptations of the human heart. Towards the end of this chapter, some clinically

P.D. Morris, BMedSci(Hons), MBChB(Hons), MRCP(Edin) (✉) •
J. Sahu, MBChB, MRCP, FACC
Department of Cardiology,
Sheffield Teaching Hospitals NHS Foundation Trust,
Herries Road, S57AU Sheffield, UK
e-mail: paulmorris@doctors.org.uk

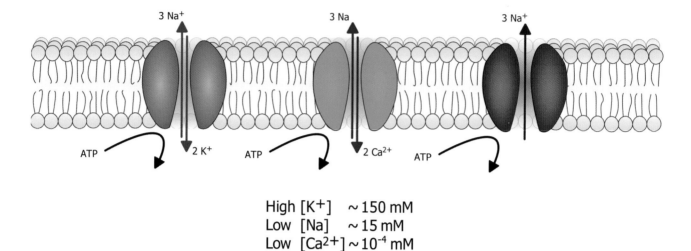

Low [K$^+$]   ~4 mM
High [Na]   ~145 mM
High [Ca^{2+}] ~2 mM

3 Na$^+$ 3 Na   3 Na$^+$

ATP   2 K$^+$ ATP   2 Ca^{2+} ATP

High [K$^+$]   ~150 mM
Low [Na]   ~15 mM
Low [Ca^{2+}] ~10^{-4} mM

Fig. 2.1 Schematic showing three of the membrane-spanning pumps which consume energy in the form of ATP in the generation of electrochemical gradients across the membrane. Approximate concentrations of the important cations are also shown in proportional format

relevant topics such as the electrocardiogram, pacemaker therapy, and basic electrophysiological interventions are also presented.

Cellular Electrophysiology

Resting Membrane Potential

The concentrations of charged ions across the cardiac myocyte cell membrane are unbalanced. This differential loading results in electrical and chemical gradients existing across the myocyte cell membrane. These gradients are generated by energy utilizing, active transport mechanisms, which drive ions across the membrane against their concentration gradients. The resulting equilibrium state results in the inner surface of the myocyte membrane being negatively charged relative to the extracellular fluid (i.e., the polarized state).

Inside the cell, the cytoplasm contains a much higher concentration of potassium ions (K$^+$) than the extracellular fluid. In the extracellular fluid, the main cations are sodium (Na$^+$) and calcium (Ca^{2+}) with the main anion being chloride (Cl$^-$). The concentration gradients are generated and maintained by the active transport of ions, counter to their concentration gradients. This process consumes energy in the form of ATP (Fig. 2.1). In order to maintain the ion concentrations across the cell membrane and thus the resting potential, three membrane-bound, energy-utilizing transport proteins are present spanning the cell membrane:

The Na$^+$–K$^+$ ATPase	Transports 3 Na$^+$ out for each 2 K$^+$ ions into the cell.
The Na$^+$–Ca^{2+} ATPase	Transports 3 Na$^+$ out for each 1 Ca^{2+} ion into the cell.
The Ca^{2+} pumps	Transport Ca^{2+} from the cell and into the sarcoplasmic reticulum (SR).

To understand the development of the resting membrane potential, one must consider the three cations (K$^+$, Na$^+$, and Ca^{2+}) and their permeability across the cell membrane. The cell permeability to K$^+$ ions is high, and as a result of the chemical concentration gradient, K$^+$ ions diffuse out of the cell through potassium channels. Intracellular negatively charged ions such as proteins and sulfates cannot cross the selectively permeable membrane and therefore remain inside the cell. The net passage of positively charged ions out of the cell creates a potential gradient across the cell membrane with the development of an increasing negative charge on the inner surface of the cell membrane relative to the extracellular fluid. Movement of potassium ions is therefore determined by a balance of forces, between the developing electrical charge, which opposes K$^+$ ion efflux, and the concentration gradient which encourages K$^+$ efflux. The point at which these two opposing forces balance is where equilibrium occurs. The electrical potential difference at this point is called the equilibrium potential (E). For K$^+$ ions, the "E_K" is −96 mV; for Na$^+$ ions, the E_{Na} is +52 mV; and for Ca^{2+} ions, the E_{Ca} is +134 mV.

The relative contribution of the individual cations to the membrane potential is not equal and is determined by the permeability or "conductance" (g) of the membrane to particular ions. Conductance is not fixed but is dynamic, and so the conductance of individual ions can vary significantly depending upon the state of the membrane (resting or active). The membrane potential (E_m) is the sum of the products of the conductance of a particular ion multiplied by the equilibrium potential of the ion, expressed as

$$E_m = \left(g_K\,E_K\right) + \left(g_{Na}\,E_{Na}\right) + \left(g_{Ca}\,E_{Ca}\right) + \left(g_{Cl}\,E_{Cl}\right)$$

Under resting conditions, the ionic conductance to potassium, g_K, is far greater than the ionic conductance to sodium, calcium, or chloride ions, and thus the membrane potential approximates the equilibrium potential of K$^+$ (E_K). A small background, inward Na current (I_b) results in the E_m being slightly higher (less negative) than the E_K. In most myocytes, this is balanced by the outward cation current (I_{Kir}) holding the resting membrane potential stable.

The magnitude of the resting membrane potential is not uniform. For ventricular myocytes, it is approximately −90 mV, whereas in sinoatrial (SA) and atrioventricular (AV) nodal cells, it is more positive of the order of −60 mV due, in part, to a relative deficiency of a particular subset of K$^+$ channels (inwardly rectifying K$_{ir}$ channels).

The direction of ionic transport depends upon the physiologic state of the cardiac myocytes. For example, there is an inward movement of Ca^{2+} ions during phase 2 of the action potential, but the ions are actively pumped out of the cell during other phases. More detail regarding the direction of ion currents is described below.

Ion Channels

Ionic transport across the myocyte cell membrane occurs through ion-specific membrane-spanning proteins. The structure and therefore selectivity of these channels does not remain static. Alterations in the intra- or extracellular electrolyte concentrations or the potential difference (voltage, mV) across the membrane may alter the conformation of channels, thus affecting conductance. This property is called gating. Cardiac channels can be divided into three classes depending upon the type of gating:
- Voltage-gated channels (the majority)
- Ligand-dependent channels
- Receptor-coupled channels

Voltage-gated channels undergo a conformational change in response to changes in the transmembrane potential. Typically this takes the form of either activation (open) or deactivation (closed). The Na$^+$ channel is typical of an "inactivating" channel, wherein application of a test potential

results in opening of the Na$^+$ channel and a rapid influx of Na$^+$ ions. Even with the maintenance of the potential, the sodium channel becomes inactivated, and so the conductance falls to zero. This inactivated state is not the same as the closed state. In order for the channel conductance to increase once again, recovery from inactivation has to occur. For a noninactivating channel, the conductance remains high for the duration of the potential, and on removal of the test potential, the conductance falls to zero. An example of noninactivating channels is the inwardly rectifying potassium channels (K$_{ir}$).

Ligand-dependent channels are highly selective. Ligands can either activate (increase conductance) or inactivate channels. An example of an activated channel is the acetylcholine (ACh)-dependent K$^+$ channel (K$_{Ach}$). Acetyl choline binds to muscarinic receptors (M2) in the myocyte cell membrane resulting in the activation of G-proteins. Dissociation and interaction of the G-protein subunits with the K$^+$ channel result in a configuration change and an increase in conductance to K$^+$ ions.

Receptor-coupled gating requires the translation of a physical stimulus into a conformational change in channel structure and a consequent change in conductance to a particular ion. Examples of such channels are stretch-activated chloride and cation channels. The former is important in regulation of cell volume, and the latter is important in cardiac dilatation.

The Na$^+$, K$^+$, and Ca^{2+} channels and their corresponding currents are responsible for the generation of a cardiac action potential and its ultimate propagation through the cardiac tissue. The organized electrical wave of depolarization that occurs is closely followed by, and coupled to, the mechanical contraction of the heart.

Although ion channels share a common basic structure with several transmembrane protein domains encircling a central aperture, there is heterogeneity in the ultrastructure and specific arrangement of the subunits and domains within the myocyte membrane. In short, ion channels vary in their level of complexity, and this determines the individual characteristics of the channel. Voltage-gated Na$^+$ and Ca$^+$ channels are composed of four (alpha) subunits, all of which are bound together into a single tetramer protein. Each of the four subunits is composed of six transmembrane-spanning domains or "motifs." Voltage-gated K$^+$ channels are similarly composed of four subunits, each with six transmembrane domains, but each subunit is not linked to the next, and so are separate. The inwardly rectifying K$^+$ channels are similar again but distinct in that each subunit is composed of only two transmembrane motifs, not six.

Sodium Channel/Current

The Na$^+$ channel is a good example of a voltage-gated, inactivating channel. This is elegantly demonstrated by performing

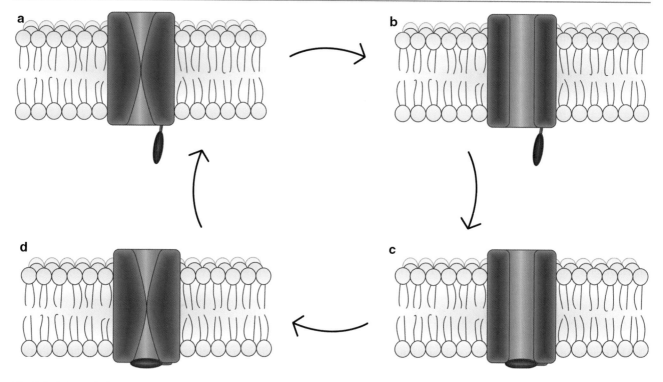

Fig. 2.2 Schematic demonstrating the sequence of activation and inactivation of the m and h gates in a cardiac myocyte Na$^+$ channel. (**a**) The *m* gate is closed during the resting state which corresponds to action potential phase 4. (**b**) The m gate opens in response to a depolarizing stimulus which brings the potential to a threshold level; this corresponds to phase 0. (**c**) After only milliseconds, the *h* gate closes inactivating the channel. (**d**) On repolarization, the *m* gate closes (**d**) and the *h* gate opens (**a**)

voltage clamp experiments. Application of a small test potential results in a small increase in Na$^+$ conductance and the generation of a small current. By increasing the amplitude of the test potential, the Na$^+$ conductance and current increases. When a threshold potential (−40 to −50 mV) is reached, the Na$^+$ channels are open, and the conductance and current is maximal. However, at more depolarized states, inactivation of the Na$^+$ channel occurs. It is proposed that this process is controlled by an activation gate (m) and a separate inactivation gate (h), respectively.

In the resting state, the channel is closed by the m gate. Partial depolarization opens the m gate allowing inward Na$^+$ ion flow and further depolarization of the cell membrane. The channel remains open for only milliseconds. At higher potentials, the h gate closes, rendering the channel inactive. On repolarization, the m gate closes and the h gate opens (Fig. 2.2). Clinically, these Na$^+$ channels can be blocked in either the active or inactivated states to treat abnormal cardiac rhythms (see Chap. 4). This model of activation and inactivation similarly applies to other currents such as the Ca^{2+} current and the transient outward K$^+$ current.

Potassium Channel/Current

This group is a very diverse collection of channels and currents. Eight types (distributed variably across cardiac

tissues) have been described with a variety of modes of gating including activation/inactivation and noninactivating, voltage gating, and ligand-dependent gating.

Potassium currents are outward currents and are important in the phases 1, 2, 3, and 4 of the cardiac action potential. The contribution of the different currents to the cardiac action potential is shown in Fig. 2.3.

Transient outward K$^+$ channels (I_{to}) occur in a relatively high density in the atria, nodal tissue, Purkinje fibers, and the epicardial myocytes. This channel contributes to some of the regional variation in the action potential duration in the heart (especially the phase 1 "spike," see below). The other major group of K$^+$ channels which is important in the development of the cardiac action potential is the delayed rectifier K$^+$ channels (K$_V$). This group includes I_{Kr} (rapid) and I_{Ks} (slow) channels. These channels are noninactivating. They are termed delayed because their activation times are relatively slow with time constants of the order of around 1 s.

The Rectifier K$^+$ Currents

Inwardly rectifying K$^+$ channels (K$_{ir}$) conduct K$^+$ inwardly at potentials more negative than E_K and outwardly at potentials higher than E_K. Therefore, they maintain ("rectify") the intracellular K$^+$ concentration at E_K, irrespective of the membrane potential. The name is slightly confusing since under

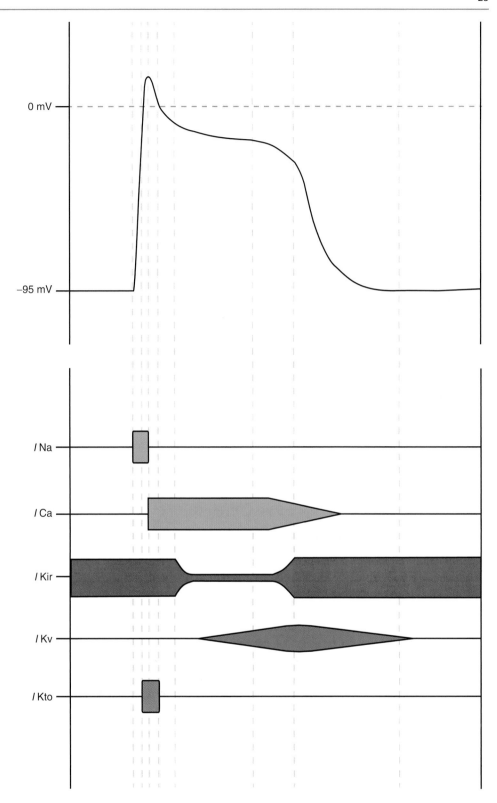

Fig. 2.3 This schematic demonstrates the timing and contribution of Na$^+$, Ca^{2+}, and K$^+$ currents through an action potential cycle. The thickness of the bars provides an approximation of how the magnitude of the currents varies through the cycle. Na$^+$ current; I_{Na}, Ca^{2+} current; I_{Ca}, inwardly rectifying K$^+$ channel current; I_{Kir}, delayed K$^+$ rectifier current; I_{Kv}, transient outward K$^+$ current; I_{Kto}

physiological conditions and during the action potential cycle, K$^+$ ion movement is outward. It is during voltage patch clamp experiments, with the application of strongly negative (hyperpolarized) voltages, when inward K$^+$ ion movement occurs. The weak Na$^+$ background current (I_b) holds the membrane potential (E_m) slightly higher than E_K, and so the K$_{ir}$ channels normally allow K$^+$ ion efflux in the resting state, along the steep concentration gradient, generating the resting membrane potential. During depolarization (phase 2 plateau), conductance through this channel is blocked by polyamines and magnesium ions. This is a useful adaptation since it conserves the intracellular K⁺ and thus reduces the overall energy consumption of the myocyte. A separate group of delayed rectifiers (K_V) are voltage gated and activate slowly during depolarization. They, therefore, activate towards the end of the action potential (phase 2, see below) and bring about repolarization back towards the resting membrane potential.

Calcium Channels/Current

Four types of Ca^{2+} channels have been identified in cardiac tissue. The two main types are the long acting (L-type) and the transient (T-type) channels.

The L-type channels are triggered by higher (depolarized) potentials and help sustain the action potential (AP) in phase 2. The L-type membrane-associated channel is the channel responsible for the majority of the calcium entry into the myocyte. The consequent rise in intracellular Ca^{2+} concentration induces calcium release from the sarcoplasmic reticulum (SR) which is vital in linking electrical excitation to the interaction of actin and myosin and thus myofibril apparatus shortening – known as "excitation–contraction coupling." These L-type channels are the target for the dihydropyridine class of calcium channel blocking drugs (amlodipine, nifedipine, etc.).

T-type calcium channels affect the rise in the resting potential (towards the depolarization threshold potential) observed in cells capable of spontaneously depolarizing without the need for an external stimulus. Thus, these channels are important in *initiating* depolarization. T-type Ca^{2+} channels are well represented in tissues with increased automaticity like the SAN and AVN. The T-type Ca^{2+} channel is an inactivating voltage-gated channel which is active at negative potentials and is inactivated by depolarization. The activation and inactivation time constants of this channel are very short. Since the conductance of the channels is relatively poor, the resulting current is relatively small.

The third type of Ca^{2+} channel occurs on the internal membrane of the SR. Ryanodine receptors on the SR detect an increase in cytosolic Ca^{2+} concentration, and this induces a release of Ca^{2+} from the SR, the so-called "calcium-induced calcium release" (CICR). Typically the Ca^{2+} ions entering the cell enter via the L-type Ca^{2+} channel. The CICR is crucial in the development of cardiac contraction. The final mechanism for Ca^{2+} release into the myocyte is an indirect mechanism utilizing inositol triphosphate (IP_3). IP_3 receptors are present in smooth muscle and the conduction system. Increased levels of IP_3 arise with both sympathetic and parasympathetic stimulation and paracrine substances such as angiotensin II.

The Action Potential

The myocardial tissues continually cycle through depolarization and repolarization, with each cycle corresponding to

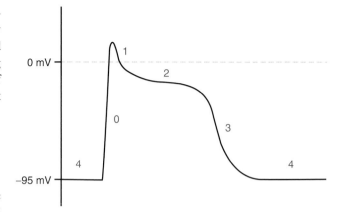

Fig. 2.4 A graphical representation of a single-action potential sequence, with the five phases illustrated

a heartbeat. This cycle or action potential (AP) is quickly conducted through the specialized cardiac conduction tissues in an organized and sequential manner to bring the wave of depolarization to the whole heart and trigger a well-coordinated myocardial contraction.

The AP follows five well-characterized phases, known as phases 0, 1, 2, 3, and 4 (Fig. 2.4). The resting membrane potential corresponds with phase 4. In general terms, the action potential sequence is similar in all cardiac cells.

Depolarization is followed by a transient partial repolarization, followed by a prolonged plateau phase before repolarization returns the membrane back to its polarized resting potential. However, it is worth considering that different anatomical areas of the myocardium serve different roles. For example, atrial myocyte function is subtly different to a ventricular myocyte which, in turn, is very different to an atrioventricular nodal or Purkinje cell function. Localized differences in the AP sequence reflect this reality. Such variability accounts for differences in action potential duration and other properties such as automaticity, as seen in nodal cells.

Similar to the neuronal and skeletal muscle fibers, cardiac myocyte depolarization is a very rapid process, taking the cell membrane from a negative membrane potential to a slightly positive membrane potential. However, the cardiac action potential is unique in its considerably longer duration (200–400 ms vs. 1–4 ms) (Fig. 2.5). This specialized adaptation is driven by prolonged inward Ca^{2+} and then Na⁺ currents which are balanced against outward K⁺ rectification currents. This accounts for the plateau in phase 2 of the action potential. The delay allows time for myocardial contraction to occur.

This section will now focus on the action potential sequence which occurs in the majority of cardiac myocytes before considering the different characteristics of the action potential in nodal cells.

Phase 4

Phase 4 is the so-called resting phase where the cardiac myocyte is held in a negative, polarized state with a resting

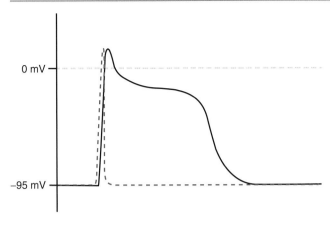

Fig. 2.5 Comparison between a neuronal-/skeletal-muscle-action potential (*red dotted line*) and a much longer cardiac myocyte (*black solid line*)

membrane potential between −90 and −95 mV. This phase corresponds to atrial and ventricular diastole. In atrial and ventricular myocytes, this phase is relatively stable (flat profile), and depolarization (usually) occurs if a depolarizing electrical stimulus is conducted to the myocyte from adjacent cells. If such a stimulus brings the myocyte membrane potential to a threshold level of ~ −60 mV, then fast Na⁺ channels open, and phase 0 commences.

Phase 0

Once the threshold potential is reached, fast Na⁺ channels open, and Na⁺ rapidly diffuses into the cell down the steep concentration gradient. This inward Na⁺ current (I_{Na}) raises the intracellular membrane potential (becoming less negative) to approximately +20 mV. Once depolarized, the voltage-gated Na⁺ channels quickly inactivate and close. The Na⁺ current is thus abruptly terminated.

Phase 1

Phase 1 is a phase of rapid but only partial repolarization back to a membrane potential of about zero (0 mV). It is driven by the short-lived, outward current of K⁺ ions (I_{to}). This current is very transient being activated by depolarization and inactivated very promptly by the partial repolarization.

Phase 2

During this phase, there are a number of competing but balanced ion currents. The net result is a plateau in the membrane potential. Thus, it remains depolarized for a prolonged period. The early part of the plateau is driven by the inward Ca²⁺ current (I_{Ca}). This current is conducted through L-type Ca²⁺ channels. These are activated by depolarization and, as their name suggests, remain activated for a prolonged time before slow inactivation. The latter part of the plateau is driven by the inward Na⁺ current (I_{Na}) which is, in turn, driven by the Na⁺: Ca²⁺ exchange pump. This pumps Na⁺ into the cell in exchange for Ca²⁺ ions out and is aided in its function by the relatively high intracellular calcium levels during

myocyte depolarization. Balancing these currents, the major outward current is of K⁺ ions through a variety of channels (I_{to}, I_{Kr}, and I_{Ks}).

Phase 3

Towards the end of the plateau phase, the slow K⁺ channels, also known as delayed rectifier channels, open. K⁺ efflux currents (I_{Kv} comprising I_{Kr} and I_{Ks}) begin to increase in magnitude and eventually overpower the late inward Na⁺ and Ca²⁺ currents (I_{Na} and I_{Ca}) active during the plateau phase. This results in the membrane potential becoming increasingly negative and eventually becoming polarized once again (phase 4), back to a resting membrane potential of −90 to −95 mV.

The heart is "wired" in such a way as to allow these waves of depolarization to efficiently and rapidly spread across the entire endomyocardial surface and then the myocardial wall – resulting in efficient ventricular filling (ventricular diastole) and emptying (ventricular systole).

The SAN is a collection of myocytes found in the posterior wall of the right atrium close to the entry point of the superior vena cava. These cells spontaneously generate action potentials which, via gap junctions, are propagated to the remainder of the myocardium. The wave of depolarization rapidly moves across the right and (via Bachmann's bundle) the left atria, resulting in a near synchronous atrial contraction. The atria are electrically insulated from the ventricles by the annulus fibrosis, which corresponds to the fibrous mitral and tricuspid valve annuli. The only way for impulses to reach the ventricles in the normal heart is via the AVN, which is situated in the inferior interatrial septum (see Chap. 1). Here, the wave of depolarization slows down to allow optimal ventricular filling before being transmitted down the interventricular septum through the bundle of His.

The bundle of His rapidly transmits the impulse down the septum towards the ventricular apex. The His bundle divides at the lower end into a right bundle branch and a left bundle branch. The left bundle branch separates into a left anterior and left posterior bundle. These insulated bundle fibers terminate into a vast network of subendocardial Purkinje fibers. The Purkinje fibers rapidly disseminate the wave of depolarization to the entire right and left ventricles in an endocardial to epicardial direction. Although the ventricles depolarize almost synchronously, the apex to base direction of conduction allows the apex to depolarize and contract very slightly earlier than the base. This allows the heart to expel blood in an efficient manner (Fig. 2.6).

Nodal Action Potential

Clusters of specialized cardiac myocytes arranged into the SAN and the AVN differ from other excitable tissue in that they have an intrinsic and spontaneous electrical instability (automaticity). In the healthy heart, it is these cells that act as the cardiac pacemakers, dictating the frequency of

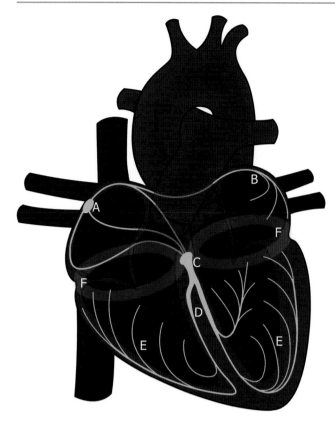

Fig. 2.6 Representation of the arrangement of the conduction tissues ("*wiring*") in the heart. (*A*) SAN, (*B*) Bachmann's bundle, (*C*) AVN, (*D*) bundle of His dividing into right and left anterior and left posterior bundles, (*E*) Purkinje fibers, (*F*) insulating fibrous annular ring around the mitral and tricuspid valves

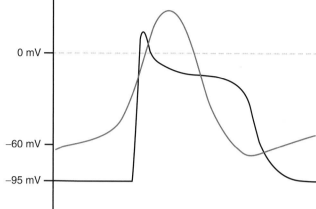

Fig. 2.7 A comparison between a ventricular or atrial action potential (*black line*) and a nodal action potential (*blue line*). Note the less-negative and upwardly drifting phase 4 membrane potential, the slower phase 0, and lack of plateau in the nodal action potential

depolarization and repolarization of all the other myocytes and hence the heart rate. In health, the SAN cells serve this function, but as a fail-safe mechanism, a hierarchy of other areas (AVN, His bundle, and Purkinje cells) can act as subsidiary pacemakers to prevent asystole if the sinus node fails. However, these subsidiary pacemakers have slower rates of discharge. As a general rule, the anatomical distance from the SA node is associated, inversely, with the frequency of action potential generation. Consequently, subsidiary pacemakers, if required to perform this function, do not always pace at a sufficient rate or in such a well-coordinated fashion.

The action potential profile of nodal cells is quite distinct from that of other myocytes. Polarization is not as prominent in these cells since there is a relative deficiency of the rectifier K$^+$ channels (K$_{ir}$). The "resting" membrane potential is therefore less negative than previously described, at approximately −60 mV, and is thus held closer to the threshold potential. The "resting" membrane potential does not really exist in such cells since the potential in phase 4 is constantly rising towards depolarization. Instead of the relatively stable, flat profile of phase 4 previously described, the membrane potential is constantly drifting upward (becoming less negative) and bringing the myocytes towards the threshold potential

which will trigger depolarization (Fig. 2.7). The quicker the rise in membrane potential in phase 4, the quicker the rate of discharge and, thus, the quicker the heart rate. These phase 4 "pacemaker potentials" are generated by several unbalanced ion currents. In addition to the slow inward background Na$^+$ current (I_b), the "hyperpolarization-activated" or "funny" current (I_f) allows Na influx at potentials more negative than −50 mV. The channel and its corresponding current are known as "funny" since it is, rather unusually, activated by hyperpolarization and not depolarization. The I_b and I_f currents result in the *initial* rise in membrane potential in these cells.

When a threshold of −50 mV is reached, activation of transient (T-type) Ca^{2+} channels occurs. Nodal cells possess a high density of these channels. The resulting Ca^{2+} ion influx further depolarizes the membrane potential and brings the cell to approximately −40 mV. At this point, the L-type Ca^{2+} channels become activated. This is the major current of phase 0 in nodal myocytes and is quite distinct from atrial and ventricular myocytes. The kinetics of these currents are relatively slow in comparison to the fast Na$^+$ current which accounts for phase 0 in non-nodal myocytes. As a consequence, the slope of the phase 0 depolarization in nodal cells is much gentler and the conduction velocity slower in these cells. The currents that cause repolarization in nodal tissues are similar to the non-nodal cells (i.e., the delayed rectifier K$^+$ currents, I_{Kv}).

The spontaneous depolarization or "automaticity" that is seen in nodal tissue (phase 4) is actually not unique. The rate of spontaneous depolarization in the SAN is greater than that of the AVN. The origin of the cardiac depolarization therefore arises from the site with the fastest rate of spontaneous depolarization. In the normal, healthy heart, this occurs in the SAN. If this node, the natural pacemaker site of the heart, is affected from some disease process, then subsidiary pacemaker sites such as the AVN may take over as the site of origin of cardiac depolarization. A good example of this is in complete heart block, where there is no electrical communication between the atria and the ventricles. In this situation, the heart relies on cells below the atria to generate action potentials; otherwise, ventricular asystole would occur. Depending on the precise level of the block, cells in the AVN, His bundles, or Purkinje fibers can, therefore, take over the role of pacemaker. However, the "escape" rate of spontaneous depolarization in these tissues becomes progressively slower, often resulting in symptomatic bradycardia and the requirement of a pacemaker.

Modulation of the Pacemaker Function

The intrinsic rate of SAN depolarization is approximately 100–110 beats/min (bpm). However, at rest, the adult heart normally beats at around 60 bpm, and during significant exercise, the rate can be closer to 200 bpm. The pacemaker rate is therefore modulated by a variety of factors, the most important of which is the autonomic nervous system.

The parasympathetic nervous system, via the vagus (X) nerve, has the effect of slowing the pacemaker rate, the speed of conduction, and the duration of the action potential. Its nerve fibers are mainly concentrated in the nodal and conduction tissues. The sympathetic nervous system (T1–T5, sympathetic chain) innervates relatively more of the myocardial tissues including the ventricular myocardium, and activation has the opposite effect. Since the inherent rate of the SAN is 100 bpm, at rest, the predominant effect is from the parasympathetic system.

Noradrenaline (NA) released from sympathetic nerve fibers and adrenaline (A) from the adrenal medulla bind to beta adrenoreceptors, of which the beta-1 adrenoreceptor predominates. Receptor binding results in activation of adenylyl cyclase via a G-protein-coupled signal transduction pathway. Adenylyl cyclase catalyzes the conversion of ATP into cyclic adenosine monophosphate (cAMP). cAMP has the effect of activating the "funny" channel in nodal cells and also of activating protein kinase A (PKA). Activation of the funny current (I_f) accelerates the rise in phase 4 of nodal cells and so accelerates "pacemaker potentials" and increases heart rate (positive chronotropic effect). Activation of PKA has several desirable effects. PKA activates L-type Ca^{2+} channels which also accelerate the phase 4 pacemaker potentials in nodal cells. L-type Ca^{2+} channel activation results in an amplification of the depolarization and plateau magnitude currents. The resulting increased inward Ca^{2+} flux increases intracellular Ca^{2+} concentration, and this increases contractility (positive inotropic effect) which is usually appropriate under sympathetic activation. PKA also augments the function of the

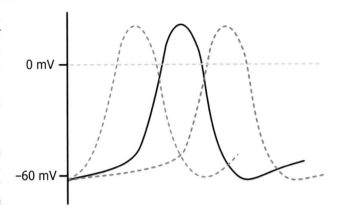

Fig. 2.8 The effect of the autonomic nervous system on nodal pacemaker potentials. A "normal" nodal action potential is shown in *black*. Sympathetic nervous stimulation increases pacemaker potentials in phase 4 and causes a steeper rise in the phase 4 potentials. The threshold potential is therefore reached sooner, and thus, an action potential is triggered earlier (*blue dotted line*) resulting in a more frequent rate of discharge. Parasympathetic stimulation has the opposite effect and causes a slower rise in potential in phase 4. The threshold is reached later, and so the action potential is delayed (*green dotted line*) resulting in a slower rate of discharge

delayed rectifier currents, and this shortens phases 2 and 3 of the action potential. Another effect of PKA is a faster clearance of Ca^{2+} back into the sarcoplasmic reticulum following systole. This results in quicker relaxation of the myofibrillar contractile apparatus (positive lusitropic effect).

With predominant parasympathetic activity, acetylcholine (ACh) binds to muscarinic M_2 receptors and, via the release of inhibitory G-protein subunits, inhibits adenylyl cyclase. This results in a reduction in cAMP. The effects of parasympathetic activation are therefore to oppose the mechanisms and currents described above. The rate of rise of the membrane potential in phase 4 is therefore reduced, thus delaying the development of the next action potential. Spontaneous pacemaker activity is thereby reduced with a consequent reduction in heart rate (Fig. 2.8).

Once a cardiac myocyte has depolarized, further stimulation cannot generate an action potential for a defined period of time. This is called the effective or absolute refractory period (ARP). This period includes phases 0, 1, and 2 and the first part of phase 3. The short remaining period of time to completion of repolarization is the relative refractory period (RRP) (Fig. 2.9). During the RRP, a stimulus of sufficient energy may generate another cardiac action potential. This is one of the mechanisms which may cause polymorphic ventricular tachycardia.

Effects of Electrolyte Disturbance and Disease

Disturbances in intra- or extracellular electrolyte concentrations can have deleterious effects on the action potential and

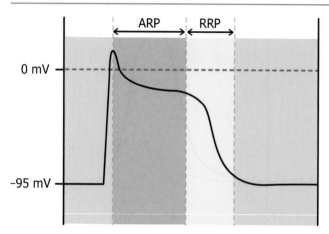

Fig. 2.9 The absolute refractory period (*RRP*) and the relative refractory period (*RRP*)

therefore the rhythm of the heart. Since the resting membrane potential is influenced more by K⁺ (E_K) than any other ion, alterations in the concentration of this ion have more impact than any other.

Significant hyperkalemia impacts on the E_K and has the effect of increasing the resting membrane potential (becoming less negative). Na⁺ channels can be activated (phase 0), inactivated (phase 1–3), or closed but excitable (phase 4). At less negative potentials, Na⁺ channels are more likely to be inactivated, and although the membrane potential is "closer" to the threshold potential, this results in a weaker and more delayed phase 0. Hyperkalemia also augments the function of the delayed K⁺ rectifier channels which results in stronger repolarization currents and ultimately in more rapid repolarization. The effect of hyperkalemia is therefore a reduction in myocardial excitability and a reduction in the speed of onset, duration, and magnitude of phase 0 of the action potential, along with a brisker repolarization phase. Overall, the action potential duration is shortened. Profound hyperkalemia can result in cardiac arrest due to bradycardia or asystole.

Conversely, hypokalemia induces hyperpolarization, and this results in an increase in the number of Na⁺ channels held in the activated state. This results in more excitable myocardium. Hypokalemia inhibits the function of K_{ir} channels leading to a delayed repolarization phase and a prolongation of action potential duration. This can predispose to re-entrant tachycardias – such as ventricular tachycardia (VT) which may degrade into VF or asystole.

Magnesium is required for Na–K ATPase function and for the partial blockade of the rectifying K⁺ channels during plateau phase 2. Hypomagnesemia, therefore, results in reduced polarization (less negative in phase 4), intracellular K⁺ depletion, and prolonged repolarization. In extreme cases, hypomagnesemia can result in re-entrant arrhythmias like polymorphic ventricular tachycardia (PVT) also known as Torsade de Pointes (TdP).

Profound hypocalcemia results in a prolonged plateau phase, whereas profound hypercalcemia shortens the plateau phase. Hypercalcemia also reduces the action potential conduction velocity and reduces the ARP. Thus, the net effect of hypercalcemia is a shortening of the action potential duration and predisposition to AVN block. The net effect of hypocalcemia is a prolongation of the action potential duration with a corresponding lengthening of the refractory period which may have an antiarrhythmic effect.

In chronic heart failure and conditions associated with myocardial fibrosis (e.g., after a myocardial infarction), myocytic expression of certain K⁺ channels (predominantly K_{to}) may be reduced leading to a delayed repolarization phase. The prolongation of the plateau phase results in a prolongation of the action potential duration and higher intracellular Ca⁺ levels which may predispose to afterdepolarizations. Afterdepolarizations and prolongation of repolarization (and thus refractory period) may both result in malignant ventricular arrhythmia. This helps explain the higher rates of sudden arrhythmic death seen in this population. Acute ischemia induces the K_{ATP} channel, which is a subtype of K_{ir} channel. This increases rectifying currents and overpowers the inward cation currents during the phase 2 plateau. This results in a shortening of phase 2, more rapid repolarization, and less Ca²⁺ influx. This has a negative inotropic effect, which is desirable in that it helps, at least in part, limit the ischemic burden.

Cardiac Conduction and Excitation–Contraction Coupling

Conduction of Electrical Impulses

Cardiac myocytes are arranged and connected longitudinally. The junction between two cardiac myocytes is called the intercalated disk. Adjacent myocytes are connected by anchoring proteins called desmosomes. Efficient cardiac contraction (systole) and relaxation (diastole) relies upon the atria and subsequently the ventricles contracting synchronously as single units. The wave of depolarization and repolarization must therefore propagate across the myocardium rapidly with little resistance to ionic flow between cells. Ion currents, and therefore impulse transmission, are made possible by the presence of gap junctions between myocytes.

Gap junctions are membrane-spanning conduits that allow ions to flow between adjacent myocytes freely. Each gap junction or "connexon" is constructed of six-protein subunits ("connexins") arranged into a membrane-spanning tubule. Connexons join end-to-end with connexons from adjacent cells. This arrangement results in the cytoplasm of each myocyte being in direct continuity with the cytoplasm of, not only adjacent myocytes, but also the remainder of the myocardium. The density of these gap junctions varies in the adult with a relatively high density along the orientation of the fiber and a relatively sparse density orthogonally. As a result, the conduction velocity along the fiber orientation is relatively rapid with conduction velocities at other angles being reduced.

Certain loci, such as the SAN and AVN, have a relatively low density of gap junctions with a consequent slowing of action potential conduction. Within healthy myocardium, there is variability in conduction velocity between different myocardial regions. Conduction velocity is proportional to the density of gap junctions and relates to the predominance of either fast (non-nodal myocytes with Na^+-dependent phase 0) or slow (nodal myocytes with Ca^{2+}- dependent phase 0) response fibers.

In pathological situations, for example, when scar is present within the myocardium, the conduction velocity may be significantly impeded or even blocked, which may encourage an arrhythmia. The impulse conduction velocity may also be influenced by other factors such as the autonomic nervous system, hormones, ischemia, and drugs.

Excitation–Contraction Coupling

The wave of cardiac depolarization is quickly followed by contraction of the myocardium, i.e., "excitation–contraction coupling." The importance of rapid impulse conduction across the myocardium, in a normal heart, cannot be overemphasized. Near-simultaneous depolarization in the atria and later the ventricles results in synchronous contraction of the atrium and subsequently the ventricles.

The wave of depolarization is delayed through the AVN, and this allows time for atrial contraction to augment and optimally fill the ventricles (the atrial "kick") prior to ventricular systole. The action potential duration in cardiac myocytes is much longer than that of nerve cells and skeletal muscle fibers. However, there is another key difference between these tissues. Nerve and skeletal muscle cells release Ca^{2+} in response to the high intracellular Na^+ which occurs with depolarization. However, in cardiac myocytes, it is the rise in intracellular Ca^{2+} concentration, which occurs during phase 2 of the action potential, that is, the stimulus for calcium release from the sarcoplasmic reticulum and hence myocardial contraction. This is termed as calcium-induced calcium release (CICR).

Contraction of the myocardium occurs during phase 2 of the cardiac action potential. Ca^{2+} enters the myocyte during this phase via Na^+–Ca^{2+} exchange and the L-type Ca^{2+} channel. The L-type Ca^{2+} channels are clustered in the transverse tubules, close to the junctional regions of the sarcoplasmic reticulum (SR) (see earlier Chap. 1). The L-type channels are activated during phase 2 (plateau) of the action potential, and the resulting inward Ca^{2+} current causes a relatively small increase in the local Ca^{2+} concentration around the junctional SR. The rise in Ca^{2+} concentration, in turn, activates the ryanodine channels (also known as calcium release channels) in the junctional SR membrane, leading to a release of Ca^+ from the SR into the cytoplasm with a corresponding large increase in the cytoplasmic Ca^{2+} concentration. Towards the end of systole, the myocyte expels the Ca^{2+} back into the SR via Ca ATPase pumps and back into the extracellular space via Na^+–Ca^{2+} exchange proteins, a process known as restitution.

The Ca^{2+} released into the cytoplasm interacts with the troponin–tropomyosin binding on the thin actin filaments causing a conformational change which exposes the myosin binding site on the actin filaments. Cross-bridges can therefore form between the myosin heads and the actin binding sites. This is an energy-utilizing process with a single molecule of ATP being used to "cock" the myosin head prior to the force being applied and contraction. The contraction involves troponin-mediated movement of the actin over the thick myosin filament, a mechanism known as the sliding filament mechanism (Fig. 2.10). Disengagement of the myosin head from the actin binding site also requires energy and utilizes another molecule of ATP. Thus, both contraction and relaxation are energy dependent.

Under resting conditions, the rise in intracellular Ca^+ is sufficient to activate approximately 30–40% of the available actin–myosin cross-bridge binding sites. Under increased physiological stress, more Ca^+ is released from the SR. This results in more actin–myosin cross-bridges being recruited, which has a positive inotropic effect (increased contractility). The contractile force is therefore increased in proportion to the rise in cytoplasmic Ca^{2+}.

Beta-adrenergic receptor stimulation by NA or A achieves this effect by increasing the amplitude and duration of phase 2 Ca^{2+} currents. Myocardial stretch increases the myocyte's sensitivity to Ca^{2+} ions, and this forms the basis of the Frank–Starling mechanism, whereby increased myocardial stretch (during diastolic filling) results in increased contractile force. Therefore, cardiac output is maintained under times of physiological stress and when there is an increase in diastolic filling pressures or prolonged filling times.

The Electrocardiogram (ECG)

Having been invented over 100 years ago, the ECG has been in routine clinical use for the last 50 years. It is quick and cheap to perform this bedside test, with many automated devices now in existence. The ECG can provide a wealth of diagnostic information as an adjunct to the clinical assessment of the patient. While entire textbooks are dedicated to the subject, here, the basics are provided, with further reading suggested later.

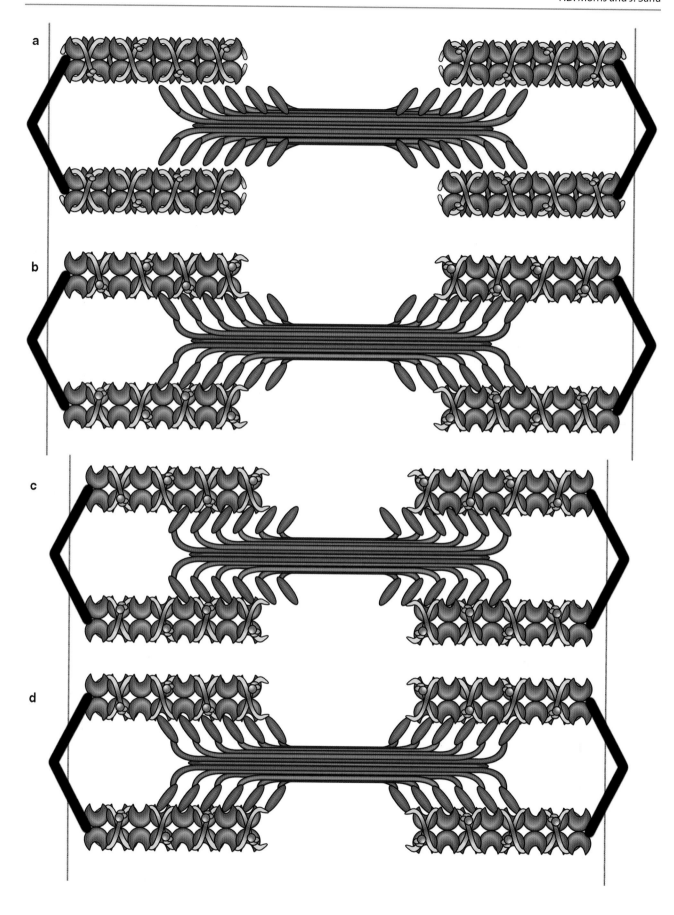

The ECG noninvasively evaluates cardiac electrical activity via external transducers placed across the body surface. This is made possible by the fact that cardiac electrical signals are conducted through the body's fluid and tissue compartments. It is important to note from the outset that the electrical signals recorded at the body surface onto an ECG tracing represent a *summation* of all the electrical impulses from all the tissues of the atria and the ventricles. This means that not all individual currents are seen on the ECG trace. Larger currents may "cancel out" or "hide" the effects of any smaller currents as the wave of depolarization sweeps across the surface of the heart.

By using 10 electrodes (1 of which acts as earth) on the surface of the body, 12 different representations of the electrical activity of the heart can be displayed (i.e., the "12-lead" ECG). The 12 "leads" do not refer to 12 individual transducers but to the 9 unipolar and 3 bipolar "views" of the heart which are represented in graphical form on a 12-lead ECG printout. The limb leads comprise three bipolar recordings (leads I, II, III) and three augmented (a) unipolar recordings (aVR, aVL, and aVF). These six leads look at the heart from different positions in the coronal plane to give a 2-D electrical representation of the heart.

The recordings are such that an electrical wave moving towards the electrode is represented by a positive (upward) deflection and a wave traveling in the opposite direction by a negative (downward) deflection. The electrical activity is delineated as an electrical potential plotted against time (seconds). The opposite deflections are true for a wave of repolarization. Thus, a single complex (cardiac cycle) with atrial depolarization (P wave) followed by ventricular depolarization (QRS waves) and repolarization (T wave) is shown in Fig. 2.11 with the component parts.

Leads I, II, and III are bipolar recordings. Lead I records the electrical activity of the heart as "seen" between the left arm and the right arm. The positive vector is from right to left. Lead II records between the right arm and the left leg with a positive vector from the right arm to the left leg. Lead III records between the left arm and the right leg. The positive vector is from the left arm to the right leg.

The augmented (a) leads, aVR, aVL, and aVF, are unipolar recordings. They display the summated signals from a single point, the right shoulder, left shoulder, and symphysis pubis,

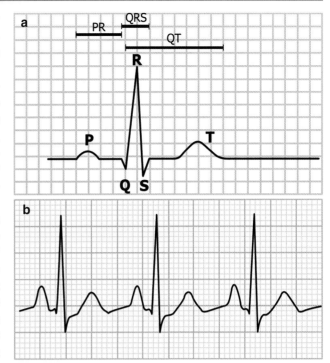

Fig. 2.11 (**a**) A single PQRST ECG complex. The PR interval, QRS interval, and the QT interval are shown. (**b**) An ECG rhythm strip demonstrating normal sinus rhythm. A P wave is followed by a QRS complex and then a T wave. The rate is approximately 80 beats per minute

respectively. The limb lead tracings may be useful in deducing the overall electrical axis of the heart, which can be influenced by various disease states, and are also useful in "looking" at the inferior surface of the heart (typically leads II, III, and aVF), for example, in diagnosing an inferior myocardial infarction. Figure 2.12 demonstrates the six limb leads and the angles from which they electrically "view" the heart.

In addition to the limb leads, there are six unipolar chest leads. These leads "view" the heart in a slightly tilted transverse plane and can be used to localize abnormalities and disease states in the right ventricular, septal, anterior, or lateral walls of the heart. If required, transducers can be moved onto the right side of the chest or to the posterior chest wall to aid the diagnosis of diseases in other territories (e.g., right ventricular or posterior territory myocardial infarction). Figure 2.13 demonstrates the arrangement of the six chest leads.

Fig. 2.10 A representation of the sliding filament theory of myofibril contraction. The diagram shows a simplified representation of a sarcomere with central myosin thick filaments surrounded by actin thin filaments which attach peripherally at the Z line. (**a**) The myosin binding sites on the actin thin filaments are blocked by tropomyosin (*yellow*). (**b**) Calcium (*purple*) causes a conformational change which exposes the myosin binding sites allowing cross-bridge formation between actin and myosin. (**c**) The myosin heads are "cocked" back which is an energy-utilizing process consuming a single molecule of ATP. Note that this has the overall effect of sliding the actin along relative to the myosin and shortening the sarcomere. (**d**) The myosin heads have "ratcheted" on to the next binding site. Disengagement of the myosin heads also requires energy via ATP

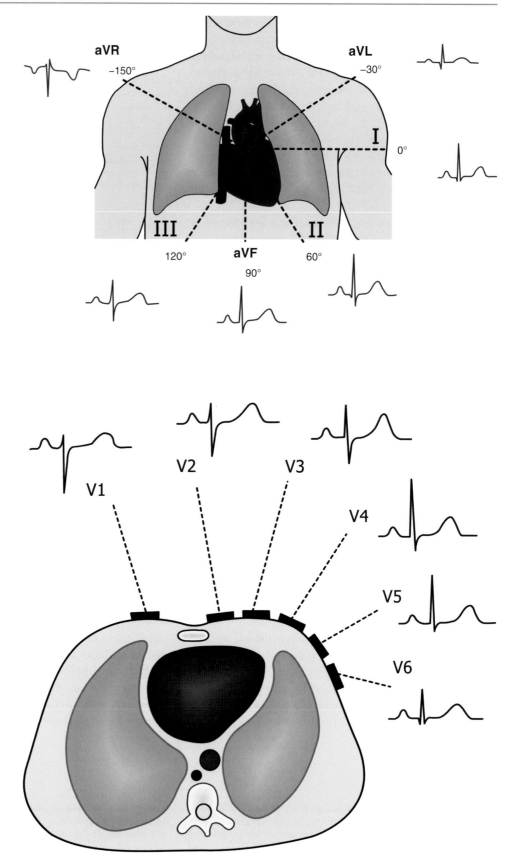

Fig. 2.12 The six limb leads and the angles from which they "view" the heart's electrical activity. Coronal section

Fig. 2.13 The six chest leads as viewed from below in CT scan style. Note V1–2 correspond to the RV, V3–4 correspond to the septal region, and V5–6 correspond to the left ventricle and lateral wall

Fig. 2.14 An example of first degree heart block with a prolongation of the PR interval

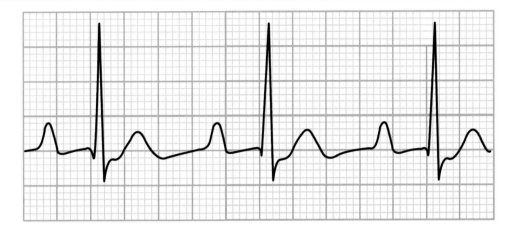

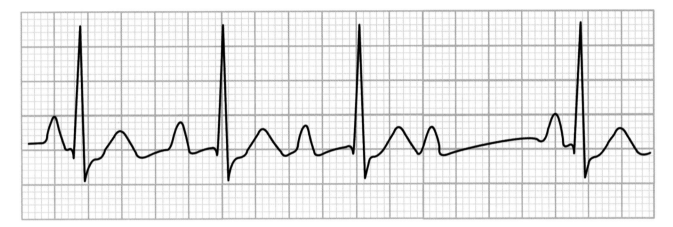

Fig. 2.15 An example of second degree heart block, Mobitz type 1 (Wenckebach). Note the progressively prolonging PR interval culminating in a dropped beat

Taken together, the 12-lead ECG can thus be appreciated to illustrate the equivalent of a 3-D view of the electrical activity of the heart. A standard ECG is performed at a paper speed of 25 mm/s and calibrated with a 1-cm deflection per 1 mV. The P wave represents total atrial depolarization, and the QRS complex represents ventricular depolarization. The T wave represents ventricular repolarization. Atrial repolarization does occur, but this is usually hidden by the ventricular depolarization which occurs at the same time. In health, a small Q wave represents septal depolarization (from left to right). A larger (pathological) Q wave mostly represents an established myocardial infarction in a particular territory denoted by the lead involved.

For a healthy individual, at rest, the ECG should be within the following normal limits:

PR interval	120–200 ms
QRS interval	<120 ms
QT interval[a]	<450 ms in men
	<460 ms in women

[a]Should be corrected for rate

The data presented on a 12-lead ECG can be assessed quantitatively and qualitatively. Both aspects are important.

The components of the cardiac cycle have values within a population-based normal range. Abnormalities on an ECG could indicate either anatomic or physiologic problems, or both. Disease of the conduction tissues may result in delay or blockade of the normally efficient propagation of the wave of depolarization from SAN to ventricular myocytes. This can be identified on the ECG in various guises (Figs. 2.14, 2.15, 2.16, and 2.17).

Other cardiac diseases can result in fast heart rates (tachycardia circuits) developing. Tachycardia which originates abnormally from somewhere in the atrial tissues still results in normally coordinated conduction down the His–Purkinje system to depolarize the ventricles in a normal fashion. This leads to a normal, narrow QRS complex on the ECG. Since the focus is above the ventricles, this is known as a supraventricular tachycardia (SVT) and is also know as a "narrow complex tachycardia." Examples of SVT (Figs. 2.18 and 2.19) include sinus tachycardia, atrial tachycardia, atrial flutter (which are usually regular rhythms), and atrial fibrillation (which is irregular in rhythm).

When the tachycardia originates from the ventricular tissues, the flow of depolarization is poorly coordinated resulting

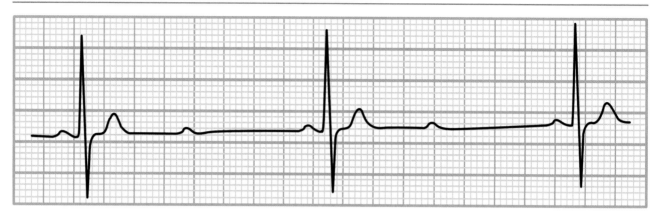

Fig. 2.16 An example of second degree heart block, Mobitz type 2. Not every P wave is conducted to the ventricles. This example shows 2:1 atrioventricular block

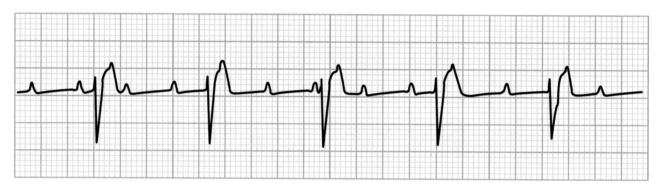

Fig. 2.17 An example of complete heart block. No electrical activity is transmitted from the atria to the ventricles. The P waves are regular, and the broadened QRS complexes are regular. However, the atria and ventricles are functioning independently of each other, and there is no electrical relationship

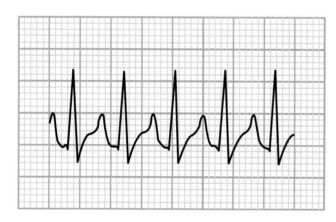

Fig. 2.18 An example of SVT. Regular narrow complex tachycardia

in a lengthening of the QRS complex duration on the ECG. This is known as ventricular tachycardia (VT) or a broad complex tachycardia (Fig. 2.20). In a structurally abnormal heart, VT is an unstable and malignant rhythm and can lead to cardiac arrest itself or can degrade to ventricular fibrillation (VF). In a structurally normal heart, VT is much more stable and rarely results in cardiac arrest. VF (Fig. 2.21) is not com-

patible with a cardiac output. VF is treatable with prompt electrical defibrillation but without successful therapy, results in death.

As well as disturbances in rhythm, much can be deduced from the morphology of the complexes on the ECG. A wide variety of abnormalities and variations in cardiac structure, physiological stresses, electrolyte disturbances, hereditary "channelopathies," and drug effects may result in specific and nonspecific patterns represented on the 12-lead ECG. For example, acute myocardial ischemia may result in vertical shift in the S–T segments or in inversion of the T waves (altered repolarization). Electrolyte disturbances can also affect the morphology of the complexes.

Hyperkalemia, as already discussed, will cause variations on electrophysiological events for cardiac myocytes. It may result in tall T waves with the reverse being true of hypokalemia. Hypocalcemia may prolong the cardiac cycle (prolonged QT interval), whereas hypercalcemia may hasten it (shortened QT interval). For a more detailed review of electrocardiography, one is advised to consult specialist texts and books – as suggested in the reading list at the end of this chapter.

Fig. 2.19 An example of AF. Narrow complex tachycardia which is irregular in rhythm. Note the absence of P waves (no coordinated atrial activity)

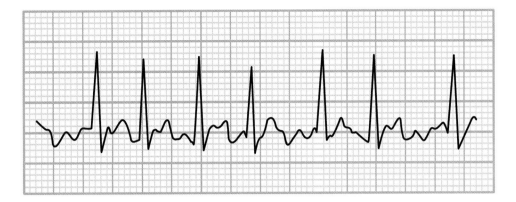

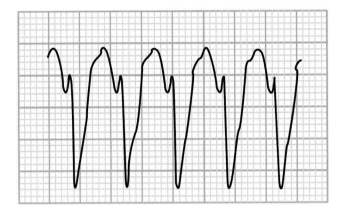

Fig. 2.20 An example of VT. Broad complex, regular tachycardia

Cardiac Arrhythmogenesis

In the most basic terms, electrical abnormalities of the heart may be due to an inadequacy of electrical activity resulting in too slow heart rhythm (bradycardia), or an excess of activity resulting in too fast heart rhythm (tachycardia). In both situations, the underlying cellular mechanisms have a similar basis and can broadly be divided into three groups:

- Disordered automaticity
- Triggered activity
- Disordered impulse conduction

Disordered Automaticity

Automaticity normally occurs in the SAN, AVN, Bachmann's bundle (an atrial conduction pathway), and potentially in the His–Purkinje system. These sites are all potential pacemaker sites. It is recognized that the tissue with the fastest rate of spontaneous depolarization dictates the rate and pattern of cardiac depolarization. In a normal heart, this occurs from the SAN. A hierarchy exists in subsidiary pacemaker sites dependent on the differential automaticity of these sites. An increase in automaticity arises as a normal physiologic response. Sympathetic nervous stimulation and/or circulating catecholamines cause the I_f and I_{Ca} currents to increase in the SAN. This causes an acceleration of phase 4 diastolic depolarization. Threshold potential is therefore reached earlier, and thus depolarization occurs more frequently (see Fig. 2.8).

Disordered automaticity refers to one of two situations. The first involves spontaneous depolarization occurring at nonpacemaker "ectopic" sites. The second involves depolarization at pacemaker sites but not in response to a normal physiologic trigger. Abnormal automaticity at nonpacemaker sites may be precipitated by partially depolarized tissue (enhanced automaticity) or secondary to triggered activity. Myocardial tissue may be relatively depolarized during phase 4 (diastole). This less-negative resting membrane potential is therefore held closer to the threshold potential. Common causes include hypoxia, ischemia, electrolyte disturbance, and acidosis. Such abnormal automaticity may occur in atrial and/or ventricular myocardium corresponding with atrial or ventricular tachycardias.

Increased automaticity affecting nodal tissue or the His–Purkinje system may be caused by nonphysiologic triggers. Clinical examples include inappropriate sinus tachycardia, postural orthostatic tachycardia syndrome, or junctional tachycardia (in children). Changes in automaticity may also result in bradycardia. In this situation, automaticity is reduced. This may affect the SAN and give rise to sinus pauses and/or sinus bradycardia. The mechanism underlying the reduced automaticity relates to a reduction in I_f and/or I_{Ca}. Hyperpolarization caused by I_{KACh} may also reduce the automaticity. Primary sinus node problems due to, for example, fibrosis may result in a reduction in I_f and I_{Ca}. Parasympathetic nervous system (PNS) activity may secondarily cause reduced automaticity of the SAN and sinus bradycardia. PNS activity causes a reduction in I_f, and the acetylcholine (Ach) released by the PNS causes hyperpolarization by acting on I_{KACh}. It also reduces I_{Ca} because of a reduction in cAMP. PNS activity may be physiologic, for example, during rest or

Fig. 2.21 An example of VF. Complexes are completely irregular in rhythm, magnitude and polarity

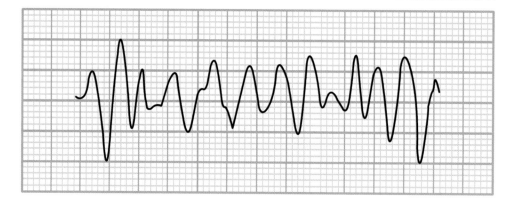

sleep, or may be non-physiologic, for example, in cardio-inhibitory reflex syncope or carotid hypersensitivity.

Triggered Activity

Triggered activity refers to depolarizing oscillations in the membrane potential, subsequent to a preceding action potential. Spontaneous secondary oscillations in membrane potential may occur during the phase 2 plateau, phase 3 repolarization, or during phase 4 diastole. Depolarizing oscillations during phases 2 and 3 are known as early afterdepolarizations (EADs). During phase 4, they are known as delayed afterdepolarizations (DADs). If triggered activity reaches the threshold potential, an action potential is generated, and depending on the timing, this can result in tachyarrhythmia. Prolongation of the action potential duration is an important factor in the development of EADs. EADs may arise when there is an imbalance between the normal inward and outward ion currents in phase 2 and 3. An increase in the inward Na^+ or Ca^{2+} currents or a reduction in outward K^+ current results in a prolongation of phase 2 resulting in an accumulation of Ca^{2+} in the SR. This, in turn, can result in abnormal and spontaneous Ca^{2+} release from the SR. The consequent rise in intracellular Ca^{2+} levels activates Na^+/Ca^{2+} exchange. This results in depolarizing oscillations in the membrane potential and may trigger a premature action potential if the potential reaches threshold. Particular clinical conditions which may promote EADs include inherited and acquired forms of the long QT syndrome, bradycardia, hypokalemia, and hypomagnesemia.

DADs result from oscillations in membrane potential during phase 4 of the cardiac action potential. If the threshold potential is reached, a depolarization occurs. The underlying mechanism involves acquired or inherited abnormalities in the SR Ca^{2+} release channels (ryanodine and IP3 channels) or in the corresponding accessory proteins (e.g., calsequestrin). These "gain of function" abnormalities result in Ca^{2+} leak from the SR into the cytosol. Ca^{2+} overload triggers Na^+/Ca^{2+} exchange, and the consequent increase in cytosolic Na^+ and

potential results in DADs. Factors which enhance intracellular Ca^{2+} load such as sympathetic activation may promote DADs. This mechanism is important in catecholaminergic polymorphic ventricular tachycardia (CPVT) where sympathetic nervous system activation, triggered by emotional or physiological stress, can precipitate VT. In the failing heart, Na^+/Ca^{2+} exchange channels are upregulated, and rectifying K^+ channels are downregulated, thus encouraging DADs. Other conditions associated with DADs include digoxin toxicity, myocardial ischemia, use of beta-adrenergic agonists (positive inotropes), and hypercalcemia.

Impulse Conduction Disorders

Disorders of impulse conduction may result in either tachycardic or bradycardic arrhythmias. If the propagating wave of depolarization is held up or slowed at any point along the conduction system, bradycardia or heart block can occur. The precise nature of the rate and rhythm depends on the level and the magnitude of the block. For example, partial blockade in or around the AVN results in first or second degree heart block with a prolongation of the PR interval or with more than one P wave to each QRS complex, respectively (see Figs. 2.15 and 2.16). If the degree of conduction block is severe, complete block may occur, and no electrical activity is conducted between the atria and the ventricles (see Fig. 2.17). However, in this example, a subsidiary pacemaker (His/Purkinje) would normally take over the role of pacemaker to pace the ventricle and prevent asystole and death.

Subsidiary pacemakers may also dictate the heart rate and rhythm if the SAN becomes abnormally slow for any reason. For example, if the frequency of SAN discharge is too slow, the AVN's inherent rate of automaticity may become the next fastest pacemaker and will thus take over control of the rate and rhythm. When this occurs, it is known as a nodal escape rhythm. Occasionally, conduction tissue copes adequately at rest but struggles at higher pulse rates due to delayed recovery from the refractory period. This is observed in some patients who have narrow QRS complexes at rest but develop bundle branch block patterns (broad QRS complexes) at higher pulse rates. This is known as "tachycardia-dependent block."

Disorders of impulse conduction can also result in tachyarrhythmia due to a mechanism involving re-entry. As has already been described, all myocytes are effectively in continuity with each other. As a wave of depolarization is conducted across the myocardium, it spreads rapidly to depolarize all areas in a coordinated and efficient manner (see Fig. 2.6). Once an area of myocardium has received a depolarizing stimulus, the wave front can only travel in one direction. The wave of depolarization cannot go backward over the territory it has just depolarized since this tissue will now be refractory. The wave can therefore only travel forward to the nonrefractory areas of myocardium which remain excitable.

However, for re-entry to occur, in relationship to a focal abnormality in conduction in a specific area of myocardium, the conduction properties of the two limbs around the abnormality should differ significantly (anisotropic property). Typically, forward conduction varies, with one limb exhibiting faster conduction (and a relatively long refractory period) and the other limb exhibiting relatively slow conduction (and a short refractory period). Subsequent antegrade block, occurring in the "fast" limb in response to an extrastimulus, and slow conduction via the "slow" limb may allow for retrograde conduction up the "fast" limb setting up a re-entry circuit and tachycardia.

Re-entry circuits therefore depend on the following:

- There must be adjacent areas of myocardium, with different electrophysiological properties with respect to conductivity and refractoriness.
- These regions must be connected distally and proximally, and each limb must be able to conduct in either direction.
- Unidirectional block in one limb allows adjacent areas of myocardium to depolarize normally.
- The distal region of the blocked limb remains excitable and can depolarize in the retrograde direction.
- If the proximal part of the nonblocked limb has recovered excitability then as the retrograde wave front reaches it, it will depolarize again antegradely, and a circuit of electrical activity is established. Therefore, retrograde conduction in the (unidirectional) blocked pathway must be slow enough to allow the normal pathway to recover excitability again.
- The impulse thus cycles continuously.

This mechanism explains re-entry within a focal area of myocardium (often around scar tissue). However, re-entry can occur on a more global cardiac scale if there is an abnormal connection between the atria and ventricles, as in the Wolff–Parkinson–White syndrome (see Table 2.1). Re-entry mechanisms are responsible for many common symptomatic and serious rhythm disturbances. Table 2.1 outlines the mechanisms responsible for several common rhythm disturbances.

Any pathology which results in unidirectional blockade of action potential conduction may result in re-entry tachycardia circuits. Although the maintenance of a tachycardia often relies upon re-entry circuits, the initiation of an arrhythmia is often secondary to enhanced automaticity and triggered activity. The initiation and propagation of arrhythmia are therefore dependent on a combination of all three described mechanisms. Any arrhythmia which results in instability of cardiac output requires urgent direct current cardioversion (DCCV) therapy – in the form of a "defibrillator shock." Pharmacological management of arrhythmias is covered in the Chap. 4.

Pacemakers

The heart rate can be modulated pharmacologically. Drugs such as beta-adrenoreceptor antagonists (beta-blockers) and certain calcium channel blockers can be used to limit the heart rate and are used in everyday clinical practice (see Chap. 4). In addition, there are drugs used in the short term to cause an increase in the heart rate. Their use, however, is limited by proarrhythmic effects and route of delivery. They are not suitable for chronic use, and consequently, chronic conditions associated with significant bradycardia are treated with pacemaker therapy.

Exogenous pacing techniques rely on the application of an external current, which acts as the stimulus required to trigger phase 0 of the action potential, and thereby myocardial contraction. Temporarily, this can be achieved by applying a current across the heart by external pacing pads attached to the chest wall. Alternatively, in an emergency situation, manual percussion to the precordium delivers just enough energy to trigger an action potential (i.e., percussion pacing). A more permanent solution involves the insertion of a permanent pacemaker (PPM) device. A PPM is composed of a pacing lead (or leads) which is/are inserted into the chambers of the heart via a vein. The leads are connected, at the proximal end, to a generator box. Normally, the cephalic, axillary, or subclavian veins are utilized. The distal end of the lead (electrode) rests against the ventricular and/or atrial endocardium. Ventricular leads are usually secured in the trabeculations of the right ventricular apex or to the interventricular septum if more physiological pacing is desirable. Atrial leads are usually secured in the right atrial appendage. Modern lead tips transiently elute steroid in order to reduce the acute inflammatory response associated with lead implantation. This helps to avoid problematic rises in pacing threshold which may result in a failure to pace.

Leads are fixed to the endocardium with either *passive* or *active* fixation techniques. Passive fixation involves placing

Table 2.1 Common rhythm disturbances

Arrhythmia	Mechanistic considerations
Atrial flutter (AFL)	Typical" AFL is due to a clockwise or counter-clockwise re-entry circuit in the right atrium, dependent on the tricuspid valve annulus anteriorly and the crista terminalis posteriorly. The pathway has a predictable cycle length of ~200 ms (i.e., ~300 cycles/min), and so the corresponding ventricular response rate will be divisible into 300. "Atypical" AFL, refers to any other pattern of AFL and tends to represent sequelae of previous surgery, ablations, fibrosis, and scarring
Atrial fibrillation (AF) (see Fig. 2.19)	AF is characterized by a fragmented wave front which results in multiple small random re-entry circuits and wavelets with no overall organized electrical or mechanical activity. The focus and stimulus for this may arise from disease in the atria or commonly from myocardic sleeves within the pulmonary veins. The initiation of AF is thought to be secondary to a combination of enhanced automaticity, triggered activity, and re-entry mechanisms
Wolff–Parkinson–White syndrome (pre-excitation syndrome) leading to atrioventricular re-entry tachycardia (AVRT)	In this syndrome, there is an abnormal electrical connection between the atria and ventricles. This may result in the ventricles becoming excited earlier than the AVN would normally allow. The abnormal connection is known as an accessory pathway. Depending on whether or not the accessory pathway has the requisite properties (see text), it may allow re-entry in an antegrade (orthodromic) direction (ventricle–atria–AVN–His–Purkinje–ventricle) with a resultant narrow complex tachycardia or in a retrograde (antidromic) direction which circuits in the opposite direction
Atrioventricular nodal re-entry tachycardia (AVNRT) (see Fig. 2.18)	AVNRTs are archetypal re-entry tachycardias and arise due to abnormalities in the conduction properties of the tissues immediately surrounding the AVN. The combination of a slow pathway with a long refractory period and a corresponding fast pathway with a short refractory period may result in the more common "slow–fast" AVNRT or in the less common "fast–slow" AVNRT. A slow–slow pathway is also recognized
Ventricular tachycardia (VT) (see Fig. 2.20)	Re-entry mechanisms account for sustained VT. Both micro re-entry and macro re-entry (around scar tissue) occur, as can re-entry involving the bundle branches. Non-re-entrant mechanisms of VT also occur and are thought to involve the "channelopathies" along with combinations of EADs, DADs, and abnormalities of automaticity
Catecholaminergic polymorphic ventricular tachycardia (CPVT)	CPVT is an inherited condition characterized by abnormalities in the Ca^{2+} channels and accessory proteins which may result in triggered activity (DADs) and VT in response to sympathetic activation
Ventricular fibrillation (VF) (see Fig. 2.21)	VF is characterized by disorganized, fragmented, asynchronous electrical activity that is not associated with any effective myocardial contraction and results in death unless urgent electrical defibrillation restores a rhythm compatible with a cardiac output. The mechanical result is more of a quiver than contraction. The ECG trace reflects this since it is devoid of any uniformity with respect to the magnitude, timing, and direction of currents detected. Fragmented depolarizing waves result in multiple small re-entry circuits which perpetually interact with surrounding currents and circuits. The initiation and propagation of VF is dependent on re-entry, enhanced automaticity, and triggered activity

the lead tip onto the endocardium and relying on small teeth/"tines" to anchor the lead tip in place. Active fixation offers a greater range of placement sites and utilizes a small "corkscrew"-type mechanism in the distal tip of the lead which screws into the myocardial tissue. The leads conduct electrical impulses but are well insulated along their length. The proximal end of the lead lies outside the vein and connects to the pulse generator box. The pulse generator contains a chemical cell/battery (typically lithium iodide) along with all the necessary hardware and circuitry required for sensing and pacing. The box is placed into a pre-/subpectoral pouch, which is fashioned by the physician at the time of implantation, and sutured in place.

Since the first human PPM implantation in 1958, the size of the generator box has become progressively smaller while the technology and functionality of the hardware housed within has become more sophisticated (Fig. 2.22). The scar, and often the generator box, can usually be identified in PPM patients just below the lateral left or right clavicle. Rarely, in more complex cases where venous access is restricted

(thrombosed veins or complex congenital heart disease), epicardial pacing leads can be used. However, this requires more invasive surgical implantation techniques, and when performed, the generator box is usually positioned under the anterior abdominal wall. Numerous parameters can be programmed into the generator box. Modern generator boxes also contain a small amount of read only memory (ROM) and random access memory (RAM) which can store data regarding any detected arrhythmia. The device can be interrogated, downloaded, and reprogrammed remotely by a separate device.

A standard antibradycardia PPM is indicated for *symptomatic bradycardia* (i.e., any condition where the patient is symptomatic secondary to a bradycardia or pause in the heart rhythm or if the heart rate fails to rise appropriately with exercise). Symptoms usually include light-headedness, syncope, or presyncope. Detailed, up-to-date guidelines regarding the indications for permanent pacing are published by the joint European and American Cardiology Societies and Associations (see further reading). Some of

Fig. 2.22 Modern pacemakers are of small size nowadays, even those with defibrillator function

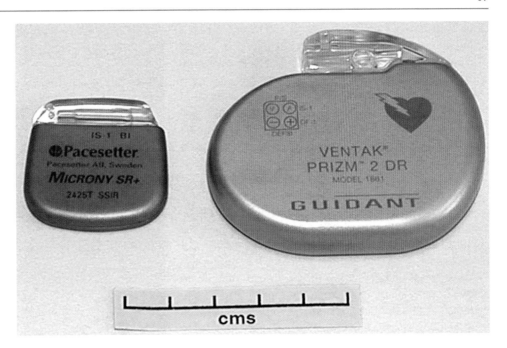

the more common indications where PPM implantation is of benefit include

- Symptomatic sinus bradycardia
- Symptomatic sinus node dysfunction (also known as sick sinus syndrome)
- Symptomatic second degree heart block
- Complete heart block (also known as complete atrioventricular block), intermittently or persistent
- Atrial fibrillation with slow ventricular response
- Atrial fibrillation with complete heart block
- Chronotropic incompetence (inability to increase heart rate in response to exercise)

Comprehensive lists of indications for permanent pacing are long but can, in general terms, be summed up by including "any condition which results in a patient being symptomatic of bradycardia or pauses in the heart rhythm where there is no readily reversible cause." If a patient is symptomatically bradycardic due to prescribed drugs, and there is no appropriate alternative, then PPM implantation should be carried out to allow drug therapy to continue. Some conditions where PPM implantation is not of benefit and may be of harm include

- Asymptomatic sinus node dysfunction
- Asymptomatic first degree heart block
- Asymptomatic bundle branch block without atrioventricular block
- Transient heart block postmyocardial infarction where the patient is asymptomatic and there is no bundle branch block
- Vasovagal syncope without demonstrable bradycardia

Modern pacemakers operate "on demand" and only pace the heart *if* the system fails to sense endogenous electrical activity (according to individually programmed parameters). Therefore, the battery life is long in patients who rarely rely on their pacemaker and more limited in those who are pacemaker dependent. When the battery has come towards the end of its life, the generator box is replaced (normally under local anesthetic), with a new box unit being attached to the existing lead/s.

For a pacemaker to operate "on demand," it must be able to perform two distinct functions: it must be able to *sense* the heart's endogenous electrical activity, and it must be able to *pace* the heart when required. It is important that both of these functions operate efficiently since problems with either can result in pacemaker malfunction. PPM-related complications can result from problems associated with implantation or lead positioning or from problems with the programming of the device. Procedure-related complications include

- Pneumothorax. Reflecting pleural damage.
- Cardiac perforation. Surprisingly, this is uncommonly of any major clinical consequence. Perforation often seals spontaneously since it involves the low-pressure right ventricle. One should aim to exclude pericardial tamponade in any patient who becomes hypotensive following PPM implantation – since this would require drainage.
- Bleeding. PPM pocket hematoma is relatively common but rarely requires evacuation.
- Lead dislodgement. This results in failure to pace or sense and requires reimplantation of the lead.
- Infection. Of all of the PPM-related complications, infection is the most feared (Fig. 2.23). Infected devices require prolonged courses of antibiotic therapy (in the same fashion as valvular infective endocarditis) along with extraction

of both the box and lead/s. Lead extraction can be a difficult and prolonged procedure requiring a general anesthetic. Sepsis associated with PPMs is associated with a significant morbidity and mortality.

The "pacemaker syndrome" is characterized by shortness of breath, malaise, and syncope. It is associated with single lead PPMs which result in atrial contraction against closed atrioventricular valves in patients with a still functioning atrium. A pacemaker-mediated tachycardia (PMT) can also occur, but this is usually amenable to reprogramming of the device settings.

Modern PPM systems contain sophisticated algorithms designed to avoid PPM-related complications (e.g., PMT), avoid arrhythmia (e.g., anti-AF algorithms), and have the ability to adapt the pacing rate appropriate to the level of physiological stress and physical exertion. Rate-responsive PPMs increase the frequency of pacing in response to detected movement (accelerometers) or by detecting increased respiratory rate (variations in impedance between lead and box). To avoid confusion, the nomenclature used to describe PPM systems has been standardized into a five-letter code (Table 2.2).

A VVIR PPM is therefore a single-lead PPM which will pace the ventricle if the device does not sense any endogenous activity (i.e., it is inhibited by sensing). The "R" means that it will detect surrogate markers of physical exertion and raise the pacing rate if deemed appropriate. A VVI device carries out the same function but lacks the rate responsiveness and will pace (if not inhibited) at a preset programmed rate. A DDDR PPM has both atrial and ventricular (dual) leads. It can pace and sense both chambers. The dual responsiveness (III code letter) relates to the ability of the device to be inhibited by sensing in one chamber while being triggered in another. For example, the atrial lead may sense atrial activity and thus be inhibited while the ventricular lead is triggered by failing to sense a subsequent ventricular depolarization. An atrial and a ventricular lead will be required in heart block since the atrial activity can be resynchronized with ventricular activity, whereas only a V lead is warranted in atrial fibrillation since there is no organized atrial activity to be detected. The fifth code letter (V) is reserved for devices with a third lead such as cardiac resynchronization therapy (CRT) devices.

More recently, devices have been designed to do more than just pace the heart during times of bradycardia. CRT has been shown to improve outcomes in heart failure associated with prolonged QRS duration on the ECG. This system relies on a third lead that paces the left ventricle. This third lead is secured in an epicardial coronary vein (see Chap. 5). The coronary veins are accessed through the coronary sinus in the right atrium. By programming the device to pace the right and left ventricles more synchronously, cardiac output can be optimized.

Other devices (e.g., the implantable cardioverter-defibrillator, ICD) have the ability to sense malignant ven-

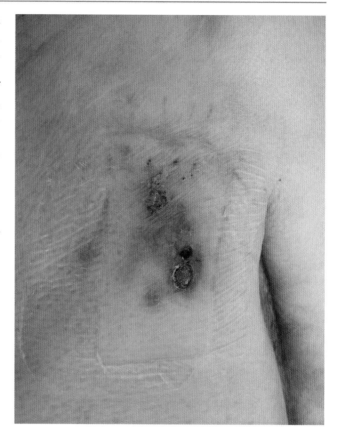

Fig. 2.23 An autopsy case of infective endocarditis associated with an infected generator unit site. Note the skin discoloration from subcutaneous abscess formation

tricular arrhythmia (VT and VF) and attempt therapeutic antitachycardia pacing or internal cardiac defibrillation, if deemed appropriate. Antitachycardia pacing algorithms aim to pace the heart faster than the sensed arrhythmic rate in order to "capture" the rhythm and then abruptly stop pacing. This often, but not always, terminates the arrhythmia, without the need for defibrillation. This is desirable since defibrillation is a painful and unpleasant experience for a conscious person.

ICDs have a capacitor in the generator box, which stores enough energy to defibrillate through one or two coils in the ventricular lead. These devices are inserted for primary prevention in high-risk individuals and for secondary prevention following VT/VF arrest (see further reading). Devices with antitachycardia pacing algorithms and the ability to defibrillate can be programmed on an individual basis to tailor the device parameters to the patient's needs. For example, the zones at which the device detects VF or VT can be manipulated as can the number of attempts at antitachycardia pacing before the device attempts defibrillation. If a CRT device has the ability to defibrillate, it is known as a CRT-D, as opposed to a CRT-P which paces but cannot defibrillate. Although effective at treating malignant ventricular arrhythmia, ICDs do not, directly, reduce the chance of arrhythmia. Thus, the

Table 2.2 The North American Society of Pacing and Electrophysiology/British Pacing and Electrophysiology Group (NBG/BPEG) generic code for antibradycardia, adaptive rate, and multisite pacing systems

I	II	III	IV	V
Chamber paced	Chamber sensed	Response to sensing	Rate responsiveness	Multisite pacing
O (none)	O (none)	O (none)	O (none)	O (none)
A (atrium)	A (atrium)	T (triggers pacing)	R (rate responsive)	A (atrium)
V (ventricle)	V (ventricle)	I (inhibits pacing)		V (ventricle)
D (dual, A&V)	D (dual, A&V)	D (T&I)		D (dual)

importance of optimal medical therapy for the underlying cardiac abnormality should not be underestimated.

Cardiac Electrophysiology

Cardiac electrophysiology (EP) involves the study, diagnosis, and management of heart rhythm and conduction disorders. In addition to drug- (see Chap. 4) and device- (PPM, CRT, ICD) based therapy, EP doctors perform invasive intracardiac electrophysiological studies (EPS) in order to identify and assess arrhythmic substrate. Furthermore, once elucidated, areas of abnormal conduction or enhanced automaticity can be treated with catheter ablation to permanently terminate arrhythmia. In many cases, this cures the patient, negating the need for long-term drug therapy. In appropriate patients, ablative strategies offer much higher rates of success (>95% cure in most SVTs) than standard drug therapies. Since the development of invasive EP techniques in mid-1970s, the field of EP has evolved hugely, and EP is now considered a cardiac subspecialty.

After a thorough clinical assessment, the electrophysiological study (EPS) is the first step in this invasive approach. During an EPS, the physician inserts a number of electrical catheters into the heart, usually via a femoral vein approach into the right atrium and ventricle, under fluoroscopic control. Although some left-sided pathways can be identified by placing a catheter in the coronary sinus. Ablation of left-sided pathways and ventricular arrhythmias often requires a retro-aortic approach or transseptal puncture (i.e., through the interatrial septum). These catheters contain electrical transducers, capable of detecting the heart's endogenous electrical activity and also pacing the heart. A large control screen in the catheter laboratory relays the nature and timing of electrical activity detected from each transducer. The screen also provides a 2- or 3-D anatomical representation of the heart in order to guide the position of the catheters during the procedure along with hemodynamic data and an external surface. Three or four catheters are usually deployed, one in the superior right atrium, one in the RV apex, a third resting across the tricuspid valve (to obtain a His recoding), and a fourth in the coronary sinus. The elec-

trical activity detected by each transducer, known as an "electrogram," provides very localized information on the electrical activation of that area of myocardium. This is in contrast to an ECG which provides summated data from the entire heart.

The study usually begins with an assessment of the conduction intervals (e.g., P–R, QRS, QT, atria–His, and His–ventricle). Programmed electrical stimulation (PES) allows the study of the conduction and refractory properties of different areas of the heart. PES can be used to assess the automaticity and refractoriness of myocardial tissues and is designed to stimulate arrhythmia. One type of PES involves delivering premature electrical stimulus, after either an endogenous beat or after an exogenously paced "drive train" of beats. This is known as extrastimulus stimulation. The duration between the paced or spontaneous beat and the extrabeat is reduced sequentially until the stimulus no longer results in a depolarization; thus the absolute refractory period can be deduced. Another type of stimulation, known as burst stimulation, involves a "drive train" of paced beats with a low-cycle length (higher frequency than the endogenous rate), and this is useful in inducing arrhythmia. Arrhythmia can also be induced pharmacologically, and drugs can play a vital role in the EPS. Drugs used include

- Adenosine to block the AVN and to reveal an atrioventricular accessory pathway or to check the success of an ablated accessory pathway.
- Atropine, which is used to increase conduction through the AVN and can be used to precipitate re-entrant pathways involving the AVN.
- Isoproterenol. This beta-adrenoreceptor agonist increases automaticity, reduces refractoriness, and stimulates arrhythmia.

Data generated by the EPS is used to "map" the electrical activation properties of the myocardium and to locate areas of abnormal conductivity, accessory pathways, abnormal circuits, and/or substrate for arrhythmia (e.g., scar). Once an abnormal pathway or circuit has been identified, it can be stimulated. If it is demonstrated that this is the likely cause for the patient's arrhythmia, the operator can use the intracardiac catheters to ablate the area of abnormality. Pathways are ablated by applying either a burn (radio-frequency energy) or freeze (cryoablation) to scar the myocardium and thus break the abnormal circuit, terminating the arrhythmic focus or current. Once ablation has been performed, the operator will attempt to stimulate the arrhythmia in order confirm success.

Ablative procedures have high rates of curative success

- In excess of 95% for most SVTs
- In the order of 90–95% for VT ablation in a structurally normal heart
- Approximately 70–80% for VT ablation in ischemic cardiomyopathy and structurally abnormal hearts

These cure rates are significantly higher than with pharmacological therapy alone. Major complications are uncommon. However, patients should be warned about pericardial effusion which may need drainage and a risk of inducing heart block by inadvertently ablating the conduction tissues (generally less than 1%).

AF ablation is slightly different. In AF, the focus of abnormal electrical activity often arises in the pulmonary veins. For this reason, an AF ablation involves ablative isolation of the pulmonary veins. Curative success rates for EP AF ablation are lower, of the order 70–80%, and patients may require one or two repeat procedures to achieve cure. AF can also be treated surgically with the pulmonary veins being isolated during open cardiac surgery. Via a median sternotomy, the surgeon can scar the atria in a maze-like pattern in order to eliminate the multiple atrial macro re-entry circuits required for the propagation of AF. During the full Cox-maze procedure, along with scarring the atria, the pulmonary veins are isolated, and the atrial appendages are removed. Although the original procedure used a "cut and sew" technique with a scal-pel and full thickness incisions, modern techniques are less aggressive and utilize radio-frequency and/or cryothermy ablation. Long-term success rates (freedom from AF) are high and are comparable to the curative success of EPS ablation (generally 70–80%).

Further Reading

Berne RM, Levy MN. Cardiovascular physiology: Mosby's physiology monograph series. 8th ed. St. Louis: Mosby; 2000.

Bonow RO, Mann DL, Zipes DP, Libby P. Braunwald's heart disease. A textbook of cardiovascular medicine. 9th ed. Philadelphia: Elsevier Saunders; 2011.

Camm JA, Luscher TF, Serruys PW. The ESC textbook of cardiovascular medicine. 2nd ed. Oxford: Oxford University Press; 2009.

Ellenbogen KA, Wood MA. Cardiac pacing and ICDs. 5th ed. Malden: Blackwell publishing; 2008.

Ellenbogen KA, Wilkoff BL, Kay N, Lau CP. Clinical cardiac pacing, defibrillation and resynchronization therapy. 4th ed. Philadelphia: Elsevier Saunders; 2011.

Epstein AE, Dimarco JP, Ellenbogen KA, Estes NA 3rd, Freedman RA, Gettes LS, Gillinov AM, Gregoratos G, Hammill SC, Hayes DL, Hlatky MA, Newby LK, Page RL, Schoenfeld MH, Silka MJ, Stevenson LW, Sweeney MO; American College of Cardiology/ American Heart Association Task Force on Practice; American Association for Thoracic Surgery; Society of Thoracic Surgeons. ACC/AHA/HRS 2008 guidelines for device-based therapy of cardiac rhythm abnormalities: executive summary. J Am Coll Cardiol. 2008;51:2085–105.

Josephson ME. Clinical cardiac electrophysiology: techniques and interpretations. 4th ed. Philadelphia: Lippincott Williams & Wilkins; 2008.

Levick JR. An introduction to cardiovascular physiology. 5th ed. London: Hodder Arnold; 2010.

Zipes DP, Jalife J. Cardiac electrophysiology: from cell to bedside. 5th ed. Philadelphia: Elsevier Saunders; 2009.

Cardiac Imaging

3

Abdallah Al-Mohammad and Peter W.G. Brown

Abstract

Imaging of the heart has many modalities; ranging from the simple chest radiograph using X-rays, through to sophisticated digital imaging of cardiac function and metabolism, using magnetic resonance or advanced nuclear techniques of positron emission tomography. There are both invasive and noninvasive techniques. The vast majority of the tests are diagnostic, attempting to elucidate any pathology, some aim to assess cardiac function and structure. Other techniques form the foundation for therapeutic interventions. Advances in cardiac imaging have enabled the health-care profession to access the heart with enhanced diagnostic skills and to gather vital information for planning the management of cardiac disease.

Keywords

Imaging • Diagnosis • Pathology • Measurement • Functional assessment • Therapeutic intervention

Introduction

The last 100 years has seen startling progress in the diagnosis and assessment of heart disease, and fundamental to this have been advances in cardiac imaging.

The first images of the heart were by chest radiography followed by fluoroscopy. This came shortly after the discovery of the effects of the X-rays by Röentgen near the end of the nineteenth century [1]. Invasive assessment of the heart using X-rays was pioneered by Werner Forssmann in the 1920s [2].

A. Al-Mohammad, M.D., FRCP(Edin), FRCP (Lond)
Department of Cardiology,
Northern General Hospital,
Sheffield Teaching Hospitals NHS Foundation Trust,
Herries Road, Sheffield, South Yorkshire S5 7AU, UK
e-mail: a.al.mohammad.87@googlemail.com

P.W.G. Brown, MBChB, FRCS(Ed), FRCR (✉)
Department of Diagnostic Imaging, Sheffield Teaching Hospitals
NHS Foundation Trust, Sheffield, UK
e-mail: peter.w.brown@sth.nhs.uk

He confirmed the feasibility of cardiac catheterization. He catheterized his right atrium using a sterile urinary catheter via his left basilic vein. By the 1940s, the first attempts of contrast aortography were undertaken [3]. The coronary arteries were "erroneously" catheterized and directly visualized without any serious consequences. Thus the modern era of selective coronary angiography was born [4].

In the 1950s, Edler and Hertz realized the potential of ultrasound in medical imaging [5]. They used the technique to obtain images of the human heart. A few decades later, echocardiography and Doppler imaging became essential in the assessment of cardiac disease.

Since the 1970s, nuclear cardiac imaging has become increasingly important in the assessment of ventricular function, myocardial perfusion, myocardial metabolism, and viability. Currently, there are two main cardiac nuclear imaging techniques: single-photon emission computerized tomography (SPECT) and positron emission tomography (PET) [6].

Most recently, two further techniques have become available for cardiac imaging. Cardiac computed tomography (CCT) and cardiac magnetic resonance (CMR) are being

S.K. Suvarna (ed.), *Cardiac Pathology*,
DOI 10.1007/978-1-4471-2407-8_3, © Springer-Verlag London 2013

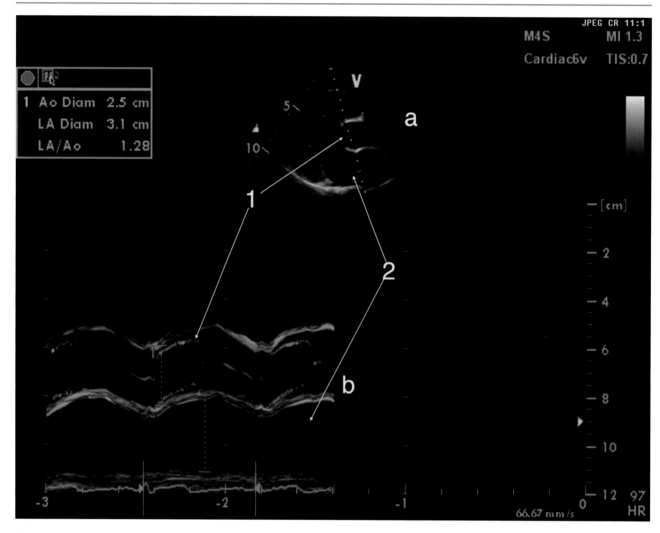

Fig. 3.1 TTE views in a normal heart: (a) 2D long axis parasternal view. (b) M-mode view through the aortic valve (*1*) and the left atrium (*2*)

used for the noninvasive assessment of cardiac disease and are expected to be increasingly important in the twenty-first century [7, 8].

Echocardiography

There are a number of modalities of echocardiography, used singularly or in combination in different clinical situations. The basic principle is the production of ultrasound waves either mechanically or electronically, which are reflected differently by various tissues and interfaces. The reflected waves are detected by a probe, analyzed and displayed in variable format, as below.

M-Mode Echocardiography

In this modality, ultrasound waves are transmitted and received along a linear track. The outcome is displayed

against time and appears as an undulating line (Fig. 3.1). Current echocardiography machines use two-dimensional (2D) echocardiography images to guide the orientation of the M-mode curser through the desired plane or section. The resulting M-mode images are useful in the measurement of the size of cardiac chambers and large vessels and in the assessment of the excursion of valve leaflets against time [9]. M mode can also study the timing of contraction and relaxation of the different parts of the left ventricle, thus determining the degree of intraventricular dyssynchrony.

2D Echocardiography

2D echocardiography (2D echo) is the most commonly used type of echocardiography and specialized cardiac imaging investigation. Transthoracic echocardiography (TTE) provides information on the anatomy and physiology of the heart's chambers (Fig. 3.2), native and prosthetic valves, great vessels, and ventricular dyssynchrony. It provides direct visualization of blood flow, turbulence, gradients, shunts, and pressures in different parts of the heart. 2D TTE is also used to assess the presence of abnormal pathology, for example, tumors (primary and secondary), vegetations, and thrombi. It is helpful in detecting complications of endocarditis and myocardial infarction such as paravalvular abscesses, ruptured chordae, and ventricular septal defects.

Doppler imaging, using the principle of analyzing a change in frequency when sound is reflected from a moving interface, is combined with 2D TTE to assess blood flow, as well as the movement of valves and myocardium. New applications of Doppler allow analysis of myocardial performance during the cardiac cycle, using tissue Doppler imaging (TDI) (Fig. 3.3). Quantitative data derived from 2D TTE, e.g., measurements of ventricular systolic function and volumes, can be misleading as geometrical assumptions are made. More accurate results can now be obtained by the recent introduction of three-dimensional (3D echo) echocardiography.

Three-Dimensional Echocardiography (3D) Echo

3D echo is superior to 2D echo in the assessment of chamber size, shape, and volume. It is more accurate in the assessment of cardiac masses and capable of detailed structural assessment of the valves (particularly the mitral valve) and in the assessment of the interatrial septal and interventricular septal anomalies.

Transesophageal Echocardiography (TEE)

This technique is based on using an ultrasonic transducer mounted on a steerable fibroscopy probe (instead of a scoping camera), allowing imaging of the heart and central vessels via the esophagus and stomach. The main advantages of TEE over TTE are clearer images and better visualization of cardiac and central vascular structures/chambers particularly if partly hidden by acoustic shadows created by mechanical prostheses. In adults, various structures can be evaluated and

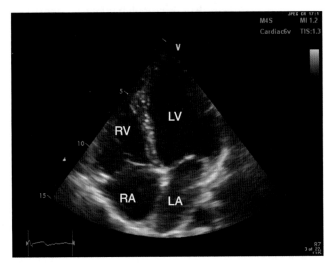

Fig. 3.2 TTE apical four-chamber view in a normal heart (*LV* left ventricle, *RV* right ventricle, *LA* left atrium, *RA* right atrium)

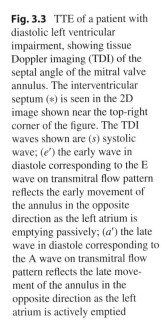

Fig. 3.3 TTE of a patient with diastolic left ventricular impairment, showing tissue Doppler imaging (TDI) of the septal angle of the mitral valve annulus. The interventricular septum (*) is seen in the 2D image shown near the top-right corner of the figure. The TDI waves shown are (*s*) systolic wave; (*e'*) the early wave in diastole corresponding to the E wave on transmitral flow pattern reflects the early movement of the annulus in the opposite direction as the left atrium is emptying passively; (*a'*) the late wave in diastole corresponding to the A wave on transmitral flow pattern reflects the late movement of the annulus in the opposite direction as the left atrium is actively emptied

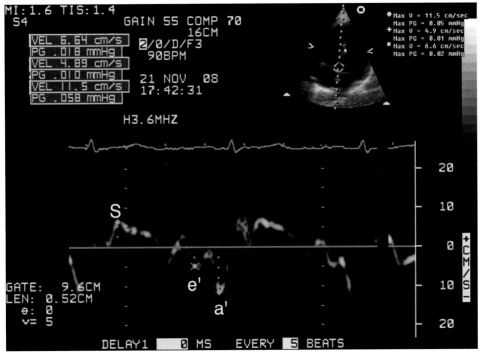

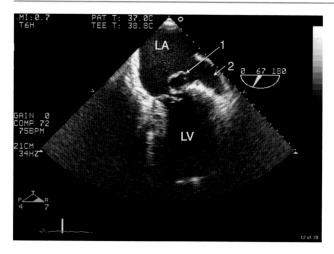

Fig. 3.4 Transesophageal echocardiography (TEE) of a patient with anterior mitral valve leaflet prolapse (*1*). It also shows the left atrial appendage (*2*) (*LV* left ventricle, *LA* left atrium)

imaged better with TEE, including the aorta, the pulmonary artery, pulmonary veins, valves, the atria, the interatrial septum, and the left atrial appendage (Fig. 3.4). In experienced hands, TEE has sensitivity and specificity as high as 95–100% for detecting left atrial and left atrial appendage thrombi [10]. The main modality used by TEE is 2D echo and more recently 3D technology.

Stress Echocardiography

With this technique, patients either exercise (by treadmill, bike, or bed-mounted bike) or the heart is stressed by pharmacological means (intravenous dobutamine or adenosine). Possible stress responses include augmentation of contraction and recruitment of segments that were either hypokinetic or akinetic at rest. The technique can also identify worsening of contraction in cases of critical ischemia, or as a part of the dual response of impaired (but hibernating) myocardium.

Contrast Echocardiography and Perfusion Imaging

Contrast echocardiography (using agitated saline microbubbles or specific echo contrast) may be used to visualize borders between different cardiac tissues or chambers. Improved wall delineation allows excellent assessment of chamber size and contraction. In addition, contrast opacification of the myocardium provides an evaluation of myocardial perfusion both at rest and on stress.

Nuclear Cardiac Imaging

The principle of nuclear cardiac imaging is creation of an image using a specialized camera detecting radiation activity emitted from the heart following an intravenous injection of radioactive material.

Radionuclide Ventriculography, MUGA (Multiple-Gated Acquisition) Scan

The first pass of the radionuclide through the cardiac chambers allows assessment of ventricular function. A MUGA scan provides a reproducible assessment of left and right ventricular systolic function (Fig. 3.5).

Myocardial Perfusion Scan (MPS) and Combined Myocardial Perfusion and Metabolism

After blood passes through the coronary arteries, the radionuclide uptake, by the myocardial cells, produces images that reflect cellular function and integrity.

Using exercise, or pharmacological stress by dipyridamole, adenosine, or dobutamine, the patient is injected with a radiopharmaceutical based on Thallium-201 m [^{201}Tl] or Technitium-99 m [^{99}Tc]. The patient is imaged by a single-photon emission computerized tomography (SPECT) scanner. Data is acquired from multiple angles allowing the reconstruction of a 3D image. The radiopharmaceutical is taken up by the myocardium in proportion to myocardial perfusion. The test is then repeated without stress, and the two sets of images are compared. Areas of reduced perfusion are said to have perfusion defects. The defects can be either reversible with rest (ischemia) or irreversible (possibly scarred). Although the sensitivity and specificity of MPS in detecting coronary artery disease are 91% and 87%, respectively [11], the presence of ischemia by MPS is not synonymous with the presence of coronary artery stenosis. In addition to predicting significant coronary stenosis, this technique provides prognostic information. The predicted risk of ischemia and of general cardiac risk depends on the extent and severity of the perfusion defects (Fig. 3.6).

Another advance is positron emission tomography (PET). Biologically active molecules labeled by positron emitting tracers (such as C^{14}, O^{15}, F^{18}, and N^{13}), introduced intravenously or by inhalation, are taken up into myocardial cells. The tracers emit pairs of rays, which can be detected, and 3D images of the concentration of tracer are constructed. This is used to study aerobic and anaerobic metabolism and myocardial perfusion. This technique can detect myocardial ischemia, myocardial stunning (reduced myocardial contraction

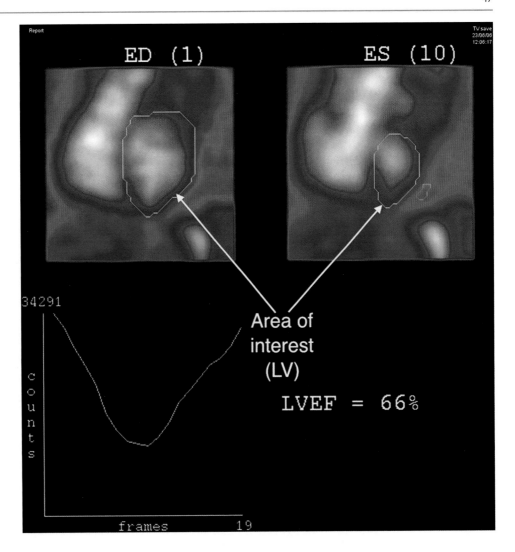

in a recently ischemic segment despite restoring myocardial perfusion), and myocardial hibernation (reduced myocardial contraction in an area of reduced perfusion with continuing metabolic activity) [12]. By acquiring the images in an ECG-gated mode, both SPECT and PET images can also be utilized to assess myocardial contraction.

Imaging of the Sympathetic Innervation of the Heart

Using a radio-labeled neurotransmitter analog ^{123}I-Meta-iodo-benzyl-guanidine (MIBG), imaging of the sympathetic innervation of the heart and the ratio of its uptake by the heart to the mediastinum (HMR) provides prognostic information in heart failure patients and may help to identify candidates for specialized pacing [13].

Cardiovascular Magnetic Resonance Imaging

Cardiovascular magnetic resonance (CMR) is an important investigation for many types of cardiac disease. It is now the procedure of choice for quantifying ventricular volume and mass, providing accurate reproducible measurements [14]. It is used to assess myocardial viability, to evaluate cardiomyopathies, and to follow up patients with congenital heart disease especially after surgery. CMR is also used to evaluate cardiac tumors, the pericardium, the thoracic aorta, and the pulmonary vessels.

Magnetic resonance imaging (MRI) is based on the principle of nuclear magnetic resonance and is a multiplanar technique capable of acquiring images in any orientation. Images are derived from signals produced by protons (H^+), which are abundantly present in the body. Each proton behaves like a small magnet when placed in a magnetic field.

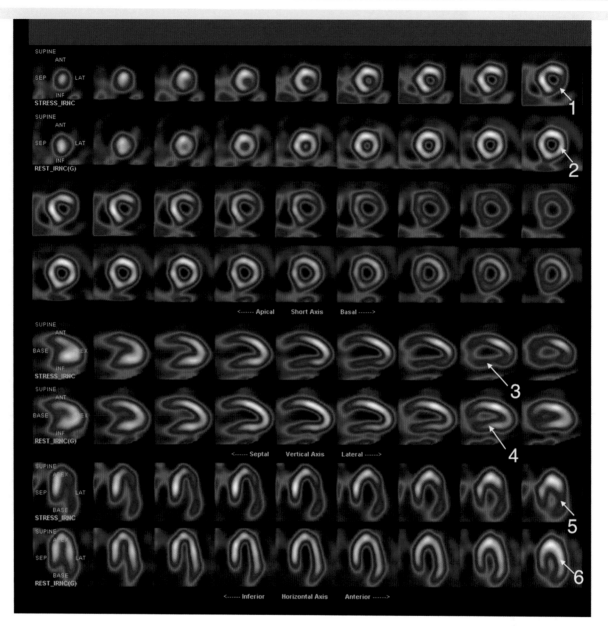

Fig. 3.6 Myocardial perfusion scan (MPS) using myoview single-photon emission tomography (SPECT). The images are arranged in four sets of rows. Each set is composed of an *upper row* of images during pharmacological stress and a *lower row* of images during rest. The first two sets (*four rows*) are short axis views of the left ventricle, fol-lowed by a set (*two rows*) of vertical long axis views of the left ventricle, and finally a set (*two rows*) of horizontal long axis views of the left ventricle. There is a moderate perfusion defect in stress affecting the inferolateral wall (*1, 3,* and *5*), with complete recovery of perfusion during rest (*2, 4,* and *6*); suggestive of ischemia

It aligns with the field and precesses at a given frequency that depends on the field strength. Protons will align parallel or antiparallel to the magnetic field with a small excess of parallel protons, causing a net magnetization vector. This vector can be altered by the application of a radiofrequency pulse. When the pulse is switched off, the vector returns to its former position, giving rise to a radio-signal detectable by a receiver. The relaxation of the vector is attributable to two distinct but simultaneous processes referred to as longitudinal (T_1) and transverse (T_2) relaxation. In order to localize the signal within the body, additional magnetic fields are applied termed gradient fields. An MRI image merely represents the spatially resolved signal arising from the relaxing protons.

Different tissues are highlighted by applying radio-frequency pulses of various types and duration, termed pulse sequences. The basic pulse sequences for CMR are spin echo and gradient echo. These have been developed into more complex sequences which are faster, allowing cine imaging via steady-state free procession (SSFP).

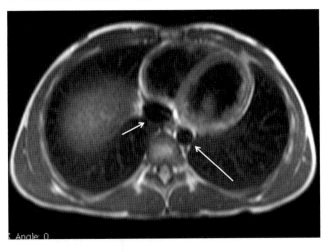

Fig. 3.7 Axial spin echo "black blood" image of the heart, aorta (*long arrow*), and inferior vena cava (*short arrow*)

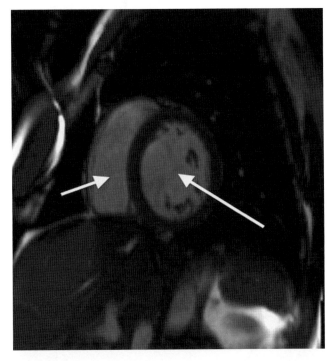

Fig. 3.8 Still frame from cine short axis SSFP image of the left (*long arrow*) and right (*short arrow*) ventricle

ECG gating is essential for CMR to coordinate the acquisition to the correct phase of the cardiac cycle. Spin echo sequences are used for the assessment of morphology, and flowing blood typically appears black (Fig. 3.7). Gradient echo and SSFP sequences are used for physiological assessment of function, and blood is usually white (Fig. 3.8). Blood flowing across a magnetic gradient can also be analyzed and encoded to quantify flow, which is important in the assessment of valvular heart disease. Further information can also be obtained by the use of Gadolinium-based contrast for the assessment of myocardial perfusion, viability, fibrosis, and

infiltration [15]. Contrast is also useful in MR angiography of the aorta and pulmonary arteries.

Having a cardiac pacemaker and/or a defibrillator is a contraindication to using CMR. Claustrophobia is a problem in about 2% of the patients. It should be remembered that cardiac dysrhythmias interfere with synchronized data acquisition.

Cardiac Computed Tomography

The introduction of spiral multidetector CT scanning has dramatically shortened acquisition times and increased spatial and contrast resolution. With ECG gating, it is possible to achieve clear images of the heart. This has resulted in a rapid expansion of the use of cardiac CT (CCT). The main use of CCT is noninvasive imaging of the coronary arteries and the exclusion of coronary disease in low-risk patients [16]. It is also useful for coronary imaging, if the patient is too high risk for invasive angiography or where catheterization had either failed or produced an incomplete data [16]. CCT is excellent at assessing the course of anomalous coronary arteries, as well as the patency and course of coronary bypass grafts [16]. Other indications include the assessment of structural heart pathology and pulmonary vein mapping [16]. There is some overlap with cardiac magnetic resonance (CMR) in the assessment of congenital heart disease, tumors, and pericardial disease.

CT scanners acquire a number of rotating thinly collimated X-ray beam projections obtained at different angles around the patient. An axial image is acquired by computer back projection. The quality of the image depends on the speed of tube rotation and the degree of overlap of the projection data. Use of multiple detectors and movement of the patient through the bore of the scanner allow a series of slices to be acquired and used for volume-rendered and multiplanar reconstruction.

The image quality is affected by several factors. The spatial resolution is less than invasive coronary angiography. The temporal resolution can be improved if the heart rate is slowed. The radiation dose is relatively high because overlapping slices are needed for accurate data reconstruction but can be reduced using ECG gating. ECG gating allows acquisition of images in specific phases of the cardiac cycle (usually late diastole) if the heart rate is relatively low. CT data is acquired over a few seconds during a breath hold. An irregular heart beat (e.g., atrial fibrillation) can degrade image quality. As technology advances, it may be possible to reconstruct images from a single heart beat. Iodinated contrast is injected intravenously during the scan.

Computer postprocessing techniques allow the reconstruction of volume-rendered images of the heart (Fig. 3.9) as well as multiplanar reformats (Fig. 3.10). The cardiac

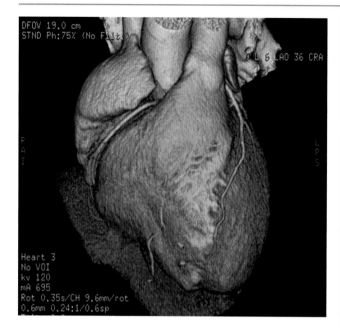

Fig. 3.9 Volume-rendered CT image of the heart

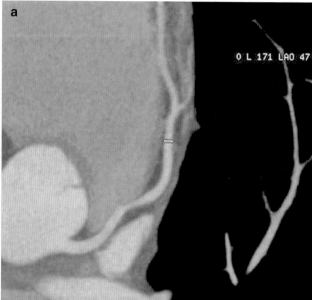

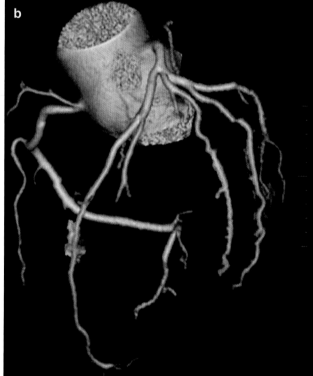

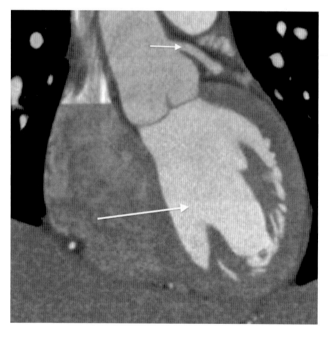

Fig. 3.10 CT multiplanar reformat of the heart showing the left ventricle (*long arrow*) and left coronary artery origin (*short arrow*)

Fig. 3.11 Postprocessing techniques allow detailed CT evaluation of the coronary arteries allowing accurate vessel analysis (**a**) or a "tree view" of the coronary arteries (**b**)

chambers, myocardium, and structures surrounding the heart are well demonstrated. If data is acquired throughout the cardiac cycle, cine images of the heart can be reconstructed to assess the wall motion and the valves. Quantitative data are less accurate than those obtained by CMR. Postprocessing software enables accurate evaluation of the course and pathology affecting the coronary arteries (Fig. 3.11) and assessment of stenotic plaques.

Selective Invasive Coronary Angiography

Cardiac catheters are passed to the aortic root from the femoral, radial, or brachial arteries and are selectively engaged into the coronary ostia before contrast is injected to delineate the coronary lumen and course. The technique has high spatial and temporal resolution, enabling accurate diagnosis of luminal stenosis (Fig. 3.12), which is used to determine the most appropriate revascularization strategy. Using a similar approach, percutaneous coronary interventions can be performed.

Coronary angiography cannot reliably assess early coronary disease and eccentric plaques unless they are calcified. However, the technique enables accurate measurement of pressures, flow, and resistance in the heart and great vessels. It allows accurate assessment of valvular lesions and ventricular contraction.

Examples of Disease Processes and Appropriate Imaging

Assessment of Morphology and Function

Transthoracic echocardiography (TTE) is the most commonly used imaging modality to assess cardiac morphology and function. It is widely available, relatively cheap, and reproducible. Not all patients can be imaged easily by TTE. TEE is a more invasive alternative, whereas CMR is more time consuming and expensive.

Left Ventricular Systolic Dysfunction
All types of 2D and 3D echocardiography and CMR assess the size and the contraction of the left ventricle and can determine if the left ventricular systolic dysfunction (LVSD) is focal or global (Figs. 3.13 and 3.14). 3D echo, MUGA, and CMR are capable of accurately measuring left ventricular volumes. The calculated left ventricular ejection fraction (LVEF) varies in the same patient according to the utilized technique.

Left Ventricular Diastolic Dysfunction
Parameters of myocardial relaxation are well developed using 2D echocardiographic Doppler techniques such as pulsed wave Doppler to study blood flow through the mitral valve and the pulmonary veins, and tissue Doppler imaging (TDI) to assess the systolic and diastolic performance of the myocardium, strain, and strain rate. Almost half the patients with heart failure do not have reduced LVEF but have abnormal diastolic parameters (see Fig. 3.3).

Left Ventricular Hypertrophy
This is measured with reasonable accuracy by 2D and 3D echocardiography (Fig. 3.15). If the echocardiographic views

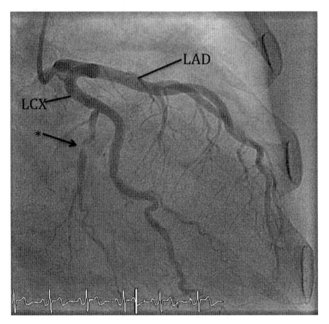

Fig. 3.12 Selective coronary angiography showing luminal stenosis (*) of a branch of the left circumflex artery (*LCX*) (*LAD* left anterior descending artery)

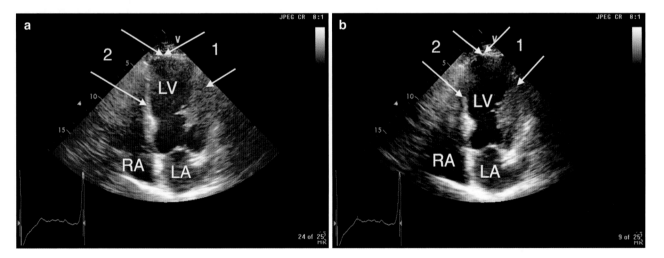

Fig. 3.13 Focal LVSD on TTE, showing a large anteroapical scar extending into the septum and lateral wall. Note that there is no difference in the size of the distal left ventricular cavity between diastole (**a**) and systole (**b**). The area defined between the *arrows* is the scarred myocardium

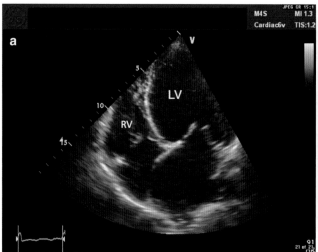
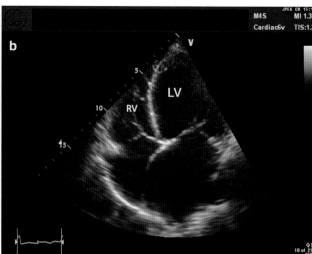

Fig. 3.14 TTE in the apical four-chamber view of a patient with severe heart failure due to dilated cardiomyopathy, showing the global impairment of the left ventricle with its remodeling. Note the little change in the shape and volume of the left ventricle between diastole (**a**) and systole (**b**). (*LV* left ventricle, *RV* right ventricle)

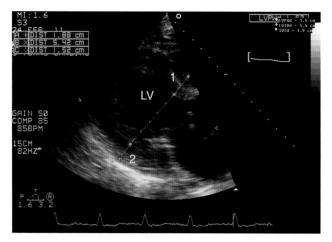

Fig. 3.15 TTE showing left ventricular hypertrophy with the interventricular septum (*1*) measuring 1.88 cm and the posterior wall (*2*) measuring 1.52 cm (*LV* left ventricle)

are poor, then it is assessed by CMR. Both techniques allow accurate assessment of the extent and symmetry of the hypertrophic process.

The Atria

Assessment of atrial size is an important measurement during echocardiography. The identification of other atrial abnormalities such as atrial thrombi, tumors, congenital remnants, and anomalies is also possible (Fig. 3.16). Assessment of the atrial function by echocardiography overlaps with the assessment of the diastolic ventricular function. It also includes pulse-wave Doppler assessment of flow in the left atrial appendage. TEE provides more accurate information about the atria than TTE, especially of the interatrial septum

and the atrial appendage. In addition, 3D echo and CMR are more capable of measuring atrial volumes. The pulmonary venous return pattern and pulmonary venous anomalies are detectable by TEE, but structural pulmonary venous anomalies are more readily assessed by CMR and CCT.

The Right Ventricle

The structure of the right ventricle is complex and difficult to evaluate. Imaging of the right ventricle is increasingly important with the realization of the effects of dysfunction on prognosis. The most common abnormalities are structural and related to dilatation of the cavity as a result of increased volume or pressure load on the right ventricle. Possible causes include pulmonary hypertension, pulmonary stenosis, right ventricular outflow tract obstruction, tricuspid regurgitation, and significant left to right shunts (such as patent ductus arteriosus [PDA] or atrial septal defect [ASD]) (Fig. 3.17). The right ventricular response to increased pressure load includes right ventricular hypertrophy.

CMR is judged the noninvasive reference standard in conditions where accurate follow-up measurements are crucial, such as follow-up of congenital heart disease or cardiomyopathy [17].

Congenital Heart Disease

Modern surgical techniques have improved the quality of life and survival of patients with congenital heart disease. Careful follow-up including imaging is essential, as complications can develop and may require prompt medical and surgical intervention. Echocardiography is the main imaging method, but CMR is also useful.

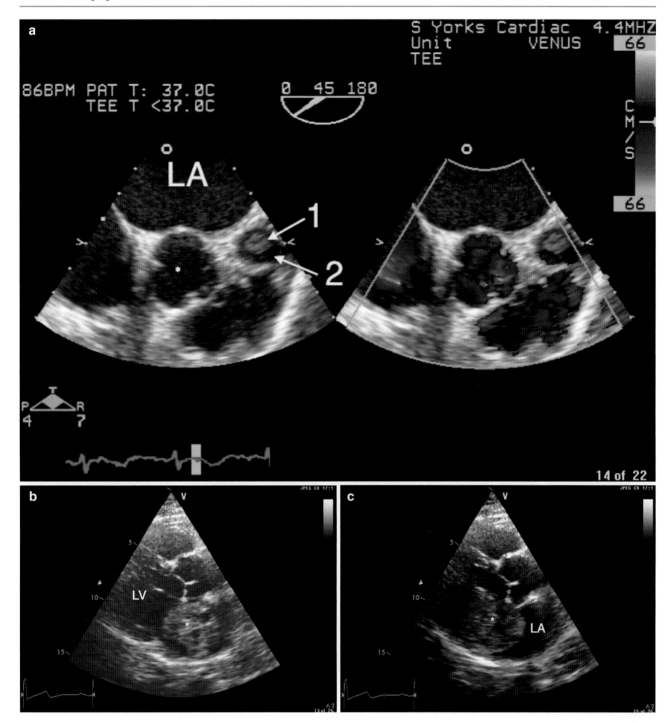

Fig. 3.16 (**a**) TEE showing a thrombus (*1*) in the left atrial appendage (*2*) on a short axis view at the level of the aortic valve (*). (**b**) Left atrial mass (*) on TTE long axis parasternal view. The mass is seen in the left atrium. (**c**) Left atrial mass (*) as in (**b**) is prolapsing through the open mitral valve into the left ventricle (*LV* left ventricle, *LA* left atrium)

Assessment of the Atria, Interatrial Septal Defects, and Pulmonary Venous Anatomy

Common congenital abnormalities seen in the atria on echocardiography include the Eustachian valve, Chiari network (Fig. 3.18), and the crista terminalis. Interatrial septal defects can be demonstrated on TTE but are best seen on TEE. A secundum ASD is the most common (see Fig. 3.17). If there is a sinus venosus defect, then anomalous pulmonary venous drainage may be visualized (Fig. 3.19). A primum ASD involves the atrioventricular junction and AV valves (Fig. 3.20). Demonstrating a patent foramen ovale with or without contrast is particularly important where paradoxical

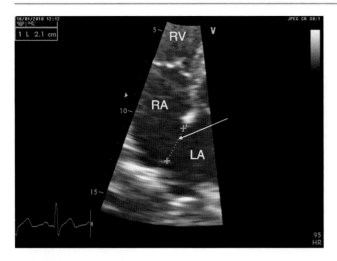

Fig. 3.17 Apical four-chamber view on TTE concentrating on the secundum ASD (*arrow*) (*RV* right ventricle, *RA* right atrium, *LA* left atrium)

embolization is suspected (Fig. 3.21). TTE and CMR may provide additional data on shunt size. Accurate calculation of the shunt can also be made during cardiac catheterization. In patients with sinus venosus ASD, accurate assessment of pulmonary venous anatomy is important. The pulmonary veins and sinus venosus defect may be visualized on TEE, CMR, or cardiac CT (see Fig. 3.19).

Valvular Abnormalities

Bicuspid aortic valve is the most common congenital valvular abnormality. It is clearly visualized by 2D TTE and TEE (Fig. 3.22). In a few patients, CMR is useful for confirmation. Bicuspid aortic valves degenerate causing stenosis and /or regurgitation. They are also associated with aortopathy and coarctation of the aorta.

The pulmonary valve is easily evaluated by echocardiography. Pulmonary stenoses can be valvular, subvalvular, or

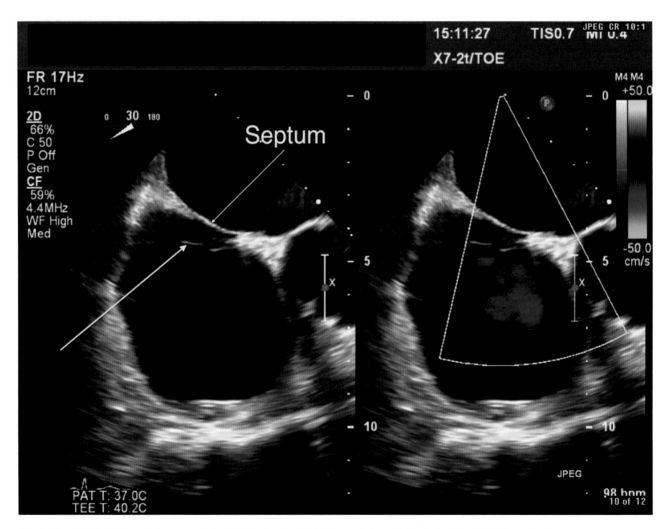

Fig. 3.18 TEE of the interatrial septum (*pointed*), also showing Chiari network (*arrow*) (*LA* left atrium, *RA* right atrium)

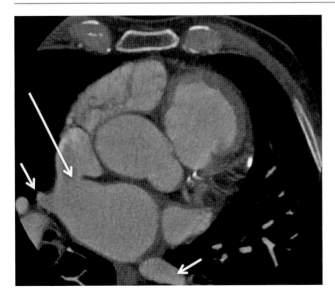

Fig. 3.19 Cardiac CT demonstrating a sinus venosus ASD (*long arrow*) and pulmonary veins (*short arrows*)

supravalvular. The stenosis may occur as an isolated abnormality or be part of a syndrome, such as Fallot's tetralogy. TTE can assist by measuring the valvular gradient. TEE provides better visualization than TTE. CMR produces even better imaging of the pulmonary valve and the right ventricular outflow tract. Other complex congenital valve lesions such as common mitral–tricuspid leaflet, Ebstein's anomaly, and subvalvular aortic lesions can be studied by 2D, 3D echo, and CMR.

Complex Anomalies of the Ventricles and Atrioventricular Connections

These complex congenital anomalies are difficult to assess with TTE. While TEE may help, CMR is the best technique for defining the morphological features of each chamber [14]. This is important in the assessment of patients with transposition of the great vessels and other complex ventricular anomalies.

Fallot's tetralogy is the most common complex cyanotic congenital heart disease. The pulmonary stenosis (or stenosis of the right ventricular outflow tract), overriding aorta, right ventricular hypertrophy, and ventricular septal defect can usually be clearly visualized on echo. CMR is most helpful in

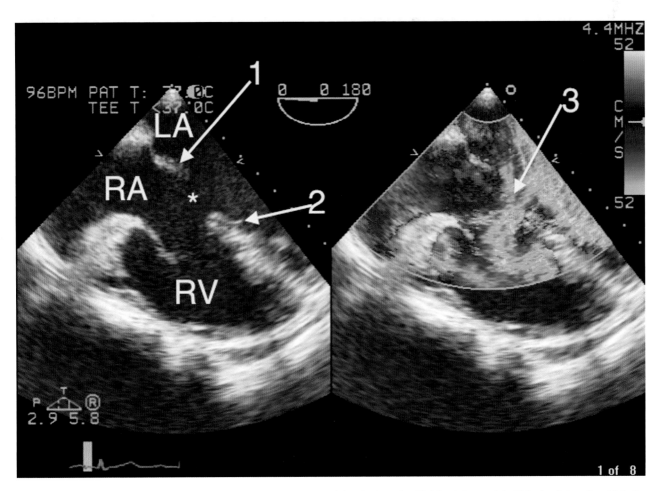

Fig. 3.20 Primum ASD with involvement of the AV valves on TEE. The defect is shown by (*). The right ventricle (*RV*), the right atrium (*RA*), the left atrium (*LA*), the common AV leaflet (2), the remnant inter-atrial septum (1) and flow on colour flow mapping showing left to right shunt (3)

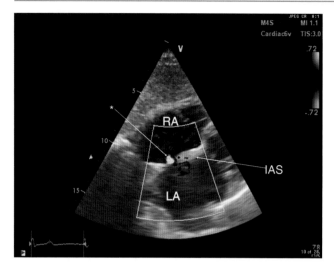

Fig. 3.21 Subcostal view on TTE of the interatrial septum (*IAS*), showing a small jet of blood (*) from the left atrium (*LA*) to the right atrium (*RA*) via a patent foramen ovale

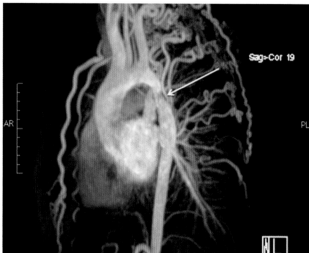

Fig. 3.23 Magnetic resonance angiogram showing aortic coarctation (*arrow*) with multiple collateral vessels

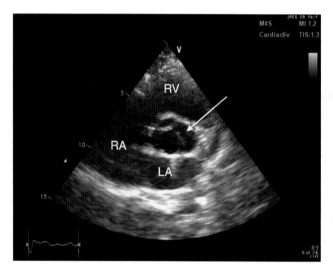

Fig. 3.22 Transthoracic echocardiogram showing a bicuspid aortic valve (*arrow*) (*RV* right ventricle, *RA* right atrium, *LA* left atrium)

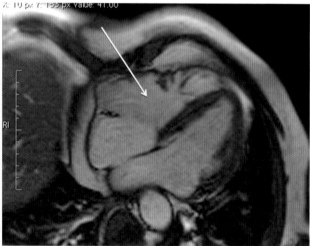

Fig. 3.24 SSFP cine image of a patient with suspected ARVD showing a dilated aneurysmal right ventricle (*arrow*) which showed focal regional wall motion abnormalities

the follow-up of postoperative patients for the assessment of pulmonary incompetence and right ventricular volumes [17].

Great Vessel Anomalies

Aortic coarctation can be readily detected by echocardiography, but both CMR and CCT can accurately define the anatomy (Fig. 3.23). The coarctation and collateral vessels can easily be visualized on both techniques, but CMR can also determine the flow velocity and thus the severity of stenosis.

Cardiomyopathies

Echocardiography is very important in the initial identification of patients who may have a cardiomyopathy, as it is readily

available and provides morphological and functional data on systolic and diastolic cardiac function. CMR can give additional information on tissue characterization, morphological definition, and ventricular contraction.

Arrhythmogenic Right Ventricular Cardiomyopathy (ARVC)

The diagnosis of ARVC is difficult and involves a number of different diagnostic criteria. The imaging criteria include regional wall motion abnormalities of the right ventricle (RV), increased RV volumes, aneurysm formation, and fatty infiltration (Fig. 3.24). The findings should be assessed alongside other non-imaging criteria. The diagnosis can be difficult on echo as the RV is poorly visualized in some patients.

Hypertrophic Cardiomyopathy (HCM)

The thickened ventricular myocardium in HCM has a distinctive appearance on echo and CMR. HCM is characterized by hyperdynamic left ventricular contraction, a wall thickness that is frequently over 15 mm, and sometimes an intraventricular or left ventricular outflow tract pressure gradient. The latter can be associated with systolic movement of the anterior mitral valve leaflet or the mitral valve chordae towards the septum. The hypertrophy may be global or focal, and the hypertrophic myocardium can be concentric or asymmetrical. It is important to differentiate other causes of hypertrophy such as systemic hypertension, aortic stenosis, and athlete's heart. All these features of HCM are detectable on echocardiography. However, CMR defines reliably the site and extent of hypertrophy and has the further advantage of characterizing the myocardium if affected by fibrosis (linked in HCM to a risk of sudden death) (Fig. 3.25) [18].

Dilated Cardiomyopathy (DCM)

DCM is a common cardiomyopathy characterized by dilatation of the ventricles, thinning of the ventricular wall, and varying degrees of impaired contraction. It can be associated with noncompaction of the ventricular myocardium. The diagnosis is usually made by echocardiography (see Fig. 3.14). To differentiate it from heart failure due to ischemic heart disease causing heart failure, coronary angiography and CMR are advised. The latter is helpful irrespective of the results of coronary angiographic findings, as CMR can distinguish true DCM from ischemic heart failure by the pattern of delayed enhancement after contrast administration [19]. Although the majority of patients with DCM show no late enhancement with gadolinium CMR, a small number show midwall myocardial uptake. Patients with severe CAD characteristically show subendocardial enhancement.

Infiltrative and Restrictive Cardiomyopathy

Infiltration of the myocardium causes reduced LV compliance and diastolic dysfunction. Where there is significant restriction, the echocardiogram will show relatively small ventricular cavities, reasonable myocardial contraction, restrictive physiology on transmitral flow pattern and tissue Doppler imaging (TDI), and significantly dilated atria. CMR may provide evidence of fibrosis and/or infiltration. The differential diagnosis includes constrictive pericarditis, where CMR and CCT detect thickening of the pericardium (Fig. 3.26).

Patients with cardiac amyloid classically have a thickened reflective myocardium on echocardiography and usually restrictive physiology. Myocardial contraction can be either normal or impaired (Fig. 3.27). CMR is helpful in supporting the diagnosis as late gadolinium imaging is very abnormal with diffuse early enhancement (Fig. 3.28).

Cardiac sarcoidosis is relatively rare, and there are no specific features on echocardiography. CMR can be useful

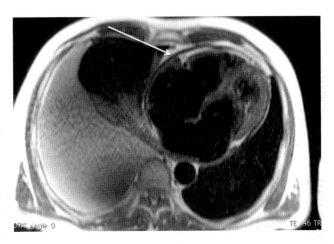

Fig. 3.26 Thickened pericardium (*arrow*) on CMR in a patient with constrictive pericarditis

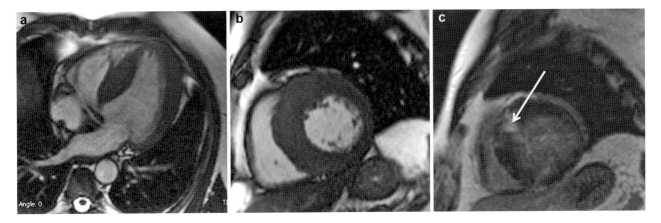

Fig. 3.25 Axial (**a**) and short axis (**b**) SSFP cine images showing thickening of the wall of the left ventricle in a patient with hypertrophic cardiomyopathy. The delayed contrast axial imaging (**c**) shows an area of focal enhancement (*arrow*) consistent with fibrosis

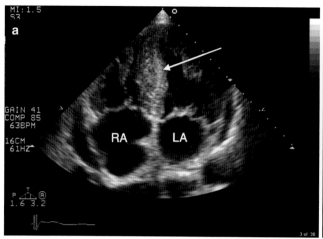

Fig. 3.27 (**a**) Apical four-chamber TTE of the heart in a patient with amyloidosis. Note the thick septum (*arrow*), the thickened valves, and the small amplitude of the QRS complex on the rhythm trace in the left lower angle of the image (*LA* left atrium, *RA* right atrium). (**b**) Short axis view of the thickened LV walls in the same patient with amyloidosis (*LV* left ventricle, *RV* right ventricle)

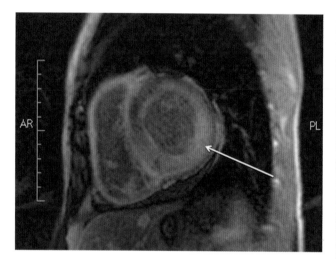

Fig. 3.28 Delayed contrast short-axis image showing extensive late enhancement (*arrow*) in a patient with amyloid heart disease

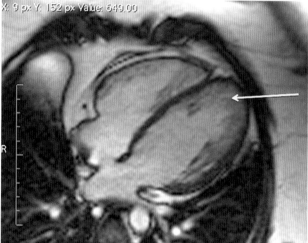

Fig. 3.29 SSFP cine vertical long-axis image of the left ventricle in a patient with left ventricular noncompaction cardiomyopathy. The ratio of noncompacted (*arrow*) to compacted myocardium is more than 2.3:1

for further assessment, and delayed enhancement is patchy, typically sparing the subendocardium.

Left Ventricular Non-compaction

This condition has become better recognized and is caused by uterine arrest of compaction of ventricular myocardial tissue during fetal growth. Patients are at risk of heart failure, arrhythmias, and embolic events. The non-compacted LV myocardium can be seen on echo particularly if contrast is administered, but the condition is particularly well demonstrated on CMR (Fig. 3.29). The diagnosis is made if the ratio of noncompacted to compacted myocardium in diastole is 2.3:1 or greater.

Myocarditis

The diagnosis of myocarditis is difficult. The ECG may show ST segment and T wave changes but are not specific. Blood tests are nonspecific. Echocardiography shows left ventricular impairment but is nonspecific. CMR provides, in addition to the wall motion abnormalities, patchy focal subepicardial or linear midmyocardial enhancement on postcontrast imaging (Fig. 3.30). The increased signal normalizes upon resolution of the inflammatory process.

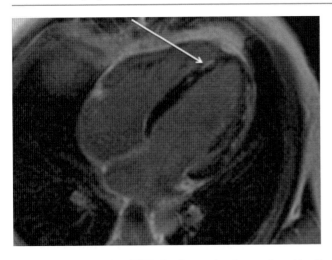

Fig. 3.30 Four-chamber SSFP cine image showing patchy midwall late enhancement (*arrow*) in a patient with myocarditis

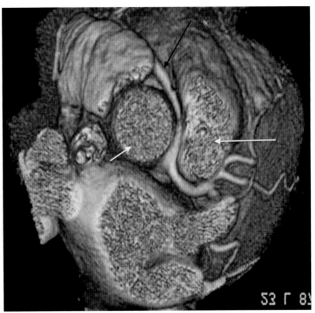

Fig. 3.31 Anomalous right coronary artery (*black arrow*) arising from the left sinus of valsalva passing in a dangerous course between the aorta (*short white arrow*) and pulmonary trunk (*long white arrow*)

Ischemic Heart Disease

Perfusion Imaging and Viability Assessment

The myocardial response to exercise or pharmacological stress (using adenosine or dobutamine) can be determined by echocardiography or nuclear medicine techniques.

Echo assessment relies on changes in myocardial contraction and thickening with stress. Echo contrast is used to enhance edge detection to improve accuracy. Myocardial perfusion can also be assessed using echo contrast but is relatively specialized. In the presence of ischemia, the myocardial segments become hypokinetic or akinetic. Low-dose dobutamine can temporarily augment contraction (positive inotropic effect) without causing ischemia. If improved contraction of a previously impaired segment is demonstrated, this suggests the presence of hibernating myocardium.

Nuclear medicine techniques assess myocardial perfusion, comparing rest and stress images, which allows the identification of reversible (ischemic) and irreversible (scarred) perfusion defects (see Fig. 3.6).

Recently, similar perfusion CMR techniques have become available.

Coronary Artery Disease

Conventional catheter angiography is the gold standard for assessing coronary disease. The technique is essential for planning revascularization and enables percutaneous revascularization. Invasive angiography carries a small risk of serious complications. The coronary arteries can also be imaged by noninvasive CCT. The role of CCT in the investigation of ischemic heart disease is evolving. CT coronary angiography has a high negative predictive value for the exclusion of coronary disease. One advantage of CCT over angiography is the characterization of plaques. However, accurate analysis of the degree of luminal narrowing is difficult if the vessel is heavily calcified. CCT is complementary to invasive coronary angiography when a vessel cannot be identified or to characterize ostial lesions. CCT is useful when angiography is deemed too high risk. The degree of coronary calcification can also be analyzed by low-dose CT scanning without iodinated contrast, providing a "calcium score" to risk stratify patients [20].

Assessment of Anomalous Coronary Arteries

Catheter angiography occasionally reveals anomalous coronary arteries but cannot depict the course of vessels in relation to other cardiac structures. CCT and CMR can demonstrate anatomical relationships of the coronary vessels and in particular identify arteries passing between the aortic root and pulmonary trunk, known to be associated with risk for sudden death in adults (Fig. 3.31).

Assessment of Graft Patency

Assessment of graft stenosis and patency following coronary artery bypass surgery is usually carried out by invasive selective angiography. Where a graft is not found, there is a role for evaluation by CCT.

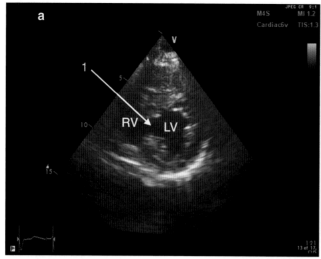

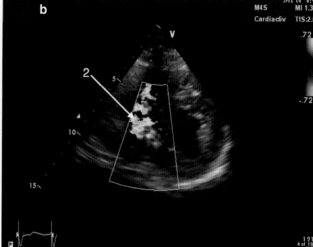

Fig. 3.32 (a) Short-axis parasternal view using TTE of a patient with an acquired ventricular septal defect (*1*) that developed 3 days following a septal ST segment elevation myocardial infarction (*LV* left ven- tricle, *RV* right ventricle). (**b**) The same view as in **a**, with color flow Doppler showing a shunt (*2*) from the left ventricle to the right ventricle

Myocardial Infarction

Echocardiography can accurately identify focal wall motion abnormalities, which occur after acute myocardial ischemia or infarction. If flow is restored promptly, there is often immediate restoration of function. Occasionally, the myo- cardial segments remain hypokinetic or akinetic and are deemed stunned. The stunned myocardial segments can recover later. Chronically, ischemic segments can be hiber- nating. These are hypokinetic/akinetic segments that regain contraction after revascularization [12]. However, when infarction is complete, there will be thinning of the akinetic segments.

Echocardiography is used to assess ventricular function after myocardial infarction and to identify complications. In addition to left ventricular systolic dysfunction, patients with ischemic heart disease may develop intraventricular thrombi, rupture of a papillary muscle/mitral valve prolapse, and ven- tricular rupture of either the free wall (usually fatal due to tamponade but occasionally causing a false aneurysm) or the interventricular septum (creating a ventricular septal defect) (Fig. 3.32).

Nuclear myocardial perfusion imaging identifies ischemic and scarred segments. CMR identifies, on delayed gadolin- ium enhancement, areas of high signal intensity denoting nonviable segments if the enhancement affects >50% of the wall thickness (Fig. 3.33). In significantly impaired left ven- tricular contraction, it is important to identify the extent of viable and hibernating myocardium as these predict the chance of improved function after revascularization. Recovery of function following revascularization is better predicted by low-dose dobutamine stress CMR than by scar

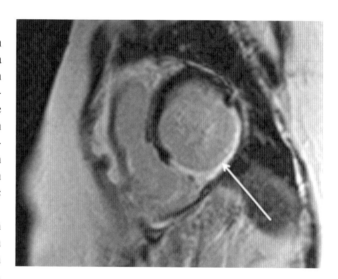

Fig. 3.33 Nonviable myocardium due to scarring demonstrated on delayed enhancement CMR as >50% enhancement on the ventricular wall (*arrow*)

imaging with CMR [21]. PET is also useful in detecting hibernating myocardium by demonstrating continuing meta- bolic activity in a hypoperfused region [12].

Valvular Heart Disease

TTE is the primary imaging modality to evaluate heart valves, and TEE is used to provide additional detail if nec- essary. Echocardiography can accurately assess valve morphology and movement. Doppler evaluation provides visual and quantitative information on valvular stenosis and regurgitation as well as turbulence and jets. CMR may complement suboptimal echocardiographic examinations.

The Mitral Valve

Mitral valve prolapse and mitral regurgitation are best assessed by TTE and TEE. Echocardiography gives valuable information on the morphology of the leaflets, their movement, and the presence of any atrial displacement or pro-

lapse. It also may detail the degree of annular dilatation, the degree of stretch of either or both leaflets due to distortion of the subvalvular apparatus, particularly in the presence of left ventricular dilatation and dysfunction. TTE and to a larger degree TEE are excellent in the assessment of the mitral regurgitant jet: its shape, direction, and severity (Fig. 3.34). Echocardiography provides functional assessment of the cause of mitral regurgitation, particularly when the mitral valve is normal, such as in hypertrophic obstructive cardiomyopathy. Mitral valve stenosis is best assessed by echocardiography, and its severity is assessed by Doppler (Fig. 3.35).

Fig. 3.34 (**a**) TEE of the assessment of an eccentric mitral regurgitation jet, using the measurement of vena contracta (*arrow*). The regurgitation is caused by prolapse of the posterior leaflet of the mitral valve (*LV* left ventricle, *LA* left atrium). (**b**) One of the elements in the assessment of severe mitral regurgitation on TEE is the demonstration of reversed S wave (*arrow*) on transpulmonary venous flow pattern

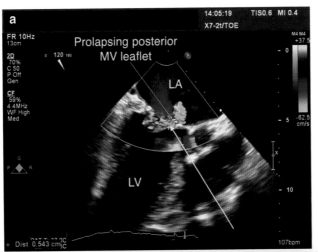
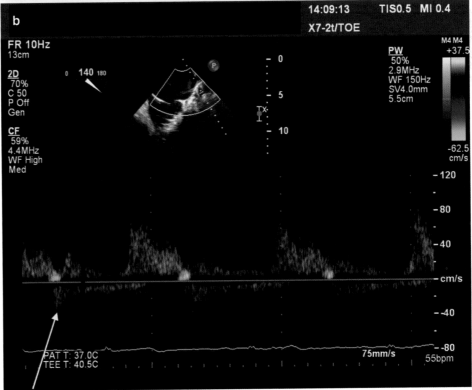

TEE provides further assessment of the left atrial appendage, which is frequently invisible on TTE.

Mitral valve vegetations are seen on TTE, but TEE provides clearer and more accurate evaluation. In particular, TEE can detect associated complications such as extension of the infective process into the annulus or perforation of one of the leaflets.

The mitral valve can be replaced surgically by biological or mechanical prostheses. Echo is used to assess stability, paravalvular leaks, vegetations, stenoses, and mechanical dysfunction. Acoustic shadowing caused by the metal stent of the bioprosthesis or by the mechanical prosthesis is problematic on TTE, and TEE is necessary in these circumstances for full evaluation (Fig. 3.36).

The Aortic Valve

Aortic valve stenosis results from morphological changes to the valve that may be either congenital or acquired. It is characteristically associated with thickening of the cusps, fibrosis, and calcification. The stenosis is associated with a progressive loss of the ability to increase the cardiac output in response to exercise. Doppler detects high-flow velocities at the valve level, and a pressure gradient can be calculated across the stenosis. The aortic valve area can also be calculated.

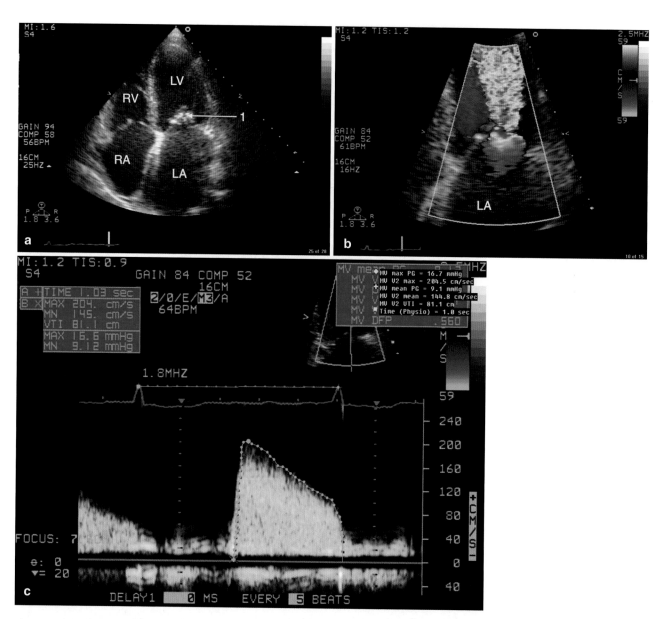

Fig. 3.35 (**a**) Apical four-chamber view on TTE of a patient with thickened, calcified, and stenosed mitral valve (*1*). Note the significant dilation of the left atrium (*LA*) (*LV* left ventricle, *RA* right atrium, *RV* right ventricle). (**b**) TTE of a stenosed mitral valve showing the increased velocity of flow of blood in diastole into the left ventricle. Note the dense jet of mitral stenosis (*LA* left atrium). (**c**) Assessment of severe mitral stenosis in a patient, who is in atrial fibrillation taken during TTE

Fig. 3.35 (**d**) In another patient who is in sinus rhythm with both E and A waves taken during TEE

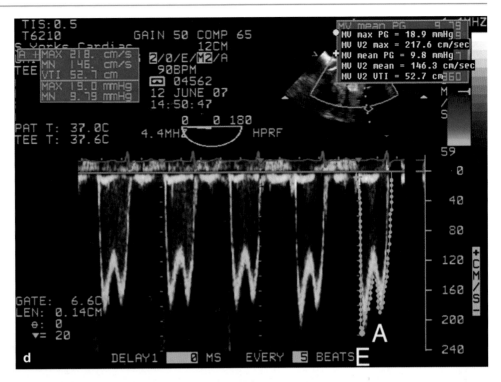

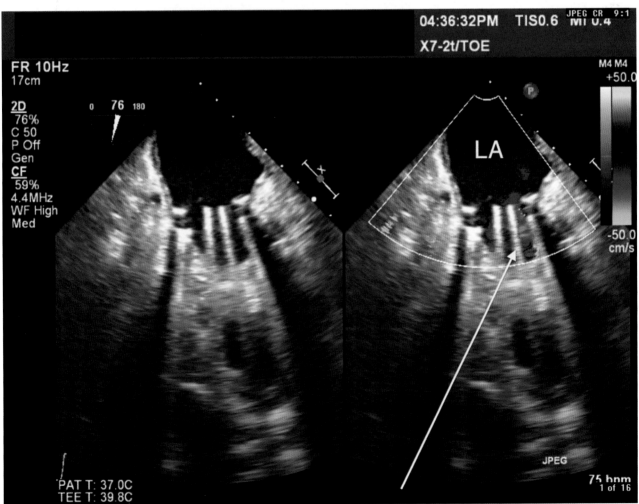

Fig. 3.36 TEE of the mechanical MV prosthesis with (*right*) and without (*left*) color flow Doppler. Note the acoustic shadows of the prosthesis leaflets obliterating the view of the left ventricle (*LA* left atrium)

Fig. 3.37 TTE study on apical four-chamber view with application of continuous-wave Doppler study of the aortic valve. The maximum peak gradient is 103 mmHg suggesting severe aortic stenosis (*AS*)

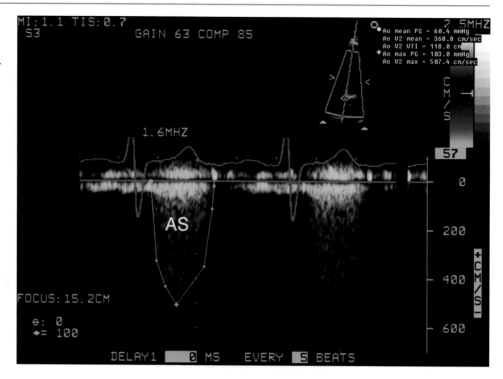

Frequently, stenosis of the aortic valve is associated with left ventricular hypertrophy. These measurements, along with assessments of the left ventricular function and the patient's symptoms, are used to determine the need for valve replacement. If the latter is delayed, left ventricular contraction becomes impaired, and the left ventricular cavity may dilate. In such cases, the gradient across the valve may become smaller despite the severity of the stenosis. All the above can be assessed by TTE (Fig. 3.37), and rarely TEE may be needed for confirmation. However, in the presence of severe aortic stenosis and a low gradient with impaired left ventricular contraction, it is crucial to differentiate between inherent myocardial disease with stenosis of the aortic valve and myocardial dysfunction that is potentially reversible by valve replacement. The latter differentiation is best made by stress echocardiography. If the gradient rises with no change in aortic valve area, the aortic stenosis is severe, and the patient should undergo aortic valve replacement. Alternatively, if there is no increase in gradient, and the aortic valve area appears to be larger due to improved myocardial contraction, then there will be no benefit from valve replacement.

TTE is excellent in the assessment of subaortic valve obstruction in the presence of hemodynamic gradient caused by hypertrophic obstructive cardiomyopathy and in the presence of fixed anatomical defects such as rings or shelves in the left ventricular outflow tract (Fig. 3.38). CMR can also be useful in the assessment of aortic valvular and subvalvular obstruction.

Aortic regurgitation is due to failure of valve closure in diastole. If untreated, it will eventually result in progressive left ventricular dilatation and dysfunction. The severity of

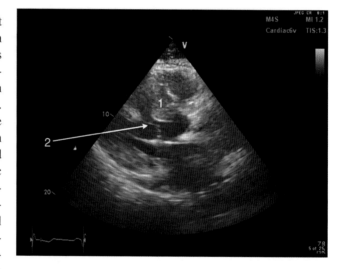

Fig. 3.38 TTE in the parasternal long-axis view of a patient with hypertrophic obstructive cardiomyopathy (HOCM). Note the significant hypertrophy of the interventricular septum (*1*) and the systolic anterior motion (SAM) of the chordae (*2*) contributing to the obstruction (*LA* left atrium)

aortic regurgitation can be assessed on echo by several methods including the distance the regurgitant jet reaches in the left ventricular cavity, the deceleration slope of the regurgitation jet on Doppler, the width of the regurgitant jet in relation to the diameter of the left ventricular outflow tract, and flow reversal in the descending aorta and arch in diastole. TTE is the main imaging modality in the assessment of aortic regurgitation (Fig. 3.39).

Vegetations of the aortic valve can be identified on TTE but are better assessed on TEE (Fig. 3.40). The latter

Fig. 3.39 (a) TTE in color flow Doppler from the apical four-chamber view, showing severe aortic regurgitation (*1*: the interventricular septum, *2*: severe aortic regurgitant jet, *3*: aortic valve). (**b**) Assessment of the severity of aortic regurgitation. Note the steep deceleration slope (*4*) of the continuous wave Doppler signal of the aortic regurgitant jet detected by interrogating the left ventricular outflow tract and the aortic valve on TTE

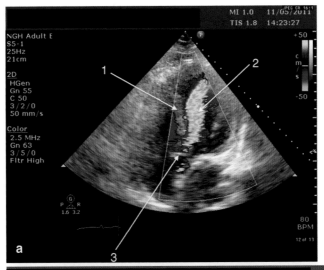

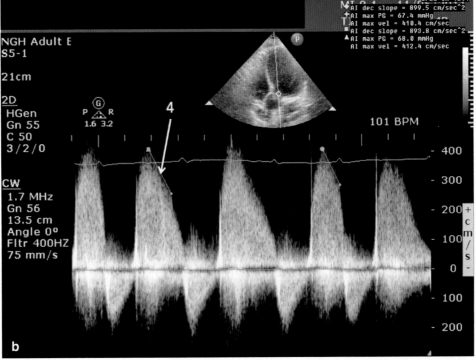

provides better visualization of the aortic root and can demonstrate destruction of valve cusps or involvement of the aortic root by inflammation and abscess formation and development of sinus of valsalva aneurysms. TEE is also used to assess prosthetic aortic valves. Rarely, CCT may be needed to clarify the anatomy in the presence of infective or postsurgical complications.

The Pulmonary Valve

Echocardiography using Doppler and color flow is used to assess pulmonary stenosis and regurgitation. Pulmonary regurgitation is common following cardiac surgery for right ventricular outflow tract obstruction. CMR is helpful for visualizing and assessing the function of the pulmonary valve.

The Tricuspid Valve

Trivial or mild tricuspid regurgitation is detected by TTE in up to 80% of people. The degree of tricuspid regurgitation can be used to calculate right ventricular pressure in systole and thus derive the pulmonary artery pressure. More significant regurgitation is usually due to dilatation of the tricuspid ring and failure of cusp coaptation (Fig. 3.41). This can be seen with either volume overload (pulmonary regurgitation, large atrial, or ventricular septal defects with left to right shunt) or pressure overload (pulmonary valve stenosis, pulmonary hypertension). Rarely, the tricuspid valve is rudimentary resulting in torrential regurgitation. Tricuspid valve disease is best assessed by echo. CMR is only indicated for assessing complex congenital anomalies.

Fig. 3.40 TEE long-axis view (**a**) of the aortic valve and the left ventricular outflow tract in a patient with infective endocarditis. The images show edema of the aortic root (*1*), vegetation (*2*) within the left ventricular outflow tract (**a** and **b**). The images in **b** are identical to **a** but with color flow Doppler, and it shows severe aortic regurgitation jet (*3*). Note also the prolapse of the infected aortic valve cusp (*4*) (*LA* left atrium)

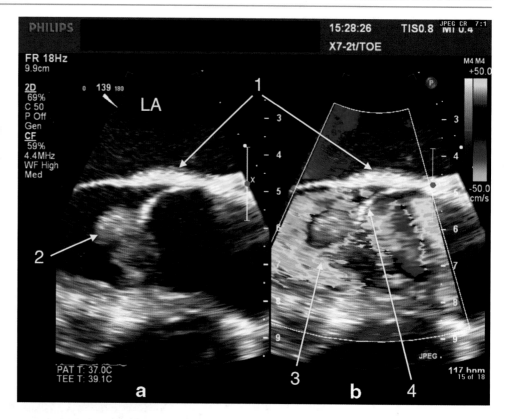

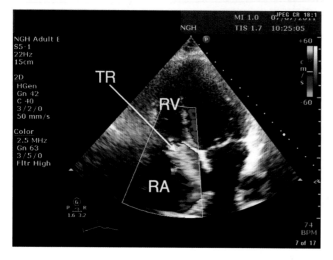

Fig. 3.41 TTE in the apical four-chamber view in a 36-year-old patient with severe tricuspid regurgitation (*TR*) (*RV* right ventricle, *RA* right atrium)

Cardiac Tumors

Primary cardiac tumors are usually detected on echocardiography (TTE and TEE). However, characterization may be incomplete, and both CMR and CCT are helpful in providing additional anatomical information, as well as evidence of extension into extracardiac structures, information about perfusion patterns, and to aid surgical planning. Certain features may assist in tumor characterization. For example, using CMR, high signal on T_1 suggests a fatty lesion, recent hemorrhage, a proteinaceous cystic lesion, or melanoma. A fat saturated sequence can confirm the presence of fat. Low signal on T_1 is seen with cystic lesions, calcification, and a signal void in a vascular malformation. Cysts have a typical high signal on T_2-weighted imaging. Fat and fluid can also be reliably detected on CCT. Tumor vascularity can also be assessed on both CMR and CCT by postcontrast imaging.

The most common primary cardiac tumor (myxoma) is easily identified by echocardiography (see Fig. 3.16b), CCT, and CMR (Fig. 3.42). Using spin echo sequences on CMR, myxomas have the same signal intensity as normal myocardium on T1-weighted images but are bright on T2 and show contrast enhancement.

Primary malignant cardiac tumors (typically sarcomas) are usually heterogeneous, broad based, large masses which occupy most of the affected cardiac chamber and may extend into other chambers and the pericardium (Fig. 3.43). There is generally heterogeneous contrast enhancement. Metastatic tumors to the heart are 20–40 times more common than primary cardiac tumors generally being seen in advanced malignant disease.

Thrombus or Tumor?

CMR is very helpful in distinguishing a cardiac tumor from thrombus, particularly if the mass is ventricular. Cardiac tumors usually enhance on perfusion imaging and may show delayed enhancement. Thrombi occur on cardiac walls which

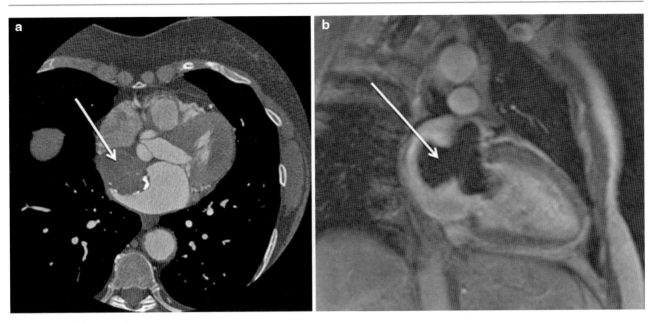

Fig. 3.42 Atrial myxoma (*arrows*) demonstrated on CCT (**a**) and CMR (**b**)

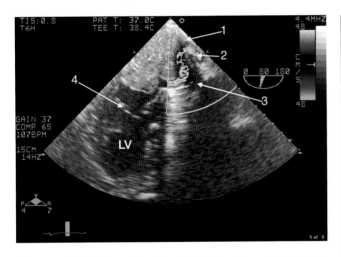

Fig. 3.43 TEE in long axis of the mitral valve, in a patient with left atrial sarcoma (*). Note the invasion (*1*) of the sarcoma into the left upper pulmonary vein (*2*). Note the left atrial appendage is hardly visible (*3*) (*LV* left ventricle, *4* posterior leaflet of the mitral valve)

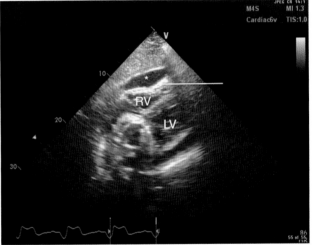

Fig. 3.44 Subcostal TTE view of the heart showing a small pericardial effusion (*), causing tamponade as demonstrated by the collapse of the free wall of the right ventricle (*pointed*) in diastole (*LV* left ventricle, *RV* right ventricle)

are akinetic and they do not enhance. However, there may be late enhancement of the underlying wall if there has been a previous infarction.

Pericardial Disease

Pericardial fluid can be easily assessed by echocardiography, CCT, and CMR and are helpful in selecting a route for effusion drainage. Echocardiography has the advantage of accurately assessing the functional and hemodynamic impact of pericardial disease, particularly in the presence of pericardial tamponade or constrictive pericarditis (Fig. 3.44). Pericardial thickening is shown well on CCT and CMR (see Fig. 3.30). The advantage of CCT is in the detection of pericardial calcification (Fig. 3.45). Although CMR can depict the septal bounce sign on free breathing scan, the best non-invasive assessment of functional abnormalities associated with the pericardial disease is provided by echocardiography. However, invasive cardiac catheterization is needed in many occasions to confirm the diagnosis.

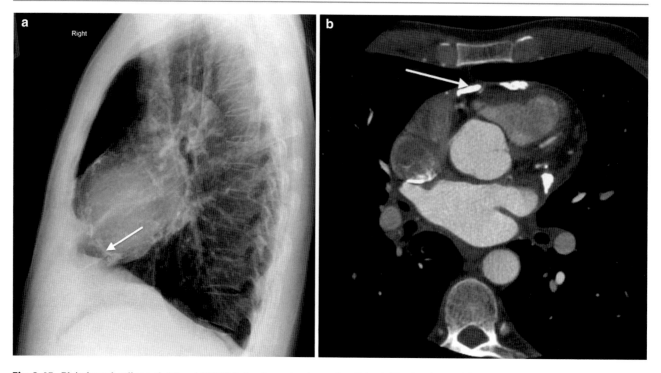

Fig. 3.45 Plain lateral radiograph (**a**) and CCT (**b**) showing extensive pericardial calcification (*arrows*) in a patient with constrictive pericarditis

Constrictive Pericarditis

This is a difficult diagnosis as there is overlap in the clinical presentation with restrictive cardiomyopathy as both conditions cause right heart failure. The hallmark of pericardial constriction is pericardial thickening (greater than 4 mm) and abnormal diastolic ventricular function. Assessment is best made by echocardiography, complemented by CMR. Invasive cardiac catheterization with simultaneous measurement of diastolic pressures from both ventricles is the most accurate way to confirm the diagnosis of constrictive pericarditis and differentiating it from restrictive cardiomyopathy. Plain chest radiographs and CCT may show pericardial calcification (see Fig. 3.45).

Pericardial Tumors

Pericardial masses are usually metastases. Primary pericardial neoplasms are rare, with the most common being malignant mesothelioma. Pericardial tumors usually present with focal or generalized pericardial thickening and a variable pericardial effusion. They are usually first detected on echocardiography but require CMR or CCT to provide additional information regarding size, location, and extent of pericardial involvement.

References

1. Novelline R. Squire's fundamentals of radiology. 5th ed. Cambridge: Harvard University Press; 1997. ISBN 0674833392.
2. Steckelberg JM, Ulietstra RE, Ludwig J, et al. Werner Frossman (1904–1979) and his unusual success story. Mayo Clin Proc. 1979;746:54.
3. Cournand A. Cardiac catheterization: development of the technique, its contribution to experimental medicine and its initial application to man. Acta Med Scand. 1975;579:7.
4. Sones Jr FM, Shirey EK. Cine coronary arteriography. Mod Concepts Cardiovasc Dis. 1962;31:375.
5. Edler I, Hertz CH. The early work on ultrasound in medicine at the university of Lund. J Clin Ultrasound. 1977;5:352–6.
6. Underwood SR, Anagnostopoulos C, Cerqueira M, et al. Myocardial perfusion scintigraphy: the evidence. Eur J Nucl Med Mol Imaging. 2004;31:261–91.
7. Fine JJ, Hopkins CB, Ruff N, Newton FC. Comparison of accuracy of 64-slice cardiovascular computed tomography with coronary angiography in patients with suspected coronary artery disease. Am J Cardiol. 2006;97:173–4.
8. Kim RJ, Fieno DS, Parish TB, et al. Relationship of MRI delayed contrast enhancement to irreversible injury, infarct age, and contractile function. Circulation. 1999;100:1992–2002.
9. Lauer MS, Larson MG, Levy D. Gender-specific reference M-mode values in adults: population-derived values with consideration of the impact of height. J Am Coll Cardiol. 1995;26:1039–46.
10. Troughton RW, Asher CR, Klein AL. The role of echocardiography in atrial fibrillation and cardioversion. Heart. 2003;89:1447–54.

11. Kapur A, Latus KA, Davies G, et al. A comparison of three radio-nuclide myocardial perfusion tracers in clinical practice: the ROBUST study. Eur J Nucl Med Mol Imaging. 2002;29:1608–16.

12. Al-Mohammad A, Mahy IR, Norton MY, et al. Prevalence of hibernating myocardium in patients with severely impaired ischaemic left ventricles. Heart. 1998;80:559–64.

13. Jacobson AF, Senior R, Cerqueira MD, et al. Myocardial iodine-123 meta-iodobenzylguanidine imaging and cardiac events in heart failure results of the prospective ADMIRE-HF (AdreView myocardial imaging for risk evaluation in heart failure) study. J Am Coll Cardiol. 2010. doi:10.1016/j.jacc.2010.01.014.

14. Pennell DJ, Sechtem UP, Higgins CB, et al. Clinical indications for cardiovascular magnetic resonance (CMR): concensus panel report. Eur Heart J. 2004;25:1940–65.

15. Godwin C, Shan K, Flamm S, et al. Role of MRI in clinical cardiology. Lancet. 2004;363:2162–71.

16. Taylor AJ, Cerqueira M, Hodgson JM, et al. ACCF/SCCT/ACR/AHA/ASE/ASNC/SCAI/SCMR 2010: appropriate use criteria for cardiac computed tomography. J Am Coll Cardiol. 2010;56:1864–94.

17. Grothues F, Moon JC, Bellenger NG, et al. Interstudy reproducibility of right ventricular volumes, function and mass with cardiovascular magnetic resonance. Am Heart J. 2004;147:218–23.

18. Moon JC, McKenna WJ, McCrohon JA, et al. Toward clinical risk assessment in hypertrophic cardiomyopathy with gadolinium cardiovascular magnetic resonance. J Am Coll Cardiol. 2003;41:1561–7.

19. Soriano CJ, Ridocci F, Estornell J, et al. Non invasive diagnosis of coronary artery disease in patients with heart failure and systolic dysfunction of uncertain aetiology, using late gadolinium-enhanced cardiovascular magnetic resonance. J Am Coll Cardiol. 2006;45:743–8.

20. Greenland P, Bonow R, Brundage B, et al. ACCF/AHA 2007 clinical expert concensus document on coronary artery calcium scoring by computed tomography in global cardiovascular risk assessment and in evaluation of patients with chest pain. A report of the American College of Cardiology Foundation Clinical Expert Consensus Task Force (ACCF/AHA Writing Committee to Update the 2000 Expert Consensus Document on Electron Beam Computed Tomography). J Am Coll Cardiol. 2007;49:378–402.

21. Wellnhofer E, Olariu A, Klein C, et al. Magnetic resonance low-dose dobutamine test is superior to SCAR quantification for the prediction of functional recovery. Circulation. 2004;109:2172–4.

Current Therapeutics for Cardiac Disease

4

Peter R. Jackson

Abstract

Drugs for the treatment and prevention of cardiovascular disease have been one of the success stories of the last half century. Consequently there are now a large number of drug classes, many with several members all in use in clinical practice. This chapter provides a scaffolding on which pathologists can build a greater understanding of the mechanisms of action, clinical uses, and toxicity of these drugs. In addition, there is a brief consideration of the adverse effects on the cardiovascular system of drugs used for the treatment of diseases in other organ systems. Such understanding will help pathologists in their interpretation of clinical cases and to provide more insightful clinical advice based on knowledge of drug action.

Keywords

Antihypertensives • Antiarrhythmics • Lipid lowering • Acute coronary syndrome • Heart failure • Antiplatelet drugs • Toxicity

Introduction

It is simplistic to expect to be able to look at a pathological specimen and fully understand the pathophysiology without adequate appreciation of the clinical scenario. There is an increasing understanding of cardiovascular physiology, and the last 50 years has seen an explosion in drug therapies. These have targeted the prevention of cardiac disease and have improved the therapy of various cardiac and vascular pathologies. Understanding of the drugs and their impact on the heart is therefore vital for a full analysis of any case.

This chapter is too brief for a full exposition of all the drugs and their pharmacology, and for this, one should consult reference pharmacology texts. Rather, this chapter aims to provide a basic working framework for the understanding of the commonly used drugs prescribed in modern cardiovascular medicine. These drugs will be found regularly in the clinical record of those dying from cardiac disease. As always, close consultation with clinical, surgical, and radiological colleagues is advocated when considering any cardiac pathology.

Antihypertensive Therapy

The fundamental factors in determining blood pressure are cardiac output and peripheral resistance. Although the former may be elevated for a short time in younger patients who develop hypertension, it is the increase in peripheral resistance which perpetuates the disorder and eventually becomes irreversible, particularly with increasing age. The replacement of elastic fibers in conduit arteries by collagen

P.R. Jackson, Ph.D., FRCP, FFPM(Dis)
Department of Pharmacology and Therapeutics,
Royal Hallamshire Hospital,
Glossop Road, Sheffield S10 JF, UK

Department of Clinical Medicine, Sheffield Teaching Hospitals
NHS Foundation Trust,
Sheffield, UK
e-mail: peterr.jackson@nhs.net

underpins the process by increasing stiffness of the arterial walls and thereby increasing resistance. The control of both cardiac output and peripheral resistance is complex, and there are many mechanisms by which drugs can be used to lower blood pressure. These are not limited simply to reversing the changes involved in the development of high blood pressure. Currently the major drug classes used include those acting on the renin–angiotensin–aldosterone system, the beta (β)-blockers, diuretics, and direct vasodilators.

Drugs Acting on the Renin–Angiotensin–Aldosterone System

The linked hormones renin, angiotensin, and aldosterone are critically involved in the control of blood pressure, and for a significant minority of patients, raised circulating concentrations of aldosterone appear to be the main driver for raised blood pressure.

Angiotensin-Converting Enzyme Inhibitors

The renin–angiotensin–aldosterone system was initially thought of as a simple linear cascade with renin produced by the kidney cleaving angiotensinogen to produce inactive angiotensin I (Ang I) which was subsequently shortened even further to the active octapeptide angiotensin II (Ang II) by angiotensin-converting enzyme (ACE). Ang II is a powerful vasoconstrictor which also stimulates adrenal release of aldosterone and thereby has a dual action in increasing blood pressure both by increasing peripheral resistance and causing sodium retention. The system is now known to be far more complex with balancing vasoconstrictors and vasodilators under independent control. Nevertheless drugs which block the conversion of angiotensin I to Ang II (ACE inhibitors such as ramipril) successfully lower blood pressure. ACE inhibitors also have important roles in the treatment of heart failure and in renal protection in patients with diabetic nephropathy. ACE not only facilitates the breakdown of Ang I but also catabolizes bradykinin and, thus, ACE inhibitors can precipitate life-threatening angioedema but more commonly cause a persistent nonproductive cough. ACE inhibition can also cause significant renal impairment particularly in patients with bilateral renal artery stenosis. In a proportion of patients (particularly the elderly or those who are sodium depleted by disease/drugs), first doses of ACE inhibitors can cause a precipitous fall in blood pressure with significant systemic perfusion consequences. Although widely advised for the treatment of high blood pressure in younger patients, ACE inhibitors are both teratogens and embryotoxic. They should

therefore be avoided in young women either planning to conceive or commencing pregnancy.

Angiotensin Antagonists

Similar beneficial effects, albeit without the production of cough or angioedema, can be achieved by direct antagonism of AT1 receptors, a drug class known as angiotensin receptor blockers (ARBs) or sartans (e.g., losartan). ARBs have a similar overall incidence of adverse effects as placebo. Importantly they can still adversely affect kidney function and are also thought harmful in pregnancy.

Aldosterone Antagonists

Aldosterone antagonists act as weak diuretics but also block the other actions of aldosterone in damaging endothelium and inducing vascular fibrosis. They have a specific role in hypertension caused by aldosterone excess (Conn's syndrome) but can be used in essential hypertension resistant to other drug treatments. The obvious adverse effects of aldosterone antagonists are hyperkalemia reflecting the antagonism of aldosterone on sodium–potassium (Na^+:K^+) exchange in the kidney with impairment of renal function. Spironolactone, the most commonly used aldosterone antagonist, may also bind to other steroid hormone receptors, particularly those for sex hormones – causing menstrual irregularity in women and gynecomastia in men.

β (Beta)-Blockers

When first introduced, β(beta)-blockers such as propranolol were not expected to lower blood pressure but were instead primarily used for the prevention of angina attacks. The discovery that they also lowered blood pressure was thus somewhat serendipitous. The precise mechanism by which they achieve this action remains unclear. Although several hypotheses have been raised, none are completely satisfactory. Indeed, it is possible that this class has a heterogeneous mechanism of action. Certainly more recently introduced drugs (e.g., labetalol and carvedilol) combine β(beta)-blockade with vasodilatation and have quite distinct hemodynamic properties. However, whether this leads to differences in clinical outcome remains unclear.

While at one time atenolol was one of the drugs most commonly used to treat high blood pressure, the role of β(beta)-blockers in the treatment of hypertension has been somewhat downgraded of late both because they appear slightly less effective at preventing stroke (particularly in the elderly) but also because of their adverse metabolic effects. Nevertheless, in patients with drug-resistant high blood pressure, or those whose high blood pressure is accompanied by ischemic heart disease/heart failure, β(beta)-blockers retain a key role. The most important adverse effect of β(beta)-blockers is exacerbation of obstructive pulmonary disease. This appears less important in patients with chronic obstructive pulmonary disease (but should not be underestimated) and surprisingly may not reduce the benefit of inhaled β(beta)-agonists. However, in asthmatics, all β-blockers, even those selective for β(beta)$_1$ receptors, are contraindicated because they can precipitate life-threatening bronchospasm.

Calcium Channel Blockers

Dihydropyridines

Dihydropyridine calcium channel blocking drugs such as nifedipine act at the L-type voltage-gated calcium channel. This is involved in stimulus–response coupling in cardiac muscle and many, but not all, smooth muscle cells. This leads to vasodilatation in some vascular beds. However, even within the circulatory system, there is considerable heterogeneity in response both between arteries and veins, between actions on blood vessels and on contractility in the heart. Calcium channel blockers (CCBs) of this class may lower blood pressure by inducing arteriolar vasodilatation, but this is often at the expense of reflex tachycardia and flushing. These symptoms often ameliorate with time, but in the long term, peripheral edema is the most common adverse effect. This is mediated by blockade of postural skin vasoconstriction which leads to capillary hyperfiltration.

Rate-Limiting Calcium Channel Blockers

By contrast, rate-limiting calcium channel blockers are more selective for the L-type channel found in cardiac tissue and therefore act as negative chronotropes and negative inotropes. Although diltiazem and verapamil are less potent vasodilators than the dihydropyridine CCBs, they block the reflex tachycardia and hence have similar blood-pressure-lowering effects. Consequently, adverse effects linked to vasodilation including peripheral edema are less frequent. However, these drugs are more likely to worsen symptoms of heart failure. In addition, reflecting their action at the atrioventricular node (AVN), rate-limiting calcium channel blockers can produce heart block – particularly if administered alongside other drugs with similar actions such as β(beta)-blockers.

Diuretics

Thiazide Diuretics

Thiazide diuretics are one of the earliest drug classes to be used in the management of hypertension. They remain important drugs, particularly in the elderly. As diuretics, they promote an increase in sodium and water loss by blocking sodium and water transport in the distal convoluted tubule of the kidney and enhance loss in the urine. It should not be assumed that the mechanism by which they lower blood pressure in the long term is a simple reduction of cardiac output, consequent upon a fall in blood volume. Certainly the initial response to a thiazide diuretic is a fall in plasma volume, but within a few days, the reduction in cardiac output triggers an increase in total peripheral resistance mediated via the sympathetic nervous system and the renin–angiotensin–aldosterone system, and within weeks, plasma volume returns towards normal. Despite this, blood pressure remains low because thiazides exert an additional vasodilatory action. Theories to account for this include a direct action on the endothelium or an indirect effect mediated by sodium loss. In support of the latter theory is the observed effect of increasing sodium intake or giving drugs which cause sodium retention which abolishes the antihypertensive effect of thiazide diuretics.

Thiazides have a number of adverse metabolic actions including increases in urate, glucose, and cholesterol, as well as the loss of potassium. This led to a drive to use lower doses in an attempt to minimize these adverse effects while maintaining the majority of their antihypertensive action. However, the most recent view is that the low doses of thiazides used in the last couple of decades may not achieve the same benefit as the higher doses particularly of drugs like chlortalidone.

Loop Diuretics

Loop diuretics cause urinary loss of sodium and water by blockade of the Na^+:K^+:$2Cl^-$ cotransporter in the ascending limb of the loop of Henle by competing with Cl^- at the luminal surface. Although loop diuretics such as furosemide produce a brisk increase in water and sodium loss in the urine at low or moderate doses, they are no more effective than thiazide diuretics in increasing 24-h sodium excretion (although at higher doses, they are more effective). In a large part, this is because the brisk diuresis they cause is followed by a period of water and sodium retention. This, along with their brief vasodilator action, makes it understandable why loop diuretics are not particularly useful for long-term control of blood pressure. In patients with significant fluid retention, following the use of vasodilator drugs, moderate doses of loop diuretics can produce dramatic falls in blood pressure.

Less Commonly Used Drugs

Alpha (α)-Blockers

Unselective α(alpha)-blockers such as phentolamine or phenoxybenzamine are rarely used in the management of hypertension, despite an increase in total peripheral resistance being important in hypertension. They cause an unpleasant reflex tachycardia, and their use is associated with a rapid development of tolerance. By contrast, selective postjunctional α(alpha)-blockers, such as doxazosin, have seen significant use, particularly in men with concomitant prostate disease. However, in clinical outcome trials, α-blockers are slightly less effective than other drug classes in lowering blood pressure and less likely to prevent end-organ damage. Consequently, they are not first-line drugs in simple hypertension. The most common adverse effects with α-blockers are drowsiness and dizziness. They also have a reputation for causing sudden and significant hypotension after the first dose.

Vasodilators

Nonspecific vasodilators such as hydralazine and minoxidil are now little used, apart from in the control of severe hypertension when minoxidil appears to have particular merit. Hydralazine is avoided because of its propensity to trigger drug-induced lupus erythematosus, but it still has a minor role in the control of high blood pressure during pregnancy. Minoxidil can cause a reflex tachycardia unless given with a β(beta)-blocker. Moreover, at higher doses, it causes intense fluid retention which can often only be controlled using substantial doses of loop diuretics.

Centrally Acting Drugs

Imidazoline Agonists
Early centrally acting drugs such as clonidine are little used in the UK because of their tendency to cause sedation, although they still find some use in the USA. Imidazoline agonists such as moxonidine are less likely to cause sedation. Both clonidine and moxonidine lower blood pressure by stimulation of central receptors which in turn inhibit peripheral sympathetic activity. This lowers heart rate, decreases concentration of circulating catecholamines, and prevents vasoconstriction. The most common adverse effects with moxonidine are dry mouth and gastrointestinal disturbance.

Hypertension Overview

In clinical practice, drugs are divided into two groups. The first includes those which work best in low renin states (favoring the elderly and Afro-Caribbeans) and includes diuretics and calcium channel blockers – which by their action tend to increase renin. The second group in contrast works best in high renin states (favoring young white Caucasians); and this group includes ACE inhibitors, angiotensin receptor blockers, and β(beta)-blockers. The majority of patients will require more than one drug to achieve good blood pressure control, and current practice is to combine drugs from the different groups above although the evidence base for this approach is slight.

Treatment for Cardiac Failure

Surprisingly, when most cases of heart failure are due to myocardial loss or damage, providing pharmacological inotropic support appears to be of little help. While positive inotropes such as milrinone are used for short-term support, clinical trials show that in the long term, such drugs actually increase mortality.

Acute Heart Failure

Inotropes

The catecholamines dopamine and dobutamine have both been used intravenously in the treatment of acute heart failure. In this context, they improve both measured hemodynamics and symptoms. They are of particular use during hospital admissions precipitated by acute worsening of heart failure where there is hypotension and end-organ hypoperfusion. Similarly milrinone, a type III phosphodiesterase inhibitor, is licensed for use in patients with heart failure unresponsive to routine therapy although there is no evidence that even short-term use improves mortality. The level of improvement in symptoms may persist for some time after the infusion ends. However, in chronic oral use, it too has been shown to cause a sizeable increase in mortality.

Chronic Heart Failure

Chronic treatment of heart failure is therefore aimed at alleviating symptoms as well as protecting the heart from further damage caused by adverse homeostatic responses of the sympathetic and adrenal systems. Left unchecked, these responses cause further vasoconstriction, tachycardia (to increase blood pressure), and fluid retention. Although apparently not reversing the primary problem, blocking these homeostatic reactions by β(beta)-blockade and ACE inhibition both improves symptoms and patient longevity. Due to the poor relationship between symptoms and mortality, it is important for both β-blockers and ACE inhibitors that drug doses are titrated to targets determined in clinical trials rather than against the extent of symptom relief.

β (Beta)-Blockers

Until recently, the use of β(beta)-blockers in patients with heart failure was anathema. Indeed, it is still the case that administering such drugs in patients with unstable heart failure can precipitate rapid deterioration, sometimes with a fatal outcome. However, if introduced cautiously in patients who have already received initial treatment with diuretics, β(beta)-blockers provide further valuable improvement in both symptoms and longevity. The mechanisms by which β(beta)-blockers achieve this result are unclear but probably include protection of the myocardium from remodeling, vasodilatation in muscle beds, by reducing cardiac work and lowering heart rate; all blocking adverse effects of counter-regulatory hormone response to the reduced cardiac output. Both β(beta)-blockers with (carvedilol) and without (bisoprolol) additional vasodilatory action have been shown to be of benefit in heart failure.

Vasodilators

Some vasodilator drugs offer benefit in patients with heart failure by "unloading" the heart. A combination of arteriolar (hydralazine) and venous (nitrate) vasodilators was the first treatment regimen to be shown to improve longevity in what was a dismal prognosis for patients with advanced heart failure. This combination is used less now because of the greater benefit seen with ACE inhibitors. However, for Afro-Caribbean patients whose response to ACE inhibitors is muted, this combination still offers some advantages. The same combination can be used in patients for whom ACE inhibitors or angiotensin receptor blockers (ARB) are contraindicated because of severe renal impairment.

Nitrates are also of use in the management of acute heart failure and, in one small trial, were shown to be more effective than loop diuretics. It is clear that the molecular mechanism of organic nitrates is via the formation of nitric oxide which activates guanylate cyclase, producing cGMP-dependent vasodilatation. The precise details as to why organic nitrates are more effective than inorganic nitrates and why some drugs affect arterioles and others veins are not clear. The production of nitric oxide following treatment with organic nitrates seems to necessitate interaction with sulfhydryl receptors, and repeated administration of organic nitrates leads to sulfhydryl depletion and tolerance. To avoid this situation, slow release preparations are given once daily and standard release nitrates in an asymmetric dosing pattern so as to leave a nitrate free interval within 24 h during which time there is some recovery from potential tolerance. Headache due to the vasodilatation is the most common adverse effect with organic nitrates. This resolves with continued use. In the long term, hypotension is the more common problem. While methemoglobinemia is seen when amyl nitrate is abused, it is an uncommon adverse effect of therapeutic organic nitrates, even when taken in overdose.

If anything, the mechanism of action of hydralazine is even less well understood, but the drug is thought to produce vasodilatation by altering calcium (Ca^{2+}) balance in smooth muscle cells inhibiting Ca release from endoplasmic reticulum and hence preventing muscle contraction. The more common adverse effects of hydralazine are those associated with vasodilatation, tachycardia, and headache, as well as, after prolonged use, fluid retention. At higher doses and particularly in slow acetylators, hydralazine can produce a lupus-like syndrome presenting with a range of vasculitides and blood dyscrasias.

Not all vasodilators benefit patients with heart failure. Thus, the calcium channel blockers are either neutral, with dihydropyridines offering neither harm nor benefit, or harmful with diltiazem and verapamil leading to a worsening of heart failure.

ACE Inhibitors

The use of ACE inhibitors in patients with heart failure did not get off to a good start. The first trial in patients early after myocardial infarction (MI) showed an increase in mortality. Subsequent studies starting the drug a few days after the MI showed benefit particularly in patients with symptomatic heart failure. ACE inhibitors are now a mainstay in the treatment of heart failure or even asymptomatic left ventricular systolic impairment. They provide an improvement in life expectancy, symptom control, and hospital stay. Of importance is that in clinical trials, drugs were titrated to a target dose rather than against symptoms, with some evidence of greater benefit in those receiving higher doses. Although working on the same pathway, the evidence for the benefit of ARBs is not quite so robust with some trials being negative. There is evidence both for escape from ACE inhibition of angiotensin-converting enzyme and the existence of pathways of angiotensin activation independent of ACE. However, adding ARBs to ACE inhibitors to avoid these additional routes does not provide additional benefit in heart failure and may be associated with added morbidity and mortality.

Diuretics

Loop diuretics remain the mainstay for initial symptom control in patients with heart failure. They are universally believed to improve both pulmonary congestion and to alleviate breathlessness and/or peripheral edema. This is despite the paucity of clinical trial evidence for benefit, whether in terms of immediate symptom control or improved longevity. The available evidence suggests that diuretics provide better symptom control than ACE inhibitors or β(beta)-blockers used alone and should therefore always be included in a heart failure regimen. Nevertheless, the evidence for a mortality gain with diuretics is also weak, and these drugs similarly should not be used alone in patients with heart failure. In acute heart failure, loop diuretics provide clinical improvement in symptoms even before diuresis occurs, and this may be because of the release of renally derived prostaglandins. Although thiazide diuretics offer similar diuresis and natriuresis to low doses of loop diuretics, this is often inadequate for patients with heart failure – hence the preference for the latter given in moderate doses.

Aldosterone antagonists (e.g., spironolactone) but not other potassium-sparing diuretics have established evidence of both symptomatic benefit and improvements in longevity in patients immediately following MI or those with established heart failure. These drugs suffer the disadvantage that when used in combination with ACE inhibitors and β(beta)-blockers, they commonly induce significant hyperkalemia.

Digoxin

For hundreds of years, this was the mainstay of the treatment of heart failure. With the advent of diuretics, digoxin's role was restricted to use for rate control in patients with atrial fibrillation. More recent data suggest that it does provide added benefit for patients with severe left ventricular impairment, even when other modern treatments are used, although this is more improvement in symptoms rather than in longevity. There is also a concern that the benefit may be gender specific, with women suffering an apparent increase in mortality, although this is based on a post-hoc analysis of clinical trial data. Unlike its mechanism in atrial fibrillation, the action of digoxin in heart failure is a direct cardiac one with inhibition of the transmembrane sodium–potassium (Na^+:K^+) pump which, via the sodium–calcium (Na^+:Ca^{2+}) exchanger, increases the availability of intracellular Ca^{2+} and therefore muscular contractility. Heart failure patients treated with digoxin may be at increased risk of arrhythmias due to diuretic-induced hypokalemia.

Heart Failure Overview

Low blood pressure is an effect of all drugs used for the treatment of heart failure apart from the positive inotropes. This hypotensive effect is surprisingly well tolerated, even in the elderly, and tends to improve with the time on drug treatment. For some patients, the hypotensive effect will be dose-limiting. The overall pathway for the treatment of heart failure centers on the use of diuretics and ACE inhibitors. Once stable, β(beta)-blockers can be introduced cautiously and titrated to target dose. If the patient is then asymptomatic, the treatment is maintained. If symptoms worsen, further treatment with aldosterone antagonists and, if necessary, digoxin is added.

Acute Coronary Syndrome Therapeutic Options

The acute coronary syndromes (ACSs) constituting unstable angina, non-ST elevation myocardial infarction (NSTEMI), and ST elevation myocardial infarction (STEMI) are caused by some obstruction to coronary blood flow – usually secondary to atheroma (often aggravated by new vaso-occlusive thrombus) in the coronary arteries. The aims of treating ACS are to provide immediate symptom relief but mainly to prevent myocardial damage by restoring coronary flow. This is usually achieved by interfering with the thrombus and prevention of further clot formation by use of fibrinolytics, anticoagulants, and antiplatelet drugs. After recovery from the acute ischemic phase, thought needs to be given to secondary treatment to prevent further vascular occlusive events, in addition to attention to the underlying atheromatous process.

Fibrinolytics

Fibrinolytic drugs convert circulating plasminogen to plasmin. This active protease, which breaks down the fibrin in established thrombus, ideally leads to lysis of the occlusion and reperfusion of downstream myocardium. In diseases such as myocardial infarction in which intra-arterial thrombosis plays a major role, fibrinolytics have been shown to provide a major reduction in mortality. Streptokinase, one of the earliest fibrinolytics, produces plasmin production throughout the circulation but also releases bradykinin. Tissue plasminogen activator (TPA) is somewhat more specific, only producing plasmin in the presence of fibrin (i.e., in the locality of thrombus), but unfortunately, this does not reduce its potential to cause hemorrhage. Adverse effects specific to streptokinase are hypotension thought secondary to the systemic production of bradykinin and allergy, with antibodies appearing within 3–4 days of use which precludes the use of repeated courses. Fibrinolytic drugs are reserved for use in patients with STEMI, but even here, they are being replaced by primary coronary intervention (PCI) with angioplasty and stenting.

Antiplatelet Agents

A range of different antiplatelet drugs can be used in the treatment of acute coronary syndrome dependent upon a patient's risk and whether intervention is anticipated. All the drugs inhibit platelet aggregation and thereby lower the ability to form further thrombus.

Aspirin

Aspirin irreversibly inhibits prostaglandin synthase in platelets and megakaryocytes preventing production of the powerful vasoconstrictor and platelet proaggregator, thromboxane A_2. Recovery from this action depends upon formation of new platelets. The onset of aspirin's action is rapid with its maximum effect achieved within 30 min following a 160 mg dose. In long-term use, maximum effect is achieved with a smaller daily dose, usually 75 mg. After acute myocardial infarction, aspirin reduces short-term risk of further cardiovascular events or death by about 30%. In long-term use in patients with previous vascular events, the relative risk reduction is slightly smaller but still worthwhile. For primary prevention (i.e., those patients at high risk of cardiovascular disease but who remain asymptomatic), the benefit of aspirin is much smaller and has to be weighed against the risk of hemorrhage – particularly gastrointestinal (GI) bleeding and hemorrhagic stroke. Further complicating this consideration is the recently described association between aspirin use and a reduction in GI and other malignancies.

Thienopyridines

The thienopyridine derivatives, clopidogrel and prasugrel, are inactive prodrugs with metabolites which bind to the $P2Y_{12}$ (ADP) receptor on the surface of platelets and thereby inhibit platelet activation. Compared with aspirin, clopidogrel is slightly more effective in preventing cardiovascular events, and the combination of the two drugs is superior to either alone. Clopidogrel is less likely than aspirin to cause GI hemorrhage, although bleeding is still its major adverse

effect. Rash and diarrhea are also common adverse effects. Ticlopidine, an early thienopyridine, is now rarely used because of its tendency to cause thrombocytopenia.

Glycoprotein IIb/IIIa Receptor Blockers

These structurally diverse drugs all block the IIb/IIIa receptor (whose role is to bind fibrinogen and provide cross-linking between platelets, necessary for aggregation and thrombus stabilization). Abciximab is a humanized mouse antibody to the IIb/IIIa receptor while eptifibatide and tirofiban are analogs of fibrinogen which compete with fibrinogen for the normal binding site on the IIb/IIIa receptor. At the doses of receptor blocker used, as many as 50% of the receptors may be blocked, and aggregation is powerfully inhibited. The effects of eptifibatide and tirofiban decline more rapidly than those of abciximab. Thrombocytopenia is a significant adverse effect of these drugs as well as the expected risk of bleeding. The glycoprotein IIb/IIIa receptor blockers are generally reserved for use in very high risk acute coronary syndrome patients, especially those about to undergo vascular intervention. When used in combination with aspirin, they can produce an additional 20% reduction in cardiovascular events.

Anticoagulants

Heparins all produce anticoagulation by a common mechanism mediated by enhancing the action of antithrombin III in modulating the activity of several of the factors in the clotting cascade. The inhibition of two of these is of greatest importance that involving thrombin and that factor Xa.

In both, a unique pentasaccharide sequence present in only 30% of unfractionated heparin molecules binds to antithrombin III producing a conformational change accelerating its inactivation of clotting factors. The inactivation of thrombin necessitates that it too is bound to the heparin molecule but at an extended polysaccharide segment. Low-molecular-weight heparins (LMWHs) contain a more homogenous range of shorter polysaccharides with far fewer molecules containing polysaccharide sequences capable of binding thrombin. Their action therefore relies much more heavily on enhancing the action of antithrombin III against factor Xa. This does not impair the anticoagulant effectiveness of LMWH in clinical practice and their more reliable pharmacokinetic profile largely excludes the need for coagulation monitoring. LMWHs are now largely replacing unfractionated heparin, apart from where rapid reversal may be necessary. In ACS, unfractionated heparin, or now more commonly LMWH, can significantly reduce adverse cardiovascular outcomes in patients with acute coronary syndrome or myocardial infarction. Since heparins bind to platelet factor 4 and can precipitate an immune response, they can produce an IgG-mediated platelet aggregation termed heparin-induced thrombocytopenia (HIT). Although this occurs less frequently following use of LMWH, routine monitoring of the full blood count is still required after 5–10 days of treatment. In long-term use, heparins can also cause osteoporosis.

Fondaparinux

Fondaparinux, a synthetic analog of the heparin pentasaccharide region that binds to antithrombin III, has a consistent chain length but is unable to bind thrombin. It therefore works entirely by binding to antithrombin III and enhancing inhibition of factor Xa alone without any direct action on thrombin. Fondaparinux may be used in place of LMWH in patients with ACS, with some evidence to suggest increased efficacy in preventing cardiovascular events along with a lower risk of bleeding. By far, the greatest risk of treatment with fondaparinux is hemorrhage, although temporary increases in liver enzymes have also been reported. Unlike LMWH, fondaparinux does not bind to platelet factor 4 and therefore does not cause thrombocytopenia.

Stable Angina

The management of stable angina is aimed at immediate symptom control of acute attacks, prophylaxis against further attacks of stable angina, and prevention of significant cardiovascular events whether in the coronary or other vascular beds.

Management of Acute Angina Attacks

Organic nitrates are still the drugs most commonly used for symptom relief during an acute episode of angina. That most frequently prescribed is glyceryl trinitrate (GTN), which can be taken either buccally as a tablet or sublingually as a spray. The advantage of these particular routes is that they provide both rapid absorption and avoid extensive hepatic first-pass metabolism. While organic nitrates such as GTN produce vasodilatation in both coronary venous and arterial beds, coronary flow actually decreases when the drug is administered suggesting that it is the reduction in cardiac work that is the most important mechanism behind the relief of symptoms. The half-life of GTN is short, such that its action is usually only sufficient to relieve pain in a straightforward attack of angina. By far, the most common adverse effect is severe headache with intermittent treatment not providing

the protection from vasodilator effects that comes with tolerance. Of practical importance is nitrate-associated hypotension, particularly if exacerbated by concomitant use with drugs such as sildenafil (Viagra).

Attack Prevention

The first-line preventive treatment of stable angina is with either a β(beta)-blocker or a rate-limiting calcium channel blocker (e.g., diltiazem or verapamil). If this alone is insufficient to control symptoms, then a drug from the other class can be added. However, the combination of verapamil with a β-blocker is contraindicated because of a high incidence of atrioventricular blockade. Only when one of these two classes is contraindicated or a patient is ineligible for intervention should one of the other classes of drugs be used.

β (Beta)-Blockers

All β(beta)-blockers including those with intrinsic sympathomimetic activity are effective in preventing attacks of angina. Importantly the shape of the dose–response curve might differ between prevention of angina and control of high blood pressure. Thus, there is little benefit in terms of blood pressure control in increasing the dose of atenolol beyond 50 mg daily while effectiveness of this drug in preventing anginal attacks might necessitate titration to doses as high as 100 mg bid.

Calcium Channel Blockers

The most effective CCBs in preventing angina are those which reduce heart rate (i.e., verapamil and diltiazem). Dihydropyridine CCBs, such as nifedipine, can paradoxically worsen angina because of the vasodilatation-induced reflex tachycardia. Indeed, immediate-release nifedipine has been linked with an increased risk of myocardial infarction. If, however, a dihydropyridine is given along with a β(beta)-blocker (to block any increase in heart rate), it does provide additional relief from anginal episodes compared with the β(beta)-blocker alone.

Nitrates

As well as being of use in the treatment of acute attacks, organic nitrates can be used to prevent angina attacks. With chronic use, tolerance is a particular issue, and once daily slow-release preparations are formulated so as to ensure that for part of the

24-h period, circulating concentrations remain low. If modified release preparations requiring a more than once-each-day administration are used, then dosing times are selected asymmetrically again to provide a nitrate free interval.

Nicorandil

Nicorandil combines the action of an organic nitrate and a potassium channel opener in the same drug molecule. Both actions produce significant vasodilatation in the coronary circulation with the nitrate moiety also producing peripheral vasodilatation and reducing cardiac work. In some studies, nicorandil has been shown to be as effective as a β(beta)-blocker or calcium channel blocker in preventing attacks of stable angina. In addition to the usual vasodilator adverse effects, nicorandil can cause focal ulceration of the GI tract (e.g., anorectal sites).

Ivabradine

Ivabradine has a novel mechanism of action, inhibiting the inward sodium–potassium (Na^+:K^+) current (I_f), which is an important component of pacemaker function in the sinoatrial node and thus reduces heart rate. It has no effect on contractility, peripheral resistance, or cardiac workload. Nevertheless, by the simple reduction in heart rate, it is an effective antianginal drug when used alone but particularly when added in either to a β-blocker or calcium channel blocker. It can produce conduction abnormalities, and in some patients, it interferes with vision.

Ranolazine

Ranolazine acts to prevent attacks of angina by a different mechanism, that of inhibiting the late myocyte sodium (Na^+) flux. Myocyte ischemia is associated with prolonged opening of the Na^+ channel following depolarization, allowing the intracellular concentration of Na^+ to rise. There are other mechanisms which may also explain the increased Na^+ concentration, but together these lead to an increase in intracellular calcium (Ca^{++}) concentration increasing contraction, even in diastole, and worsening energy consumption. Ranolazine, by inhibiting the late Na^+ flux, helps keep intracellular sodium in check and improves symptoms of angina. It can be used along with CCBs or β-blockers without adverse interaction. The commonest adverse effects of ranolazine are dizziness, headache, and constipation. Inhibitors of CYP3A4, a common drug metabolizing enzyme, may increase plasma ranolazine concentrations – and therefore when used together with verapamil or diltiazem doses should be restricted.

Secondary Prevention

Patients, either with stable angina or following an acute coronary syndrome, should receive secondary prevention with drugs to control elevated blood pressure and lower cholesterol along with an antiplatelet agent – usually either aspirin or clopidogrel. Benefits have also been demonstrated for use of β(beta)-blockers and ACE inhibitors postmyocardial infarction, even when patients do not have hypertension, angina, or heart failure.

Cardiac Dysrhythmias

Cardiac dysrhythmias reflect altered cardiac contraction rates and electrical patterns. These have an adverse physiological function in terms of body homeostasis and cardiac output. However, it has to be remembered that quite considerable variation in heart rate, albeit with a normal cardiac conduction pattern, is a normal function of daily life. This allows the individual to deal with the varying demands of work and rest. It allows the body to vary blood delivery to various organ systems with maintenance of circulation to core/critical organs (e.g., brain, kidneys, etc.).

In simple terms, cardiac dysrhythmias are classed into those with slow heart rates (bradycardias) and those with elevated heart rates (tachyarrhythmias/tachycardias). In both of these circumstances, the cardiac conduction pathway may be abnormal with initiation of the cardiac depolarization from supraventricular, nodal, and ventricular sources.

Bradycardias

Significant bradycardias (heart rates less than 60 bpm) are usually due to degenerative disease of the sinoatrial node (SAN) or atrioventricular node (AVN) although a smaller proportion are caused by extraneous causes such as drugs, raised intracranial pressure, myocardial ischemia, and so on. In the absence of a reversible cause of short-term pathology, the management of significant bradycardia is commonly dealt with by insertion of a pacemaker. In an emergency, drugs such as atropine and adrenaline (and analogs) may be used intravenously to increase cardiac output and alleviate symptoms.

Atropine, a naturally occurring alkaloid, increases heart rate by blocking the tonic action of the parasympathetic effect of the vagus (X) nerve. It is a competitive antagonist of acetylcholine at both the SAN and AVN. When administered as a bolus, therapeutic doses of atropine rarely produce the full range of anticholinergic effects but may produce dilated pupils, difficulty swallowing, hot dry skin, dizziness, and thirst.

Adrenaline is a sympathetic catecholamine secreted by the adrenals in response to stress which can be used therapeutically to increase heart rate. It binds avidly to β(beta)$_1$ adrenergic receptors in the SAN and all myocardial cells, thereby increasing automaticity, conduction through the AVN, and force of contraction. Both adrenaline and its synthetic analog isoprenaline have been used for the treatment of transient heart block, but a more common use for such sympathomimetics is in critical care when they are infused to increase blood pressure and heart rate. Since both increase cardiac work and reduce coronary blood flow, they must be used with care in patients with ischemic heart disease. Furthermore, due to their action in increasing automaticity, such drugs commonly generate abnormal heart rhythms and are not used outside the acute setting.

Tachycardias

While there are many different types (patterns) of tachycardia, the most significant are atrial fibrillation (affecting 9% of the over 80s) and ventricular tachycardia/fibrillation (implicated in cases of sudden cardiac decompensation and death). The underlying pathophysiology behind tachycardias reflects increased cellular automaticity, be that spontaneous, linked to after-depolarization of preceding contractions, or more frequently due to re-entry circuits.

Considering these underlying mechanisms, it would appear logical to develop drugs which reduce automaticity or increase the electrical refractory period after contraction. Unfortunately, blocking flux through the sodium (Na$^+$) channel (which reduces automaticity) increases heterogeneity of repolarization and promotes the development of re-entrant arrhythmias. Furthermore, prolongation of the refractory period by blockade of the I_{Kr} potassium rectifier current can precipitate the characteristic ventricular arrhythmia Torsade de Pointes (TdP). Thus, it is not surprising that antiarrhythmic drugs, introduced mainly on the basis of in vitro mechanism, are paradoxically proarrhythmic. They fail to reduce mortality and at the same time can cause significant side effects. Despite increased understanding of both the pathophysiology underlying the tachycardias and the mechanism of drug action, the clinical role of such drugs remains limited. Consequently, there is increasing emphasis on electrical intervention (ablation of accessory pathways and/or implantation of defibrillators).

A common classification of antiarrhythmic drugs by mechanism of action in isolated tissues is that of Vaughan Williams (Table 4.1).

Many drugs are now more of historical or scientific interest with few being used routinely in clinical practice. Consequently, a far more clinically useful classification is to consider the following scheme:

Table 4.1 Vaughan Williams classification of antiarrhythmic drug action

Class	Mechanism	Electrophysiological action
I	Sodium channel blockers	
Ia	Moderate	Prolongs refractoriness
Ib	Weak	No effect on refractoriness
Ic	Strong	Prolongs refractoriness
II	B(beta)-blockers	No direct effect on action potential/refractoriness
III	Potassium channel blockers	Prolongs refractoriness and delays repolarization
IV	Calcium channel blockers	Slows SA node pacemaker and AV conduction

- Drugs specifically for atrial arrhythmias
- Drugs effective against both atrial and ventricular arrhythmias
- Drugs only effective against ventricular arrhythmias

Drugs Used in the Management of Atrial Arrhythmias

Adenosine binds to a specific G-protein-coupled receptor, activating the acetylcholine-sensitive potassium current, leading to shortening of the action potential and hyperpolarization in the SAN and AVN. It also has some calcium (Ca^{2+}) channel blocking activity which, together with its primary effects, produces marked slowing of conduction through the AVN. Clinically it is used for the termination of atrioventricular (AV) re-entrant arrhythmias and to distinguish between broad complex arrhythmias arising in the atria from those derived from the ventricles. It commonly causes brief asystole, but as it is very rapidly taken up into cells, its action is brief with spontaneous recovery. Importantly adenosine can produce bronchospasm and should therefore not be given to patients with asthma.

Digoxin, a naturally occurring glycoside, is not strictly an antiarrhythmic agent. Rather, it slows the ventricular response to atrial fibrillation by increasing AV blockade. The mechanism behind the increased block is vagal stimulation, as opposed to its more commonly recognized action on the sodium (Na$^+$) pump. By contrast, at higher concentrations, its effect on the Na$^+$ pump increases cellular automaticity, and this, along with a stimulation of sympathetic activity, makes digoxin toxicity a potent cause of arrhythmias. This potentially dangerous effect is worsened by hypokalemia. In patients with a structurally normal heart, digoxin is less effective at reducing heart rate than β(beta)-blockers or verapamil, but it can be of value in patients with heart failure.

Verapamil inhibits calcium flux into cells via the slow calcium (Ca^{++}) channel in both conductive and contractile cells in the heart. As electrical activity in the SAN and AVN is dependent on calcium influx, this drug slows conduction through the AV node. It also interrupts re-entry pathways dependent upon conduction through this route. Clinically verapamil is used in the control of supraventricular tachycardias and to slow ventricular rate in atrial fibrillation. However, it is contraindicated in atrial fibrillation in association with Wolff–Parkinson–White syndrome (reflecting presence of an accessory pathway). Contrary to verapamil's effect on AVN conduction, that through the accessory pathway may be increased leading to secondary ventricular fibrillation. Its commonest noncardiovascular effect is constipation, reflecting smooth muscle effects in the gastrointestinal tract.

Drugs Used in the Management of Both Atrial and Ventricular Arrhythmias

Amiodarone, a drug structurally related to thyroxine, blocks several different ion channels in cardiac myocytes. In addition, it reduces sensitivity to circulating catecholamines by decreasing β-receptor density at the cell surface. Not surprisingly, it is one of the most effective antiarrhythmic drugs with a low propensity to cause abnormal heart rhythms. Its most common uses are in the prophylaxis of paroxysmal atrial fibrillation (PAF) and in prevention of postinfarction ventricular arrhythmias. In this latter situation, it reduces mortality. Unfortunately, it commonly causes many noncardiovascular adverse drug reactions. With its high iodine content, more than 80% patients have altered thyroid function, which can show as either significant hypothyroidism or hyperthyroidism. However, clinically more important is pulmonary fibrosis which may develop in 5–10% of patients receiving moderate or high doses of amiodarone.

All β(beta)-blockers are effective in preventing a range of arrhythmias by antagonizing the effect of circulating endogenous adrenaline, hence reducing automaticity and conductivity. The main use of β(beta)-blockers is in the prevention of paroxysmal supraventricular tachycardias and rate control in patients with atrial fibrillation. Furthermore, in patients following myocardial infarction, these drugs probably reduce ventricular arrhythmias and consequently lower mortality.

Sotalol is a β(beta)-blocker with additional type III activity. At high doses, it is probably more effective in controlling arrhythmias such as paroxysmal atrial fibrillation than other β(beta)-blockers, but this is at the expense of significant proarrhythmic activity.

Flecainide is a type Ic sodium channel blocker with activity mainly in the His–Purkinje fibers. Despite this, its main clinical use is in the prevention of supraventricular tachycardias including re-entrant tachycardias and PAF. It also has a role in pharmacological cardioversion of patients in atrial fibrillation (AF) and may also be used for the prevention of further episodes in patients identified with life-threatening ventricular arrhythmias. This latter use is limited because of the strong clinical trial evidence of increased mortality in this context. Flecainide like all antiarrhythmic drugs has a negative inotropic effect and should be avoided in patients with heart failure. The commonest adverse effects of flecainide are dizziness and blurred vision.

Propafenone is an orally active type Ic sodium channel blocker used for the prevention of paroxysmal supraventricular tachycardias. It has activity in preventing ventricular tachycardia, but because it may increase mortality in patients (as will other drugs in this class), its use is generally limited to those patients with life-threatening rhythm disturbance. It is restricted to patients whose rhythm disturbance has proved resistant to other drugs. The most frequent adverse effects are alterations to gastrointestinal motility, but like other drugs, it can cause significant bradycardia and hypotension.

Drugs Used in the Management of Ventricular Arrhythmias

Disopyramide is used for the prevention of life-threatening ventricular arrhythmias following acute myocardial infarction. Its use is limited by its proarrhythmic action and its strong anticholinergic properties.

Lidocaine (previously called lignocaine) is a type Ib sodium channel blocker, which has to be administered intravenously. Its main action is in reducing automaticity with little effect on the refractory period. Once widely used for the treatment of ventricular arrhythmias postinfarction, it is now given infrequently. Like all antiarrhythmic agents, it has a tendency to worsen heart failure and, in addition, can cause bradycardia. Noncardiovascular adverse effects usually involve the nervous system and include confusion, paresthesia, and convulsions.

Conclusions for Antiarrhythmogenic Drugs

Many drugs have been shown to prevent or ameliorate abnormal heart rhythms, but very few drugs reduce overall mortality. Indeed, several have been shown to increase mortality. There is therefore an increasing reluctance to use antiarrhythmic drugs, particularly for the control of arrhythmias arising from the ventricles.

Hyperlipidemia

Abnormal serum lipid profiles are often important risk factors for developing cardiovascular disease. The harmful abnormalities are raised concentrations of low-density lipoprotein

(LDL), cholesterol or triglycerides (TGs), or low concentrations of high-density lipoprotein (HDL) cholesterol – the latter two often occurring in combination. The source of cholesterol in such lipoproteins is both by absorption from food and de novo synthesis in the liver. The amount of cholesterol in the body may be lowered by reducing absorption, blocking synthesis, or increasing elimination. All of these are utilized in clinical practice, particularly for the reduction of LDL cholesterol. A common final pathway for this goal is the reduction of hepatocyte intracellular cholesterol concentration, which stimulates the production of surface LDL receptors facilitating catabolism of this lipoprotein.

Statins

As inhibitors of the enzyme HMG-CoA reductase, the statins have become the mainstay of treatment of most hyperlipidemias. They have been shown to reduce the risk of recurrent cardiovascular disease even in patients with normal concentrations of cholesterol. The mechanism by which they lower the circulating concentration of cholesterol is by inhibition of the enzyme HMG-CoA reductase, which converts HMG-CoA into mevalonic acid – a cholesterol precursor. The ensuing reduction in intracellular cholesterol in hepatocytes induces production of the surface LDL receptor, which then decreases circulating LDL concentration. Importantly statins also increase the concentration of HDL cholesterol and lower the concentration of triglycerides which further reduce the risk of vascular disease. The reduction in triglycerides is thought due to a fall in the concentration of very low-density lipoprotein (VLDL), consequent upon a deficiency of cholesterol ester in the liver. The rise in HDL appears secondary to an indirect activation of peroxisome proliferator-activated receptor alpha (PPARα), the same mechanism by which fibrates achieve their beneficial action on blood lipids. This causes an increase in the concentration of circulating HDL and apolipoprotein AI (Apo-I), both involved in reverse cholesterol transport.

Statins have been shown to reduce recurrence of cardiovascular events, including stroke and myocardial infarction. This appears due to a reduction in the size of atherosclerotic plaques in vessel walls although, as suggested by the appearance of clinical benefit prior to any change in the dimensions of plaques, there may be some other protective effect mediated by a different mechanism. The use of statins for primary prevention is more contentious although the evidence would suggest significant benefit in those at high risk of vascular disease. Overall, statins are well tolerated, but there is a very small risk of hepatic damage and severe muscle necrosis with rhabdomyolysis. Clinical trials showed no excess of more minor muscle problems, but patients often complain of muscle pain which they attribute to their statin. This apparent paradox has been clarified by N of 1 trials in a small number of patients where placebo and statin are supplied in blinded fashion in random order. Symptom diaries show pain occurs more commonly when the patient is receiving statin than when receiving placebo suggesting that for some patients, at least minor muscle symptoms are caused by the use of statins. This may be explained by the association of muscle symptoms in patients receiving statins with a genetic variant of the hepatic drug transporter SLCO1B1 which is linked to higher circulating concentrations of statin.

Fibrates

Fibrates are ligands at PPARα(alpha) in liver, muscle, and endothelium, which together with the retinoid X receptor modulate transcription of a number of target genes whose products are involved in lipid metabolism, the clotting cascade, and inflammatory responses. The major therapeutic effect of fibrates on circulating lipids is a 30–50% fall in the concentration of triglycerides and a rise in the concentration of HDL cholesterol of 5–15%. There may also be a reduction in the concentration of LDL cholesterol, although this depends upon the type of lipid abnormality and the pretreatment serum levels. The clinical trial evidence of benefit from treatment with fibrates is less consistent than that for statins, with many trials failing to show a significant change in their primary end point. Often subgroup analysis shows benefit in those patients with high triglycerides and low HDL cholesterol concentrations, and therefore clinical use is often focused on patients who do not respond to statins or who have this type of lipid abnormality secondary to diabetes. In patients with concentrations of triglycerides of more than 10 mmol/L, who are at increased risk of pancreatitis, fibrates may be used first line in preference to statins since they have a greater impact on triglyceride concentrations. The most common adverse effects seen in patients receiving fibrates are minor nonspecific gastrointestinal complaints. A minor increase in the concentration of liver enzymes is relatively common although there are less frequent reports of hepatitis and liver failure. The risk of myopathy and rhabdomyolysis is greatly increased when fibrates are used together with statins, and this combination should usually only be used with caution.

Inhibitors of Cholesterol Absorption

The absorption of cholesterol from the gastrointestinal tract is not a simple matter of diffusion down a concentration gradient but via a specific sterol transport pathway mediated by Niemann-Pick protein (NCPC1L1) across the enterocyte brush border membrane.

Ezetimibe

Ezetimibe binds to the extracellular loop 1 of NCPC1L1 protein preventing internalization of the receptor sterol complex, thereby inhibiting sterol absorption from the gut. There is still some lack of clarity as to why this rather nonspecific action has a selective action on cholesterol absorption rather than that of other sterols. In patients taking ezetimibe, circulating LDL cholesterol concentrations fall by around 15%, although this drug is often used in combination with a statin when a reduction in the concentration of LDL cholesterol as great as 30% may be achieved. Despite this, clinical trial results have been mixed with no strong evidence of an additional clinical benefit with the combination over the use of a statin alone. Early trials did suggest an increase in cancer risk in patients treated with ezetimibe, but this has not been confirmed. Ezetimibe used alone does not commonly produce adverse effects in excess of those seen with placebo.

Plant Stanols and Sterols

Plant stanols and sterols (although not classified as drugs) are promoted as cholesterol-lowering foods and produce a 10–15% fall in LDL cholesterol when consumed at recommended doses. Their mechanism of action appears confined to the gut with displacement of cholesterol from bile salt micelles, thereby inhibiting absorption. There is an associated increase in hepatic cholesterol synthesis, but the net effect is a lowering of circulating LDL cholesterol concentration. The sterols and stanols themselves are poorly absorbed which is perhaps fortunate as high concentrations of these agents have been linked with an increase in atherosclerosis. There is no trials showing a clinical benefit of plant stanols or sterols beyond their effect on circulating cholesterol concentrations. Similarly, in the absence of long-term structured studies in man, it is difficult to interpret the absence of major reported adverse effects of stanols or sterols.

Binding Resins

The mode of action of binding resins in lowering cholesterol concentrations is fairly simple. Bile acids are the result of the main catabolic pathway for cholesterol, and substantial quantities of cholesterol are converted to bile acids each day. The bile acids themselves have an important role in fat absorption in the gut, and as is now being explored, they also appear to have regulatory roles in glucose and fat metabolism. Bile acids undergo enterohepatic recirculation which is interrupted by the formation of insoluble complexes with binding resins which are then passed in the feces. This interruption of recirculation lowers the concentration of bile acids removing their inhibitory action on the synthetic pathway from cholesterol with a consequent increased cholesterol catabolism and fall in the circulating concentration of LDL cholesterol. Clinical trials show that use of bile acid sequestrants reduces the risk of coronary disease in patients with hypercholesterolemia. More recent studies suggest that they also lower glucose concentrations. Unfortunately bile acid sequestrants are poorly tolerated mainly because of their gastrointestinal side effects. The main complaint is constipation, although many patients also have some nausea. By contrast to the reduction in circulating cholesterol, the concentration of triglycerides may be increased. It should be noted that the use of binding resins can impair absorption of fat soluble vitamins.

Nicotinic Acid

Nicotinic acid produces beneficial changes in lipid profile by binding to the G-protein-coupled receptors HM74 and HM74A. The latter is highly expressed in adipocytes, and binding of nicotinic acid lowers the intracellular concentration of cyclic AMP leading to an inhibition of adipocyte lipolysis. This apparently straightforward mechanism reduces the fatty acid substrate necessary for hepatic synthesis of triglycerides and VLDL cholesterol particles. The net effect of nicotinic acid treatment is therefore decreased catabolism of HDL and a reduction in the transfer of cholesterol from HDL to LDL. In clinical use, nicotinic acid can produce a 13% fall in the concentration of LDL cholesterol, a 20% fall in the concentration of triglycerides, and a 16% rise in the concentration of HDL cholesterol. Despite this activity, the single trial investigating the clinical benefits of nicotinic acid alone showed only a minor reduction in the incidence of nonfatal MI. Overall mortality was not decreased during the trial itself, but the mortality was 11% lower at 15 years, long after patients had discontinued their randomized treatment regimen. The major problem with the use of nicotinic acid is the associated flush and itching which lead many patients to discontinue treatment. The side effects can be limited by the concurrent use of aspirin but more effectively by coadministration with the prostaglandin D_2 antagonist, laropiprant.

Summary of Hyperlipidemia Treatments

Reflecting their effectiveness both in terms of reduction in the concentration of LDL cholesterol and prevention of clinical events, the relatively good tolerability of statins means they are the usual first-line agents for the treatment of most hyperlipidemic states. For patients with a raised concentration of triglycerides and low HDL concentration, fibrates and nicotinic acid produce bigger changes in lipid concentrations, but outcome trials do not show any greater clinical benefit. The other drugs are therefore used mainly in patients who cannot tolerate statins or when statins alone produce insufficient reduction in cholesterol or triglyceride concentrations.

Drug Toxicity Issues

Drugs cause a wide range of adverse effects to the cardiovascular system perhaps because of the direct exposure of its components to the circulating blood. Often the mechanisms of toxicity are not as well explored as those behind the beneficial effects, as there is much less motivation to investigate these issues.

Drug-Induced Arrhythmias

Perhaps the most important drug effect on cardiac rhythm is the tendency of Vaughan Williams class III antiarrhythmics and several other drug classes (e.g., antidepressants and major tranquilizers) to produce malignant ventricular rhythms, often torsade de pointes, by inhibition of the potassium repolarizing (hERG) channel. Clinically this effect is seen as prolongation of the QT interval, and when culprit drugs are used in patients who already have a prolonged QT interval due to other factors (e.g., hypokalemia), the likelihood of arrhythmias is significantly increased. Several drugs of different classes such as grepafloxacin, cisapride, terfenadine, and sertindole have had to be withdrawn or restricted because of this tendency and screening for hERG channel effects is now part of routine drug development. This is by no means the only mechanism by which drugs cause tachycardias with digoxin toxicity probably related more to its effect on the $Na^+:K^+$ exchange pump. Catechols such as adrenaline can produce malignant arrhythmias by stimulation of cardiac β(beta)-adrenergic receptors although some of this action may be mediated by prolongation of the QT interval. Drugs can also cause symptomatic bradycardia with β(beta)-blockers and rate-limiting calcium channel blockers (CCBs), the more common culprits. However, cholinesterase inhibitors (e.g., donepezil) have a similar effect which is additive.

Drug-Induced Hypertension

Several drug classes can increase blood pressure and therefore indirectly cause damage to the cardiovascular system. Perhaps the most commonly implicated drugs are the combined oral contraceptive pill (in which estrogen probably enhances the effect of thromboxane to increase both blood pressure and clotting) and nonsteroidal anti-inflammatory drugs (when renal sodium retention appears to be responsible). Predictably sympathomimetics such as phenylpropanolamine increase blood pressure by direct stimulation of α receptors, and this cold cure was withdrawn due to an association with stroke in young women. An often overlooked cause of raised blood pressure are the specific noradrenaline

reuptake inhibitors (SNRIs) such as venlafaxine which at high doses enhance the peripheral effects of circulating noradrenaline and sympathomimetics. An alternative mechanism of inducing hypertension is exhibited by cyclosporine which enhances renin release and activates the renin–angiotensin system. Several drugs which work by modulating the vascular endothelial growth factor (VEGF) signaling pathway (e.g., sunitinib and bevacizumab) can cause hypertension, the severity of which appears strongly linked to the magnitude of therapeutic effect. The underlying mechanism appears to be by an increase in endothelin and a reduction in nitric oxide.

Drug-Induced Vasoconstriction

Vasoconstriction caused by drugs can occasionally be so severe that it presents with tissue ischemia rather than hypertension. In the era when ergot preparations were used for the treatment of severe migraine, peripheral gangrene was sometimes seen. There have also been case reports of similar ischemia with the ergot derivative, bromocriptine.

Drug-Induced Myocardial Infarction

The unexpected finding of an excess of myocardial infarction in clinical trials of Cox-II selective anti-inflammatory drugs led to the finding that most drugs from this class, whether selective for Cox-II or not, increase the risk of cardiovascular end points. In part, this adverse effect may be due to an increase in blood pressure from the effect of the nonsteroidal anti-inflammatory drugs on the kidney. However, there also appears to be an important action on the balance between prostacyclin and thromboxane production, reflecting the difference in dose–response relationships in the inhibition of prostaglandin synthase for the production of the different prostanoids – suggesting that vasoconstriction and clotting factors may also be important. Clinically chest pain is a not infrequent presentation in cocaine users, and myocardial infarction has been reported. This is probably mediated by acceleration of atherosclerosis, α(alpha)-receptor-induced coronary spasm, and direct induction of platelet aggregation by the cocaine. Rosiglitazone, a PPARγ(gamma) agonist used in the treatment of diabetes, was withdrawn because of its adverse cardiovascular actions – specifically an increase in the incidence of acute myocardial infarction and heart failure. The mechanism is not clear but may relate to inhibition of coronary vasodilatation in response to normal physiological mediators. While erythropoietin and analogs are being investigated for myocardial protection following myocardial infarction, data from earlier clinical trials suggest that use of erythropoietin potentially increases the risk of stroke and myocardial infarction. The precise mechanism is not defined, but as hematocrit is a known risk factor for cardiovascular events in the renal patient population, the drug-induced rise in blood hemoglobin levels may offer a simple explanation.

Drug-Induced Hypotension

Just as drugs can raise blood pressure, they can also be implicated in symptomatic hypotension. Some of this is the expected hypotension with antihypertensive drugs such as β(beta)-blockers and ACE inhibitors used in the treatment of heart failure. Alternatively, sildenafil causes hypotension by producing vasodilatation, an effect which is often marked when combined with blood-pressure-lowering drugs such as organic nitrates or α blockers, but has also been reported when used alone. Hypotension with L-dopa is of importance because patients with Parkinsonism are already subject to dysautonomia and postural hypotension. This may also explain the increase in mortality when L-dopa preparations are combined with selegiline. The mechanism of blood pressure reduction has been poorly investigated but is probably due to vasodilatation although there is some evidence of a reduction in brain sympathetic output.

Drug-Induced Cardiomyopathy

The drug best known to produce cardiomyopathy is the cytotoxic anthracycline, doxorubicin, but many other drugs have also been implicated in epidemiological studies. These include antipsychotics (e.g., clozapine), antidepressants (e.g., clomipramine), appetite suppressants (e.g., clobenzorex), retinoids (e.g., isotretinoin), antiretrovirals (e.g., lamivudine), as well as novel agents such as trastuzumab. The mechanisms for these varied drugs may vary, but the main contender for the common doxorubicin adverse effect is an increase in oxidative stress associated with drug-induced mitochondrial damage. The ErbB2 receptor, the site of action of trastuzumab, also appears to be associated with oxidative stress and may explain why toxicity of the two anticancer agents appears to be additive.

Drug-Induced Heart Failure

Drugs may cause heart failure either by producing myocardial damage (be that ischemic or due to apoptosis secondary to oxidative stress) or by causing fluid retention (as with nonsteroidal anti-inflammatory drugs). The heart failure induced by other drugs is not so easily explained although some association may be artifactual, such as the apparent excess of

heart failure with doxazosin which probably simply reflects a local effect on peripheral edema. Other drugs such as β(beta)-blockers and rate-limiting calcium channel blockers have a pharmacologically mediated negative inotropic effect. The excess of heart failure seen in clinical trials of the antiarrhythmic dronedarone is currently unexplained.

Drug-Induced Valvulopathy

Directly acting serotonergic drugs, such as some appetite suppressants, have been linked with valvular abnormalities similar to those seen in patients with carcinoid syndrome or with ergotamine use. Similar findings have been described in patients treated with dopamine agonists used for the treatment of Parkinson's disease or hyperprolactinemia. Animal studies have shown a key role for serotonergic receptors in heart development, and animals lacking the serotonin transporter which leads to high circulating concentrations of this transmitter have developed fibrosis involving heart valves.

Vasculitis

Many drugs are capable of eliciting immune responses which involve the body's own cells often producing damage to blood vessels usually the small arteries to the skin. Older drugs such as hydralazine have long been implicated, and such adverse reactions are perhaps one reason why they are no longer widely used. Recently ANCA-associated vasculitis has been described with the anti-TNF agents used in the control of inflammatory disorders such as rheumatoid arthritis and Crohn's disease. The mechanisms of the two classes of drug are likely to be different but currently neither is fully understood.

Final Overview

There has been considerable success in the treatment and prevention of cardiovascular disease in the past half century. However, within this advance, there are areas of strength and weakness. Of particular note are the benefits from the treatment of hypertension, hyperlipidemia, and heart failure, all of which have had a major impact on morbidity or mortality. Progress has been much less pronounced in the treatment of abnormal heart rhythms and cardiac ischemia. Unfortunately, along with this progress, we have seen an increase in cardiovascular drug toxicity, often from drugs used in the treatment of other diseases. Consequently, a reasonable, working knowledge of these drugs, and their pharmacology, is vital in the study and appreciation of cardiac disease***.

Further Reading

Brunton LL, editor. Goodman and Gilman's the pharmacological basis of therapeutics. 12th ed. New York: McGraw-Hill; 2011.

Estrada JC, Darbar D. Clinical use of and future perspectives on antiarrhythmic drugs. Eur J Clin Pharmacol. 2008;64:1139–46.

Fernandez SF, Tandar A, Boden WE. Emerging medical treatment for angina pectoris. Expert Opin Emerg Drugs. 2010;15:283–98.

McInnes GT. Clinical pharmacology and therapeutics of hypertension. Handbook of hypertension, vol 25. Amsterdam: Elsevier; 2008.

Sata Y, Krum H. The future of pharmacological therapy for heart failure. Circ J. 2010;74:809–17.

Toth PP. Drug treatment of hyperlipidaemia: a guide to the rational use of lipid-lowering drugs. Drugs. 2010;70:1363–79.

The Heart at Autopsy

5

S. Kim Suvarna

Abstract

The autopsy examination of cardiac tissues is described in detail with stepwise consideration of the individual components of the heart. The approach to common pathological processes, cases with therapeutic interventions, and specialized tests is provided. There is a stepwise photographic illustration of the dissection technique together with discussion of the appropriate histological investigations, special stains, ancillary tests, and ultrastructural analysis. The method for cardiac conduction system assessment is illustrated, and an approach to various cardiac devices is discussed.

Keywords

Heart • Autopsy • Histology • Electron microscopy • Prostheses • Stent • Pacemaker

Introduction and General Considerations

The examination of cardiac tissue at autopsy [1, 2] is not simply a matter of opening the body and looking at the heart! It must be understood that any autopsy examination requires triangulation of all relevant information that is mapped to the autopsy examination in question. Thus, consideration of the circumstances of death, antemortem clinical history, radiological tests, blood results, family history, and other investigations are of direct relevance and of assistance in any cardiac tissue examination. When considering and appreciating all of the above factors, any pathological process will be judged from all perspectives: inherited cardiomyopathy, degenerative disease, and previous medical/surgical interventions. Indeed, one could argue that without having this background/ancillary information, one can only perform a partial examination/evaluation of the cardiac specimen. It should also be remembered that an understanding of the individual's lung status/function is required in any cardiac tissue assessment.

To a degree, one could regard the heart and lungs as one single unit, although it is also clear that kidney, liver, and other organ realities and diseases may also interplay with cardiac status and function. However, when armed with all the appropriate information, one may proceed to examine the body and thereby fully appreciate the heart.

The Autopsy Procedure

The external morphology of the body is often rushed, missing the opportunity to identify peripheral indicators of cardiac disease that include clubbing, splinter hemorrhages, peripheral edema, and other phenotypic abnormalities (e.g., Marfanoid habitus) which may indicate specific abnormalities. Taking a few moments to stop and think about the features and possible cardiac realities will often be a valuable exercise.

The majority of examinations start with the standard autopsy incision exposing the chest rib cage and musculature [3]. The sternal bone and associated ribs anteriorly are cut, being removed as a plate – thereby permitting good access to the lungs, heart, and mediastinal structures. While the general autopsy often proceeds with removing all organs in groups/*en-masse*, there are cases of sudden cardiac death

S.K. Suvarna, MBBS, B.Sc., FRCP, FRCPath
Department of Histopathology, Northern General Hospital,
Sheffield Teaching Hospitals NHS Foundation Trust,
Sheffield S5 7AU, UK
e-mail: s.k.suvarna@sheffield.ac.uk

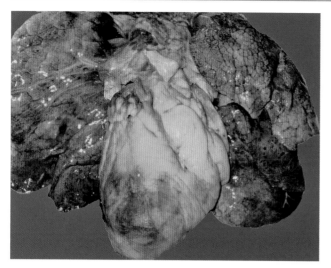

Fig. 5.1 This case of dextrocardia was evident on opening the chest but is better appreciated when displayed free from adjacent structures. Reversed lobation is noted for the lungs, and the heart points towards the right and has isomerism of the appendages

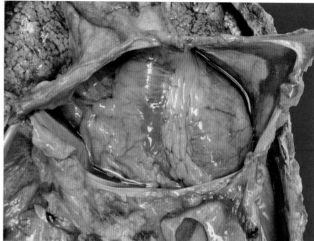

Fig. 5.2 The pericardial tissues have been opened to show the heart. The epicardial surface is normal, but there is some brown pericardial fluid adjacent which can be sampled for cytology or microbiology, if deemed necessary. The fluid volume should be quantified

when direct and immediate attention to the pericardium and heart is relevant. There is no absolute rule in this matter, but one must focus attention on the issues in the case and, only then, decide when it is best to examine the heart. This avoids disturbing/degrading any anatomical or pathological reality.

The heart is best inspected from the front initially, being enclosed in the pericardiac sac and bounded on either side by the lung tissues. The lung parenchyma should be analyzed in situ in terms of its lobation – in order to consider potential cardiac isomerism or other architectural abnormalities (Fig. 5.1). Macroscopic evaluation of lung parenchyma may also indicate underlying lung disease, which will automatically place a burden upon the right side of the heart with associated pathological effects [4–6].

It is customary to open the pericardium with an incision, often in the shape of an inverted T. It is then possible to reflect the pericardial parenchyma and remove this parenchymal membrane for greater access to the heart. The presence, volume, and nature of any fluid should be determined at this point (Fig. 5.2), with sampling for microbiological assessment – if considered pertinent. On occasion, histological and microbiological sampling of the pericardial tissue is of importance when considering disseminated neoplasia and infective agents (Figs. 5.3 and 5.4).

It is now possible to review the heart in terms of its position and gross architecture. The great vessels should be inspected for correct alignment, size, and position directly. All aspects of the tissue can be seen from the anterior viewpoint, and by lifting the apex of the heart upward and cranially, one may consider the undersurface. The coronary artery tributary pattern can also be seen at this point along with all the epicardial surfaces of the chambers. The appendages should be checked in terms of position and

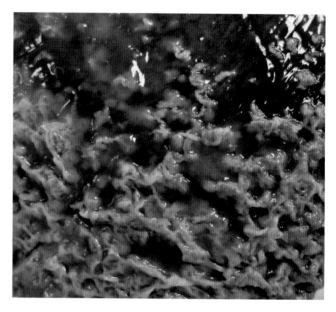

Fig. 5.3 The epicardial surface in this image shows the "bread and butter" pattern of pericarditis. Histology later proved there was a high-grade lymphoma underlying this process

structure, and one should examine the heart for focal external lesions [5, 7, 8].

Removal of the Tissues

The heart can be removed for further inspection by transection of the aorta and pulmonary artery followed subsequently by cutting the pulmonary veins and both venae cavae. It should not be forgotten that large pulmonary emboli can be semi-impacted within the proximal pulmonary artery in

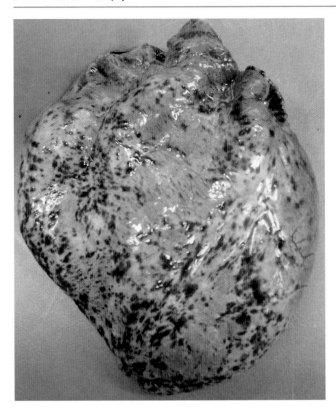

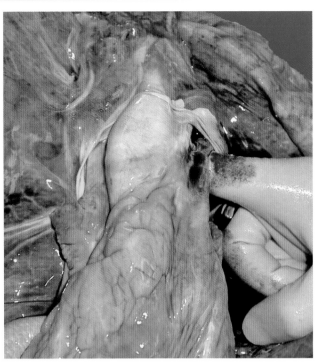

Fig. 5.5 Digital palpation of the lumen of the pulmonary artery root will identify any large thromboemboli impacted at this site

Fig. 5.4 The epicardial surface here shows widespread petechial hemorrhagic lesions, reflecting heavy bacteremia and disseminated intravascular coagulation in a case of *Neisseria meningitidis*

cases of sudden death. Careless transection of the pulmonary arteries may cause these emboli to be dislodged and lost to view, if one does not check for their presence during cardiac tissue removal (Fig. 5.5).

Having removed the heart, it should again be inspected both front and back, for the features of normality (Figs. 5.6 and 5.7). Photography is of benefit throughout, and the advent of cheap and reliable digital imaging has become a key adjunct to autopsy practice. It would be fair to state that without imaging being available, the autopsy procedure will potentially be limited. Remember that heart weight is a vital datum for recording at autopsy [9–11], but this should only be performed after opening the heart and drainage of blood/clot material. The weight of the heart ultimately should be considered against body mass and height (see Chap. 1).

Coronary Arteries

The coronary tissues should next be inspected. This author recommends starting in the midsection of the left anterior descending artery with transverse slices at 3–5 mm intervals, passing initially downward along the left anterior descending artery and thence upward towards the left main stem and aortic root (Fig. 5.8) [1, 2, 5, 12]. This downward/

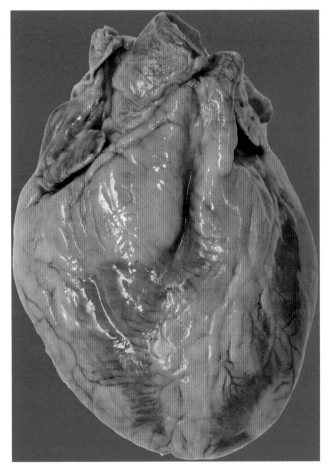

Fig. 5.6 The anterior aspect of the myocardial tissues is displayed with normal appendages and chamber layout

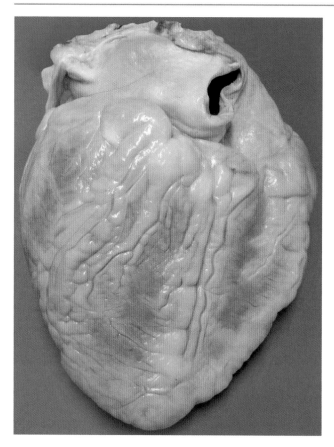

Fig. 5.7 The posterior aspect of the heart is demonstrated with the atria at the top and right and left ventricles showing normal architecture and alignment

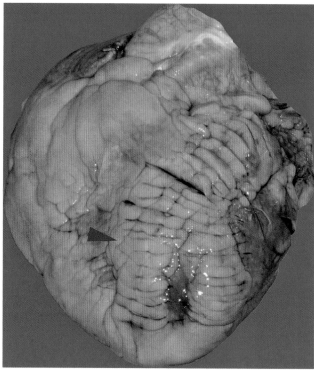

Fig. 5.8 The coronary artery tissues, starting in the mid/low part of the artery (*arrowed*), are sectioned transversely with a sharp scalpel at 3–5 mm intervals. Careful inspection of each cut aspect of coronary artery tissue is made to consider the extent of stenosis, presence of thrombosis, and/or dissection

upward sequence will allow identification of the bifurcation point for the circumflex vessel. This also requires similar transverse slices to be passed along the circumflex artery towards the upper septum of the heart posteriorly. The same attention with transverse sectioning must follow for the diagonal branch (originating from the left anterior descending artery) and the obtuse marginal arteries (arising from the circumflex vessel). The right coronary artery is examined initially by a transverse slice in the fatty tissue immediately on the right-side base of the aorta, allowing identification of the artery. Similar transverse slices are made along the length of this artery. The branch point and runoff to the acute marginal artery should be likewise evaluated. Finally, as the right coronary vessel passes onto the posterior aspect of the cardiac tissues, one should look for the anastomosis with the distal circumflex vessel and the combined runoff into the posterior interventricular branch.

Any areas of occlusion, dissection, thrombosis, or vascular defect should be noted, described, and possibly photographed (Fig. 5.9). It is common in autopsy practice to find vessels with significant atheromatous disease even if it is determined that this disease played no part in the death of the individual. Some atheromatous disease is heavily calcified. Ideal practice when faced with such calcified vessels is to

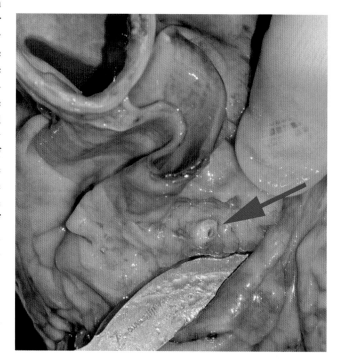

Fig. 5.9 High-grade atheromatous disease is seen narrowing the coronary lumen of the artery

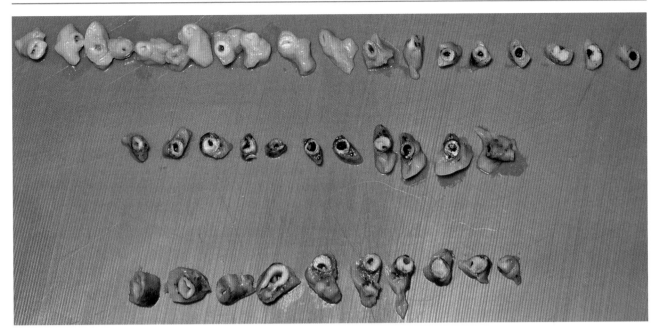

Fig. 5.10 The coronary arteries can be dissected in one strip, in their entirety along with some local epicardial fatty tissue. Once decalcified, easy sequential transverse section of heavily calcified/diseased vessels is accomplished. The samples are laid out allowing for good appreciation of the degree of disease and to enable targeted block sampling or permit ordered histology of the entire coronary tree

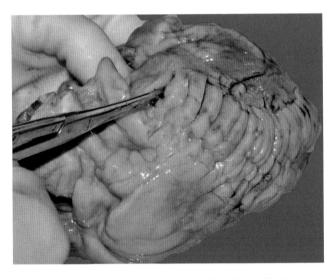

Fig. 5.11 Scissors can be used to cut across heavily calcified coronary arteries. It should be understood that this may fragment and distort coronary plaque disease

remove vessels en bloc for decalcification (Fig. 5.10). One- or two-day formic acid decalcification after fixation usually suffices to soften the vessels. Following decalcification, standard transverse sections can be made. The vessels can be arranged to demonstrate the disease status along the vessels (see Fig. 5.10). This process will facilitate block selection. However, many autopsy practitioners simply cut across partially calcified vessels using scissors (Fig. 5.11). In so doing, those using scissors have to accept the reality that this will fracture any calcified plaques and may impede accurate appreciation of the artery tissues and vessel lumens. The degree of coronary artery disease can be assessed directly by visual inspection of the artery from the regular cuts made (see Figs. 5.9 and 5.10), noting the degree of stenoses in relation to the estimated normal architecture. It has to be recognized that the human eye is an imperfect assessment tool, but one can make some fairly broad statements in terms of the presence of pinpoint stenoses or try to evaluate the stenosis in terms of percentage narrowing. On occasion, blocking of the entirety of the coronary system is of relevance when considering failed angioplasty/stenting techniques.

Coronary Artery Stents

On many occasions, coronary stents have been deployed in patients with coronary artery atheromatous disease. These metallic mesh units can be approached in several ways. Firstly, it is possible to leave intact this part of the heart (or remove epicardial soft tissue block containing the artery) and perform plain radiography (Fig. 5.12) in order to consider the stent position, deployment, and architecture [2]. This is particularly useful in cases when a poor outcome soon after/ during stent deployment occurs, mapping to a macroscopic lesion (Fig. 5.13). It is also possible to gently irrigate water from the top end of the vessel towards the stent along the length of the blood vessels. Then, by placing a cut below the stent, it is possible to observe whether water passes through the stented area. This simple (cheap and immediate) test can provide significant information in terms of the physiological function of the stent in vivo.

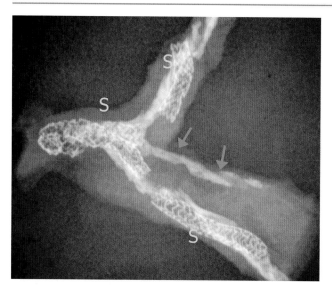

Fig. 5.12 Radiology of a stented proximal left coronary system showing native calcified plaques (*blue arrow*) stented vessels (*S*)

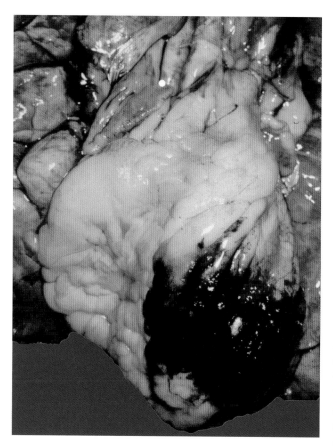

Fig. 5.13 This specimen shows a zone of epicardial hemorrhage that was associated with cardiac tamponade. The process was initiated by dissection of coronary artery during an angioplasty

However, usually one is left with a binary choice in terms of pathological stent analysis for the tissues. There are some who believe that stent should be removed en bloc together

with the artery and local soft tissues, fixed into resin, and then sectioned with appropriate knives and metal cutting microtomes [2]. This produces sections with the artery, stent, and tissues seen together (Fig. 5.14). It has to be said that this is relatively uncommon, being time consuming and expensive in terms of machinery. However, the histology of the sample cannot be underestimated as it gives a good account of the state of the artery, the device, and the lumen! The other choice, chosen by many, is simply to open the vessel longitudinally, inspect the stent, remove it, and then consider the background cardiac tissues with photography and/or histology (Fig. 5.15). This is acceptable but will always create some artifact, and be less than ideal.

The coronary veins are not normally subject to much pathology directly and are normally only inspected as a result of being blocked together with associated coronary artery tissues.

The Right-Side Heart Tissues

The cardiac tissues are best considered in terms of the chambers "as the blood flows," meaning that one starts with the right atrium and then passes to the right ventricle, left atrium, and left ventricle. However, before this process takes place, it is advisable to make sequential transverse sections across the heart, starting at the apex involving the right and left ventricle, at approximately 1 cm intervals (Fig. 5.16). This should continue to the midlevel of the ventricles, unless one knows of a congenital heart abnormality – which requires an alternate dissection protocol (Fig. 5.17). The transverse slices can be considered in terms of chamber layout/diameter, wall thickness, fatty infiltration along with the opportunity to inspect for areas of infarction and prior scarring (Fig. 5.18). The transverse diameters of the two chambers are immediately apparent. Stopping the transverse sections at the midlevel means that the apical papillary muscle and valve apparatus are preserved.

It almost goes without saying that knowledge of the normal architecture is required when one considers any of the cardiac chambers [7, 13]. However, in order to appreciate these, it is required to open the heart preserving as much of the gross architectural anatomy as possible and yet allowing easy inspection of the parenchyma. For the right atrium, there are two methods favored to open the cardiac tissues. The first starts with a cut on the posterior arterial wall in a line between the superior and inferior venae cavae (Fig. 5.19). The second method involves placing a cut from the inferior vena cava to the apex of the right auricle. Both permit good access to the chamber, thus allowing anatomical review. The evaluation of the closure or patency of the foramen ovale, the architecture of the Eustachian valve/coronary sinus, and appearance of the tricuspid valve should be made at this point. As with all

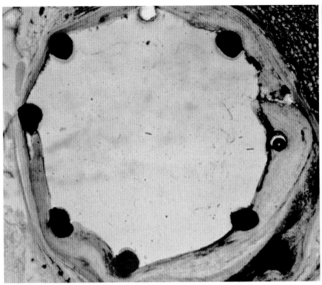

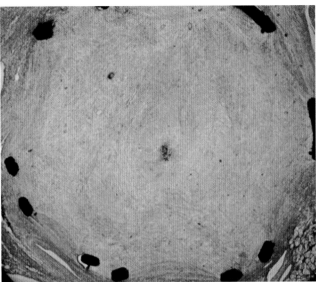

Fig. 5.14 Two resin-embedded sections of coronary artery are seen together with wire stents. The stent struts are seen in section as the black metal elements. The *left-side* view shows a well-deployed stent with a patent lumen. The *right-side* stent shows neointimal fibrous connective tissue completely occluding the lumen

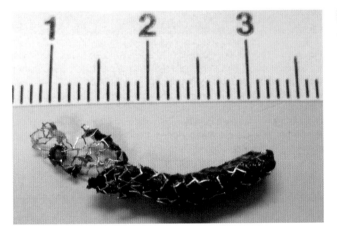

Fig. 5.15 This stent has been dissected free from the coronary framework by scalpel blade and then opening the calcified wall to allow extraction of the framework. There is a large amount of in-stent luminal thrombus occluding the lumen. There is clear evidence of partial stent disruption with this extraction technique

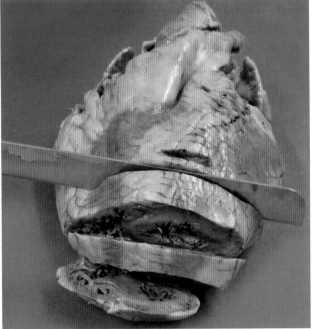

Fig. 5.16 Three transverse sections are taken across the lower part of the ventricles using a long knife to produce good transverse sections. It should be noted that prior examination of the coronary tissues has taken place, and some coronary tissue has already been reserved for histology beforehand

autopsy analysis, photography and microbiology sampling should take place as the dissection progresses – if indicated.

Following direct inspection of the tricuspid valve, one places an incision from the lower end of the inferior vena cava insertion, downward through the tricuspid valve, running 1 cm to the side of the posterior interventricular coronary artery towards the apex of the right ventricle (see Fig. 5.19). Then, turning the heart onto its back, the anterior right ventricle is incised with the cut passing up through the conus and into the pulmonary artery (Fig. 5.20). At this point, it is now possible, from both the front and back, to consider the general layout of the right atrium in relation to the right ventricle and to measure precisely the tricuspid valve, pul-

monary valve, outflow tract for the right ventricle and to consider with any focal lesions present in either chamber.

In cases where pacing wires are present, these should be traced to their point of insertion prior to transverse section of the ventricles, by following the lead(s) to the ventricular (and sometime also atrial) insertion(s). Ideally one should try to

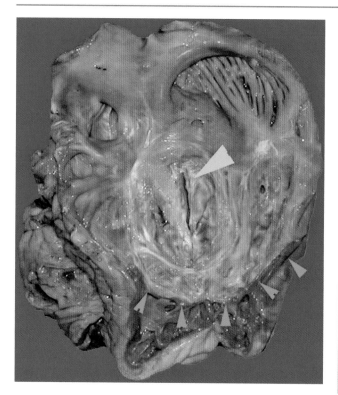

Fig. 5.17 An Ebstein anomaly within a case of sudden death in the community. The atrial tissues appeared abnormal, and transverse sectioning of the ventricles was not undertaken. Rather a single longitudinal posterior slice was made. The slit-like orifice of the valve tissue is noted (*yellow arrowhead*), and the downward displacement of the tricuspid valve is clearly demarcated (*green arrowheads*)

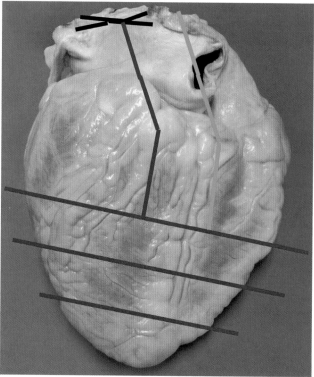

Fig. 5.19 The posterior aspect of the heart is seen with three (*red*) transverse section lines allowing ventricular appreciation. The cuts for the right atrium run from the superior to inferior vena cava, with a further cut running down through the tricuspid valve and then into the right ventricle parallel to the interventricular septum posteriorly (*green line*). A similar set of cuts can be made between the pulmonary veins for the left atrium with the cut running down the back of the left atrium and across the mitral valve into the left ventricle (*blue line*)

ventricular tissue (Fig. 5.22). Microbiology assessment of thrombi or vegetations (if present) may be needed. Following this inspection, the electrodes can be removed with associated tissues for histological sampling if necessary (Fig. 5.23). Deactivation of defibrillator pacemakers is required before any autopsy handing to avoid risk of discharge and pathologist injury [2, 16].

The Left-Side Heart Tissues

The left atrium is examined from above and behind by an interlocking set of incisions between the pulmonary veins (see Fig. 5.19). This allows direct inspection of the chamber and the mitral valve. It is not necessary to directly incise into the auricle, as this can be fully appreciated by direct vision. Again, the foreman ovale should be considered, and the gross architecture of the chamber should be evaluated, looking for thrombus formation, myxomatous tissue, and any other lesions (Fig. 5.24).

With the heart lying on its front, by passing the cut from the right inferior pulmonary vein downward across the mitral valve, it is possible to run the cut 1 cm at the side of the

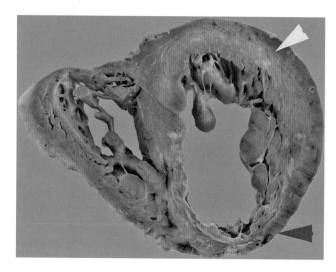

Fig. 5.18 This transverse view of the ventricles shows a large left ventricle with a dilated chamber in relation to an old fibrous scar. The anterior aspect (*red arrow*) shows aneurysmal bulging of the wall tissues in relation to muscle atrophy and fibrosis. The posterior aspect shows slight fibrosis (*yellow arrow*) and a mildly hypertrophic architecture for the left ventricle. No acute ischemic changes are seen

keep the entire pacemaker unit intact (Fig. 5.21) in the event that formal pacemaker testing is required [2, 14, 15]. Alternatively, one does not perform the transverse slices of

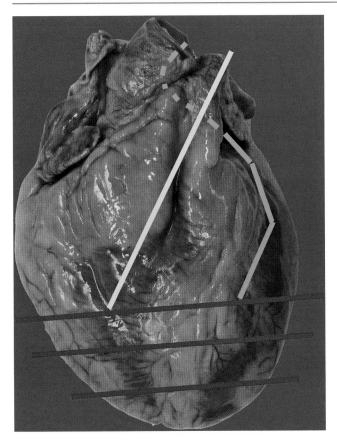

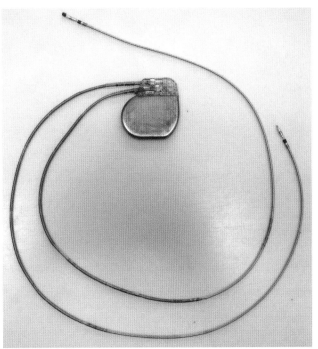

Fig. 5.21 The pacemaker unit in this case has been dissected completely free and is seen with the pacemaker unit and the two electrodes and wires. Careful inspection of the box, wires, and electrodes allows exclusion of sepsis, thrombosis, and consideration of damage to the pacemaker unit and its connections

Fig. 5.20 The dissection plane for the right ventricle outflow tract and pulmonary artery runs from the anterior right ventricle myocardium obliquely upward and through the pulmonary valve (*yellow line*). The cut for the left ventricle (*green line*) and aortic root runs parallel to the left anterior descending artery upward and towards the base of the aortic tissues. It passes behind the pulmonary outflow tract (*dotted green line*) and between the left atrial appendage and the left main stem origin allowing preservation of the mitral valve and aortic root tissues. The transverse slices across the ventricles are marked in *red*

posterior interventricular descending artery, in a manner akin to that of the right side described above towards the ventricular apex (see Fig. 5.19). The left ventricle can be considered in a similar manner from this particular incision with measurement of the mitral valve being possible.

The next incision is a matter of choice. Many autopsy practitioners, leaving the heart in this position, simply transect the mitral valve centrally in order to gain access to the aortic root and valve (Fig. 5.25). This process automatically disrupts the mitral tissue but is quick and direct. The alternative is to turn the heart onto its back and pass the cut on the anterior left ventricle wall (see Fig. 5.20) [2]. By means of knife/scissor incision, it is possible to pass a cut upward (alongside the left anterior descending artery on the front of the anterior free wall of this chamber). Entering the region of the outflow tract, one continues the incision (to the left of the mitral valve leaflet), by making a gentle turn immediately behind the left main stem and in front of the left auricle in order to enter the aortic root (Fig. 5.26). Performed

correctly, it will permit examination of the aortic root tissues without disruption of the mitral valve apparatus (Fig. 5.27). It also provides the opportunity to measure the left ventricle outflow tract and to look at the parenchyma for mitral valve impact lesions and small septal defects. The best place to consider right and left ventricular wall thickness is in the outflow tracts (1 cm below the valve) as this is easy to define. It is also without the trabeculations adding complexity to the assessment. The aortic valve can now be fully inspected, and the position and status of the coronary ostia may be checked (Figs. 5.25, 5.28, and 5.29).

In addition, at this time, the great vessels can be inspected directly for their gross architecture and the presence/absence of focal pathology. Atheromatous disease, connective tissue degenerations (Fig. 5.30), and dissections are the commonest lesions although on occasion, neoplasia can be relevant. It is now possible to weigh the heart and cross compare with standard weight charts/tables [9–11].

Fulton Index

The Fulton index [17] measurement is usually performed in order to interrogate the heart's response to coexistent lung disease rather than as a primary assessment of cardiac pathology. The method described involves the dissection of the fixed right ventricle from the left ventricle and septum.

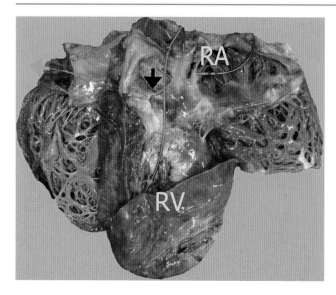

Fig. 5.22 The heart has not been opened with the transverse slices across the ventricles in order to demonstrate a modern multiple lead pacemaker and the deployment of the different leads. There is one electrode interacting with the right atrium (*RA*), one with the right ventricle (*RV*), and another passing through the coronary sinus (*black arrow*) and round the heart via the main vein (*green arrow*)

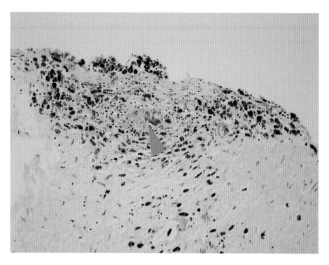

Fig. 5.23 Endocardial tissues showing iron-laden macrophages adjacent to the implantation site as well as a giant cell (*green arrow*)

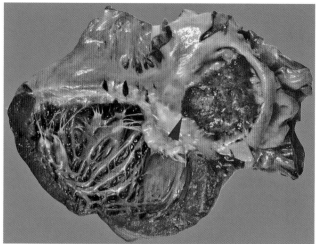

Fig. 5.24 This left atrial tissue has been exposed to reveal a large adherent thrombus (*arrowed*) partially occluding the chamber and distorting the blood flow antemortem. Some calcification was present at the base in keeping with chronicity

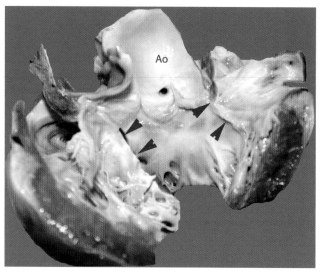

Fig. 5.25 This cardiac tissue dissection shows the mitral valve to have been divided in its middle of the anterior leaflet with direct exposure of the aortic root. The two cut edges of the mitral valve are marked by *red arrow heads*. Of note, the aortic root has only a single coronary artery ostium (right coronary artery). It is also noted that the endocardial tissues of the left ventricle are thickened and fibrotic, reflecting the other (anomalous) coronary artery origin from the pulmonary artery with subsequent left ventricle ischemic damage

The fatty epicardiac tissue and atrial parenchyma should also be removed. The ratio of the mass of the right ventricle to left ventricle/septum in normality is generally taken to be approximately 1:2.3. A raised right ventricular mass ratio is seen in cases of chronic lung disease, wherein right ventricle hypertrophy has occurred by virtue of altered pulmonary artery resistance. Similarly systemic hypertension can produce significant left ventricle hypertrophy that can be appreciated by this technique, although morphological description of concentric hypertrophy may suffice. The Fulton protocol for assessment can be performed on autopsy unfixed tissue, although separation of fat is difficult.

Nevertheless, if one does not have the permission/time to perform fixed tissue analysis, then unfixed tissue assessment is reasonable. This evaluation inevitably destroys the tissue architecture and should only be performed if there is to be no further assessment of the cardiac architecture. It should certainly not be performed on cases where one might wish to return to the cardiac tissue for further samples and certainly should not be performed in cases of congenital heart disease (see Fig. 5.17) or if the case is to later be subject to medicolegal review.

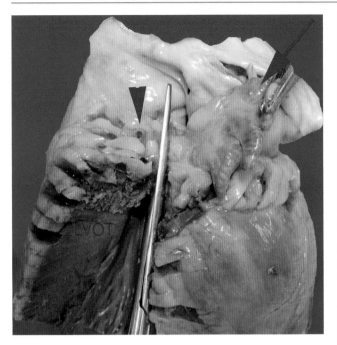

Fig. 5.26 Scissors are use to cut from the left ventricle outflow tract (*LVOT*) behind the left main stem (*red arrowhead*) and in front of the atrial appendage (*red arrow*)

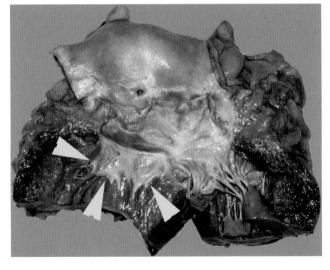

Fig. 5.27 Macroscopic view of the left ventricle outflow tract showing and impact lesion from the mitral valve in a case of hypertrophic cardiomyopathy (*arrowed*). Note that the lesion is the mirror image of the mitral valve leaflet

The Cardiac Conduction System

The sinoatrial node is found at the apex of the atrial chamber and is removed en bloc with the adjacent superior vena cava and atrial tissues. Blocks are made from longitudinal slices taken longitudinally to permit review the nodal parenchyma histology (Fig. 5.31).

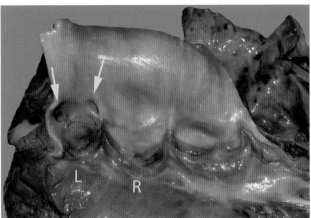

Fig. 5.28 Anomalous coronary artery origin (*yellow arrows*) from a single valve cusp in a case of sudden death. Both arteries use the left coronary sinus and the right side sinus has no artery

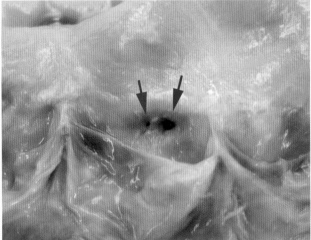

Fig. 5.29 In the base of the aorta, a small artery (*red arrow*) supplying the conus tissue, can sometimes be seen adjacent to the right coronary artery (*blue arrow*). This should not be confused with a congenital anomaly

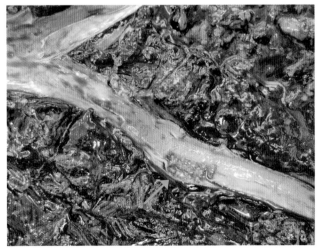

Fig. 5.30 Aortic and common iliac artery tissues are seen with focal intimal wrinkling and a dissection (*arrowed*) in a case of connective tissue disorder. Local massive bleeding has occurred

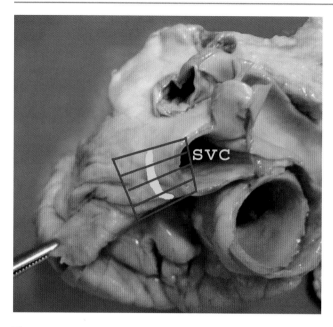

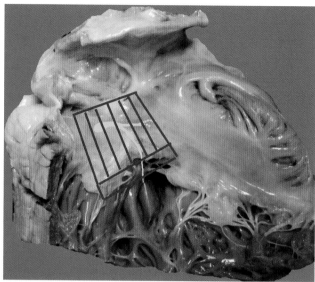

Fig. 5.31 This view of the superior aspect of the right atrium demonstrates the sinoatrial node (*yellow*). It is recommended that the blocks are taken longitudinally as indicated by the red grid (see Chap. 1 for histology of the node)

Fig. 5.32 The atrioventricular node and proximal His bundle/bundle branches (*yellow*) are best sampled with an approximately square block of tissue being removed from the right atrial aspect. This should incorporate the top part of the tricuspid valve and is best performed as one complete block extraction. Thereafter, part of the tissue block is removed transversely from the base, allowing for proximal septal tissues to be considered with subsequent longitudinal block slices (*red grid*), being taken across the bundle branches, His bundle, and node tissue in sequence

The atrioventricular nodal tissue is best dissected with a roughly square block of tissue removed from the right atrium, tricuspid valve, and ventricle septum in one large piece with the membranous septum sitting centrally. To accomplish this maneuver, one makes four sequential cuts, looking at the heart from the right side forming a square shape into the center of the cardiac tissues, to capture the nodal and bundle tissues (Fig. 5.32). Once this piece of tissue is cut free, it is recommended that the base of the block of tissue is first removed horizontally, allowing a transverse high septal block of tissue to be appreciated histologically. The remainder is blocked in longitudinal sliced fashion passing from the left through to the right side. This technique allows the ventricular bundle branches, His bundle, and atrioventricular nodal tissue to be appreciated in sequential order, although levels through individual blocks may be required for full analysis. The presence of focal lesions (e.g., cystic atrioventricular node tumor) within this important tract of tissue may be missed if only one block of tissue is taken.

Coronary Artery Bypass Graft (CABG)

Coronary bypass surgery needs a specific approach if one is to assess the graft patency and status. It is recognized that grafts show aging and arterialization phenomena, with some having progressive occlusive atheroma – akin to native vessels. Ideally, transverse section of the grafts should be used, although old grafts may be difficult to trace

through established fat/densely fibrous tissues. One must pay attention to the origin and insertion of these vessels, whether vein grafts or internal mammary artery origin (Fig. 5.33). Transverse slicing and block sampling (Fig. 5.34) the artery from across the anastomosis allow one to inspect the native vessel and any graft, together with the fibrous response at this site. Deaths very soon after grafting need very careful inspection of these anastomosis sites looking for thrombosis, suture dehiscence, and/or dissection.

Valve Prostheses

Valvular tissues are generally replaced by either tissue or metal prostheses currently. The tissue prostheses are usually animal (xenograft), or rarely human (allograft), in type. These valves are sterilized and then mounted on to a plastic polymer cage with a cloth base for easy placement/suturing. The valves can show progressive degradation with time with some fibrosis and leaflet calcification. Later perforation of the cusps can occur, with repetitive abnormal hinging degrading the tissues in long standing cases. The standard risks of infective endocarditis exist for all such prostheses. Careful exploration from above and below of the valve tissues is recommended (Figs. 5.35 and 5.36).

Metal valve prostheses currently favor a tilting disk (usually twin leaflet) mechanism with a peripheral metal ring and cloth-covered base construct. Previous varieties have included single leaflets, tilting disks, and ball-in-cage patterns to name but a few [18]. The metal valves have much

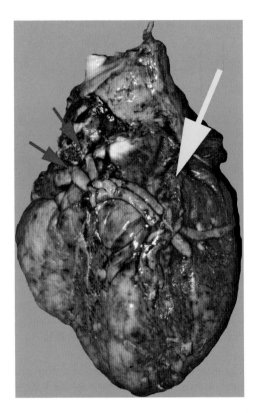

Fig. 5.33 This coronary bypass case died shortly after surgical intervention. Careful inspection of the left internal mammary artery (*yellow arrow*) and its insertion site should be made along with confirmation of lumen patency. The vein bypass grafts (*red arrows*) should be traced from their origin in the aorta down to their insertion points. After review of the grafts, the examination of the native coronary vasculature is required

longer lifetimes but require appropriate anticoagulation as well as episodic antibiotic prophylaxis for the standard risks of infective endocarditis. A similar dissection protocol should be employed when considering these cases.

Some valves are replaced with a local sleeve of Dacron mesh in order to address large artery dilation. When examining this in the aortic root, one should carefully examine the coronary (button) insertion points (Fig. 5.37) to confirm that no coronary artery occlusion has occurred.

One cannot cut across valve prosthesis with ease, and this should only be attempted if there is a particular issue to be addressed (Fig. 5.38). In general, it is recommended that

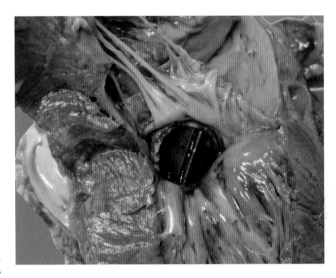

Fig. 5.35 A metal twin leaflet valve device is seen immediately adjacent to the mitral valve. Extensive dissection of the tissues has been required to see this aspect of the device. Minor hemorrhage is seen in the endocardium nearby. No thrombus is seen, and placement appears correctly positioned

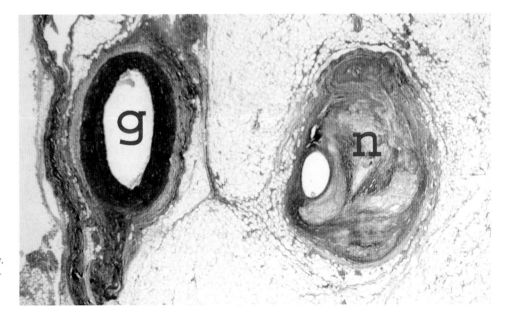

Fig. 5.34 This section shows native coronary artery (*n*) with heavy calcification, and only a small lumen is seen eccentrically. The grafted vessel, seen immediately adjacent (*g*), clearly has an open lumen

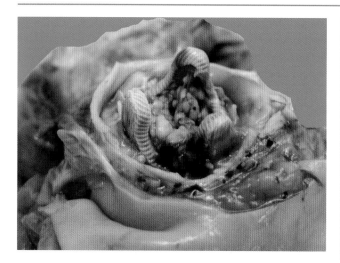

Fig. 5.36 Extensively dissected view of a xenograft showing the cloth-covered assembly. There is thrombotic material occluding the valve

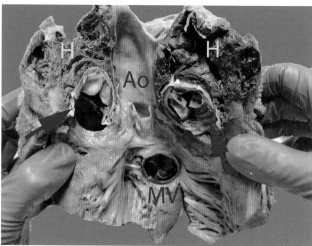

Fig. 5.38 A complicated case opened to demonstrate significant hemorrhage (*H*) around a pulmonary artery xenograft and Dacron root replacement (*red arrows*). The specimen has been opened in bivalve fashion to show the pulmonary artery root with compressive hemorrhage in relation to the valve replacement. A metallic mitral valve (*MV*) prosthesis is also present, and the aortic root can be visualized (*Ao*)

Septal Closure Devices and Materials

A variety of materials are used in cases of abnormal chamber communication (e.g., septal defects) or to reconstruct chamber blood flows. The commonest materials are synthetic (e.g., Dacron), although pericardium can be used for small patches. These are directly sutured into place and can re-endothelialize. They become incorporated within fibrous tissue and sometimes calcify with time. They have a standard risk of infective endocarditis. On occasion, metal frame devices can be employed to close septal defects by the endoluminal route (usually via the systemic veins). These are often hinged metal or expandable frames in type, and they are opened/deployed in situ under radiology guidance (Fig. 5.39).

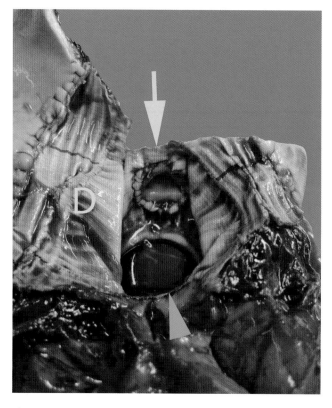

Fig. 5.37 An opened aortic root is seen with Dacron (*D*) sleeve graft replacement of the previously dilated aortic root into which are inserted the coronary artery buttons (*yellow arrow*). A metal valve prosthesis is seen at the base of the aorta (*green arrowhead*)

Other Devices

A variety of other devices can be inserted into the heart. These include variable caliber long lines to deliver drugs and to monitor pressures within the heart/pulmonary circuit. If one is faced with such cases, then some knowledge of the type of line/catheter/device is helpful. One should also try to identify the position of the line to exclude any iatrogenic pathology [2].

Large vessel stents can also be employed for major arteries and veins (Fig. 5.40). This is particularly relevant in cases of mediastinal sclerosis or tumor encroachment. The devices are often deployed by an endovascular approach, allowing

exposure of the chamber from above and below is undertaken – with photography as deemed necessary. Wide access exposure and direct visualization of the valve are required to exclude thrombotic material, infective vegetation, fibrous overgrowth of the valve cusps (pannus), calcification, or paravalvular leakage [2, 5, 6].

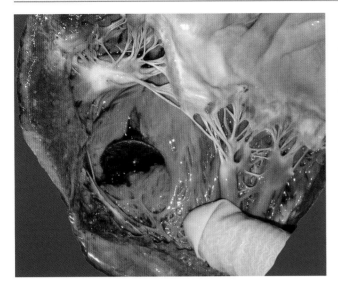

Fig. 5.39 Autopsy view of a case of sudden death during ventricular septal device deployment in an attempt to close a septal perforation after myocardial infarction. The device has not aligned fully with the ventricular walls

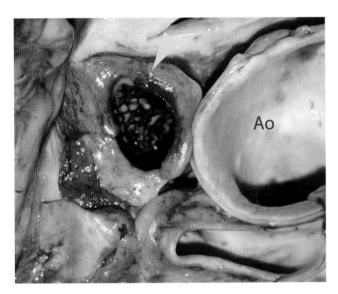

Fig. 5.40 A large vessel wire stent is seen within the superior vena cava. This maintained the lumen in a case of mesothelioma (*yellow arrowhead*) causing superior vena cava obstruction. The aorta (Ao) is seen adjacent

for appropriate symptom palliation. They are a similar structure to those of coronary stents and should be dealt with in a similar fashion.

Ultimately, knowledge of the antemortem clinical history and surgical interventions is required for maximal appreciation of devices and procedures when faced with cardiac tissues at autopsy. Reservation of implanted material/device for later analysis possibly with return to the manufacturer may be of relevance in cases of device failure.

Congenital Heart Disease (CHD)

This chapter on autopsy examination is too short for a detailed consideration of this increasingly important topic. One cannot really deal with cases of CHD without an understanding of congenital malformation patterns and syndromes, and these are discussed in detail in the later chapter on congenital heart disease. Certainly, one needs knowledge of the surgical/medical corrective therapies that have been used for these cases.

There are many CHD cases now surviving to adulthood. These often present with sudden death (often aged 25–40 years, without warning symptoms) in the community. These may have had many and various treatments. These cases of grown up congenital heart disease (GUCH) require special consideration if one is to assess, firstly, the underlying disease and, secondly, the treatments employed. Often extraction of the heart and referral to specialist center for dissection, photography, and analysis is advocated, unless one has training in this area of pathology. The dissection protocol needs to be versatile/variable depending on the case, in order to adequately demonstrate the pathology and any surgical techniques that have taken place (Figs. 5.38 and 5.41). In addition, it must be emphasized that this scenario (often needing cardiac tissue retention and detailed analysis) must take into account the relatives of the deceased. Their support and agreement for tissue retention must be sought.

Many cases of congenital heart disease will have abnormal coronary artery architecture (see Fig. 5.28), although they usually lack high-grade atherosclerosis. Tracing the coronary arteries may be complex. Careful consideration as to the origin of the coronary arteries should be made, as origins from the wrong cusp region in the lower aorta or from the right coronary artery are associated with sudden cardiac death (see Fig. 5.25). Assessment of the chamber architecture and the connections must be rigorous, and like assessment of the normal heart, the analysis is best considered with sequential chamber analysis "as the blood flows." The size and shape of the chambers must be individually considered, with attention to the wall thickness and trabeculation pattern. The identification of septal defects and surgical interventions must be a key focus, with consideration of the potential for infective endocarditis.

In many cases of congenital heart disease, the degree of histological sampling may be best limited. This allows preservation of the tissues for detailed photography. Handling the case in concert with the clinicians and radiologists may allow one to fully appreciate all the realties.

Sudden Cardiac Death Cases

These generally are seen in the young, often described as sudden adult death syndrome (SADS) cases. These cases may have an overt macroscopic pathology, such as unsuspected congenital heart disease (see Figs. 5.17 and 5.28). However,

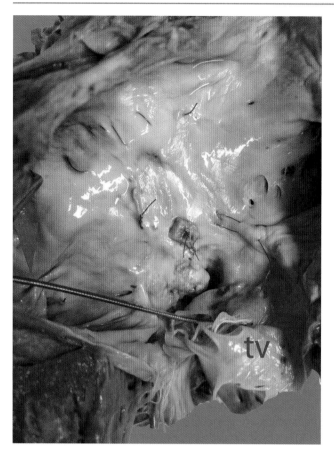

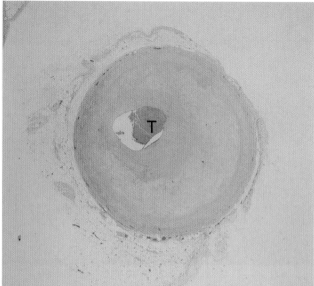

Fig. 5.42 High-grade coronary atheromatous disease is seen in a coronary artery. Focal thrombus (*T*) is seen occluding the lumen (Hematoxylin and eosin)

Fig. 5.41 This macroscopic view of the right atrium is complicated by the reality of multiple surgical interventions in life. The septal walls are seen centrally with a row of sutures superiorly and evidence of septal defect closure including a pledget. Immediately below this is a zone of calcific nodularity in relation to Dacron material. A pacemaker line (*red arrowhead*) is seen running from the superior vena cava obliquely across the distorted atrial tissues and towards the tricuspid (*tv*) leaflet

many lack any clues from the macroscopic perspective. In these circumstances, widespread sampling of coronary artery, nodal, ventricular, and sometimes valve tissues is required. Securing appropriate histology blocks, special stains and sampling of tissues for microbiology, molecular techniques, and ultrastructural analysis is mandatory. Referral of the cardiac tissues, before significant dissection, to specialist centers should always be considered. However, one should be sensitive to the needs of the relatives. Prompt and relevant communication with any legal parties should also be made in order to facilitate specimen handling.

Histology (General Principles)

Taking samples of the myocardium tissues at autopsy is a complicated task. However, some cases need no sampling – particularly after finding a diagnostic gross pathology, such as cardiac tamponade following myocardial infarction. Nevertheless, cardiac histology and other tests are of particular value in terms of fully appreciating any underlying cardiac disease. Histology may also identify occult pathology that was unsuspected by clinician and pathologist alike! In order to maximize the diagnostic information being gathered, one should have a scheme for tissue sampling [2].

Coronary Vessel Histology

The coronary artery tissues can be sampled for histology, either by means of taking the worst affected area. Alternatively, one may sample multiple samples being taken from all three major coronary vessels. Thus, a single block of an area of high-grade stenosis (Fig. 5.42) with a thrombosis could be sufficient in a case of myocardial infarction, with another block of cardiac tissue confirming the infarcted tissue (Fig. 5.43). An increased number of coronary transverse samples and blocks are required where more of the coronary tree needs assessment, such as cases of treated coronary disease. Rarely, the entire coronary tree may need sampling, but this is generally reserved for postangioplasty or medicolegal cases. The number of blocks and indeed amount of tissue required should reflect the needs of the case directly, and there is no simple rule that can be applied for all cases.

The need for resin-embedded stent section must be considered before direct sampling of the coronary tissues. Any attempt to transversely cut a stent by means of scalpel/scissors will inevitably lead to distortion and likely partial/complete crushing of the stent with fragmentation of the plaque tissue adjacent (see Fig. 5.15). This will ruin any attempts to evaluate the vascular parenchyma – and it also blunts the blade of the dissecting tool!

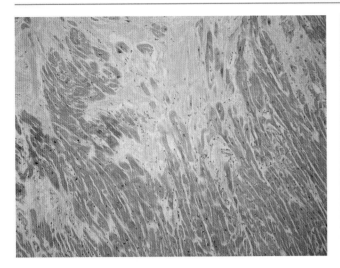

Fig. 5.43 Hematoxylin- and eosin-stained section showing dense fibrosis in a case of myocardial infarction. Dense collagenized tissue is noted with some residual viable myocytes enmeshed

Myocardium Histology

The cardiac tissues should be considered again in terms of individual chambers and specific areas [1, 2, 19]. One can sample the atrial parenchyma on both sides, although this is an infrequent task. Atrial sampling is generally a low-yield process, unless there is a focal lesion (e.g., myxoma/thrombus). However, two recommended sites for sampling in the atrial compartment are those of the sinoatrial node and atrioventricular node (and thence His bundle, etc.) tissues (see above). If necessary, one can return to the atrial tissues, as the needs dictate later.

The bulk of attention is usually focused upon the ventricular parenchyma. A longitudinal sample of the right ventricular outflow tract, merging into the pulmonary root, is advantageous, as an adjunct to the macroscopic assessment of the tissue thickness macroscopically. This block is normal taken in longitudinal fashion, along the line of the blood flow (Fig. 5.44). However, transverse sections of the right ventricle anteriorly, below the conus, are of advantage since these permit analysis of the "triangle of dysplasia" that is commonly affected with arrhythmogenic right ventricle cardiomyopathy (see Fig. 5.44) [20].

The septal tissues will be considered firstly by the block immediately below the atrioventricular node/ His bundle parenchyma (described above) (see Fig. 5.32). The tissues can also be appreciated as a separate transverse block showing both right and left ventricle aspects, ideally at midchamber level. It is helpful to either notch or ink one side in order to confirm the septal polarity.

Samples from the posterior, lateral, and anterior left ventricle wall are advisable (Fig. 5.45), thereby sampling the various coronary artery territories. Alternatively, one can extract a full ring of ventricular wall tissues and thence sample

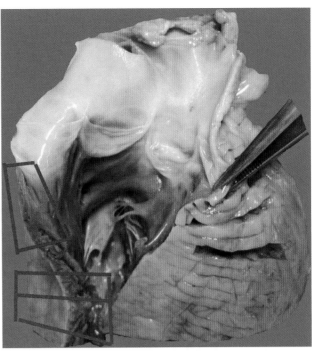

Fig. 5.44 The right ventricle outflow tract is seen with block sampling sites *marked*. The blocks should be taken from the right ventricle outflow tract along the line of the flow of blood and from the right ventricle to interface with the "triangle of dysplasia"

this into multiple standard size blocks. Another technique is to take one of the midventricular slices and to examine this in "jumbo/geographic" blocks (see Fig. 5.45). The advantage of this latter technique is the global perspective it provides for ventricular tissue. It also permits mapping of the parenchyma against clinical/radiological data in a more complete fashion. Samples from the apex of the left ventricle can be of use in some cases of cardiomyopathy. Certainly focused sampling of any lesion identified macroscopically is of direct relevance. The number of blocks should always reflect the individual case realities, but no absolute rule exists.

Examination of cardiac valves generally is not routinely undertaken. However, rheumatic valves and any infective process (Fig. 5.46) need appropriate block sampling. The valve tissues should have all the material ideally being in the same block, with the parenchyma displayed in longitudinal fashion so that the edge of the valve is evident together with the valve leaflet and base tissues in sequence. Thus, the lesion can be appreciated in terms of the geography of the valve parenchyma.

Tissue Processing and the Stains Needed

All cardiac tissue blocks for routine histology should be placed into 10% neutral buffered formalin and then processed through to paraffin blocks for subsequent routine

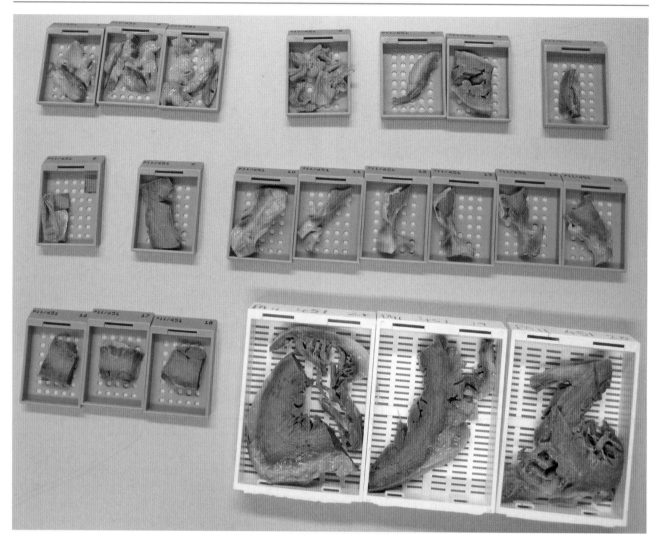

Fig. 5.45 Cardiac dissection often leads to many blocks. In this view in the *top row*, there are sections from the three coronary artery territories, sinoatrial node, right ventricle outflow tract, right ventricle tissues and right atrium. In the *middle row* there are samples of the left atrium, high septum and also six blocks of atrial/membranous septum/high sep- tal tissues which incorporate the AV node and branch ramifications. The *third row* shows samples from the posterior, lateral, and anterior aspect of the left ventricle with three large "jumbo" blocks of right ventricle, left ventricle, and septal tissues

histology. Conventional hematoxylin and eosin sections are the norm, but at least one myocardial block should have the following histology stains:

- Elastic van Gieson (EVG) and/or Masson's trichrome for connective tissues in particular collagen and elastic (Fig. 5.47)
- Perl's for iron
- Periodic acid Schiff (PAS) for carbohydrates, in particular glycogen
- Alcian blue and diastase periodic acid Schiff (ABDPAS) for mucins
- Congo/Sirius red histochemistry for amyloid (Fig. 5.48)

These stains will permit a comprehensive review of myocyte architecture and inspection of cellular fibrillar patterns. Phosphotungstic acid hematoxylin (PTAH) can be employed but is not favored by many laboratories (Fig. 5.49). These stains are an important adjunct in terms of considering the parenchyma, and they should be performed routinely. Occult and subtle pathologies can be identified using this protocol (see Fig. 5.48). In cases of sepsis (e.g., infective endocarditis), standard histochemical stains for infections (Gram, periodic acid Schiff (PAS), and Ziehl-Neelsen) may assist such case analysis.

Other Samples to Be Taken

Alongside cardiac tissue sampling, the potential for considering lung parenchyma should take place. Furthermore, at least one piece of kidney/liver is advantageous when considering any autopsy case. Accessing other tissues may also be relevant in systemic diseases of various types.

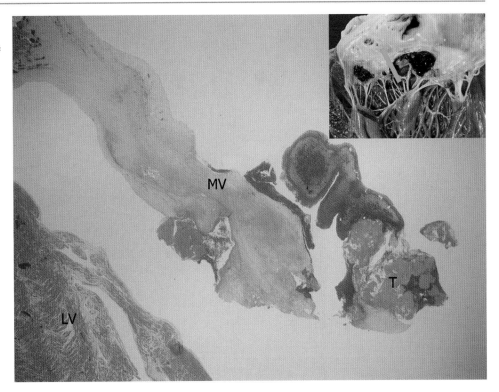

Fig. 5.46 Irregular thrombotic and hemorrhagic vegetation (mainly thrombus, *T*) affecting the mitral valve (*MV*) in a case of streptococcal infective endocarditis, seen with hematoxylin and eosin stain. The left ventricle is seen adjacent. There has been considerable destruction of valve tissue (see macro insert, *top right*). The plane of blocking is indicated by the *green bar*

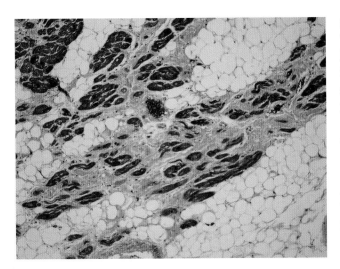

Fig. 5.47 Masson's trichrome is particularly helpful in identifying the fibrous interstitial component with fatty atrophy in a case of arrhythmogenic right ventricular cardiomyopathy

Photography

Digital photography of the dissection of cardiac tissues is a great benefit when considering cases (Fig. 5.50). Often, once dissected/sampled for histology, it is not possible to reconstruct the tissues for another person to review in the same manner as the fresh sample. Photography is a vital tool in terms of the dissection record [2]. As an adjunct or even replacement to histology, it can provide significant informa-

tion for clinicians and radiologists when reviewing cases. The ability to cross-correlate against previous tests and imaging may be of particular value in cases with medicolegal interest. Furthermore, this modality of tissue consideration allows images to be e-mailed/sent to other experts/interested parties for consideration (see Fig. 5.38).

Microbiology

As with other tests above, the assessment will need to reflect the individual case specifics. However, general autopsy sampling of blood and potentially infected tissues should be encouraged in cases of putative sepsis, and any focal infective lesion should be sampled for microbiological assessment [2, 5, 19]. The need to consider atypical infective agents, particularly in the era of cancer treatments and immunosuppressive disease, is important. Furthermore, consideration of potential viral diseases should be made especially in suspected myocarditis cases.

Molecular Studies

It is possible to reserve some heart parenchyma for DNA and equivalent studies, in particular for inherited cardiomyopathies [21]. However, it should be borne in mind that a 2-cm cube-sized sample of spleen tissue is a better substrate, given the higher density of DNA per unit volume tissue. This can

Fig. 5.48 Cardiac amyloid demonstrated by Sirius red (SR) histochemistry. The *inset* shows the classic birefringence under polarized light. It is recommended that thick sections (10 μm) are used when looking for amyloid histologically

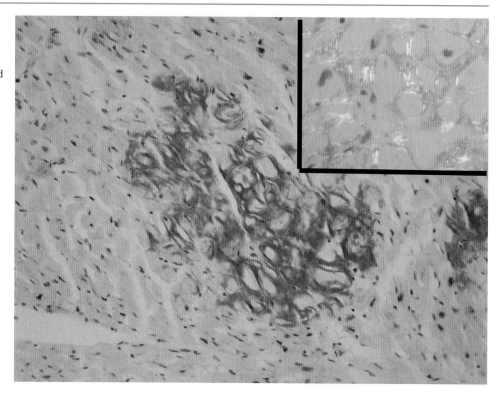

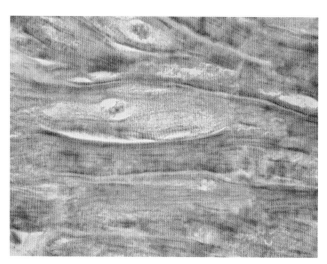

Fig. 5.49 Phosphotungstic acid hematoxylin (PTAH) stained myocardial tissues showing the striated quality of the individual cardiac myocytes

be snap frozen for storage, or DNA extraction can take place promptly after the autopsy, depending on the local autopsy practices.

Enzyme and Metabolic Studies

Rarely enzyme and equivalent tests are needed for assessment of underlying inherited/acquired metabolic errors. The amount of tissue and method for preservation/transport to the appropriate laboratory needs to be considered before starting

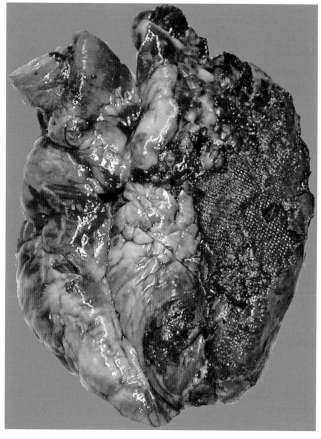

Fig. 5.50 Postoperative death case showing widespread contusion of the cardiac tissues together with hemostatic material having being applied to the left atrium and left ventricle in an attempt to arrest bleeding during the operation

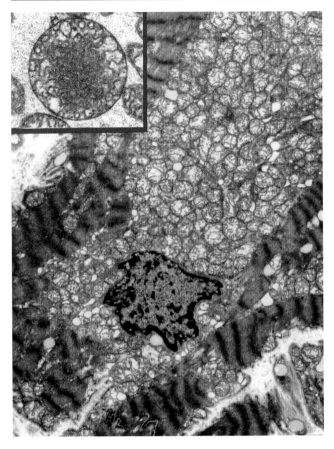

Fig. 5.51 Ultrastructural examination of myocardial tissue showing abundant mitochondria in a case of mitochondrial myopathy. The *inset* shows one mitochondrion with atypical morphology

the autopsy. The realities of the sampling and assays will reflect the clinical query being posed. One should follow the guidance/requests of the clinical biochemist/toxicologist.

Electron Microscopy

Some cardiac tissues are best considered by means of electron microscopy, particularly those with potential storage disorder realties. While it is possible to examine tissues at the ultrastructural level from formalin-fixed parenchyma, ultrastructural samples are best primarily placed in to 4% glutaraldehyde for electron microscopy assessment. They should be sectioned and seen in transmission electron microscopy format (Fig. 5.51). Freeze fracture techniques are generally not required.

Summary

It is not possible to be absolute in terms of precisely how one should examine all hearts at autopsy. There are general rules and guidelines [1, 2, 5, 13, 19] that assist the examination of cardiac tissues. This chapter provides a pragmatic and safe

approach for autopsy cases. It is emphasized that the clinical history and investigations in life may well provide significant information that will guide autopsy analysis. Similarly, the identification of macroscopic pathology will determine the selection of histology blocks and/or other sampling of tissues (e.g., microbiology, electron microscopy, molecular studies, etc.). The role of photography cannot be underestimated, particularly if detailed dissection and sampling of cardiac parenchyma is to take place. Photography also provides a record of pathology seen at various stages and will assist any second opinion review.

It is emphasized that careful histological consideration of the cardiac parenchyma is mandatory in many cases of autopsy practice. Even those with a noncardiac cause of death require diligent consideration of the heart. Prompt consideration (ideally before starting the case) of the need to refer the whole heart or part of the cardiac tissue samples to specialist centers should be undertaken as routine. Indeed, there is an argument that all cases of likely sudden cardiac death should only be examined by specialist cardiac pathologists.

References

1. Basso C, Burke M, Fornes P, Gallagher PJ, de Gouveia RH, Sheppard M, Thiene G, van der Wal A. Guidelines for autopsy investigation of sudden cardiac death. Vichow's Archiv. 2008;452: 11–8.
2. Suvarna SK. National guidelines for adult autopsy cardiac dissection: are they achievable? Histopathology. 2008;97–112:53.
3. Rutty GN, Burton JL. The evisceration. In: Burton JL, Rutty GN, editors. The hospital autopsy. 3rd ed. London: Arnold; 2010. p. 115–35.
4. Farrer-Brown G. A colour atlas of cardiac pathology. London: Wolfe Medical Publications Ltd.; 1977. p. 88–91.
5. Rutty GN, Burton JL. Dissection of the internal organs. In: Burton JL, Rutty GN, editors. The hospital autopsy. 3rd ed. London: Arnold; 2010. p. 136–58.
6. Edwards WD. Cardiovascular system. In: Ludwig J, editor. Autopsy practice. 3rd ed. Toronto: Humana Press; 2002. p. 21–43.
7. Becker AE, Anderson RH. Cardiac adaptation and its sequelae. In: Cardiac pathology. An integrated text and color atlas. Edinburgh: Churchill Livingstone; 1982. p. 1.2–1.8.
8. Silver MM, Silver MD. Examination of the heart and cardiovascular specimens in surgical pathology. In: Silver MD, Gotlieb AI, Schoen FJ, editors. Cardiovascular pathology. 3rd ed. New York: Churchill Livingstone; 2001. p. 1–29.
9. Kitson DW, Scholz DG, Hagen PT, Ilstrup DM, Edwards WD. Age-related changes in normal human heart during the first ten decades of life. Part II. Maturity: a quantitative anatomical study of 765 specimens from subjects 20–99 years old. Mayo Clin Proc. 1988;63: 137–46.
10. Lucas SL. Derivation of new reference tables for human heart weights in light of increasing body mass index. J Clin Pathol. 2011;64:279–80.
11. Gaitskell K, Perera R, Soilleux EJ. Derivation of new reference tables for human heart weights in light of increasing body mass index. J Clin Pathol. 2011;64:358–62.
12. Sheppard M, Davies MJ. Cardiac examination and normal cardiac anatomy. In: Practical cardiovascular pathology. London: Arnold; 1998. p. 1–16.

13. Anderson RH, Becker AE. Normal cardiac anatomy. In: Anderson RH, Becker AE, Roberts WB, editors. The cardiovascular system. Part A: General considerations and congenital malformations. Edinburgh: Churchill Livingstone; 1993. p. 3–26.

14. Raasch F. Pacemaker post-mortem. In: Wecht C, editor. Legal medicine annual. Boston: Butterworth, 1997, p. 97–100.

15. Suvarna SK, Start RD, Tayler DI. A prospective audit of pacemaker function, implant lifetime and patient cause of death. J Clin Pathol. 1999;52:677–80.

16. Prahlow JA, Guilleyardo JM, Barnard JJ. The implantable cardioverter defibrillator. A potential hazard for autopsy pathologists. Arch Pathol Lab Med. 1997;121:1076–80.

17. Fulton RM, Hutchinson EC, Morgan Jones A. Ventricular weight in cardiac hypertrophy. Br Heart J. 1952;14:413–20. doi:10.1136/hrt.14.3.413.

18. Schoen FJ. Approach to the analysis of cardiac valve prostheses as surgical pathology or autopsy specimens. Cardiovasc Pathol. 1995;4:241–55.

19. The Royal College of Pathologists. Guidelines on autopsy practice 2005: Scenario 1: Sudden death with likely cardiac pathology. www.rcpath.org/resources/pdf/AutopsyScenario1Jan05.pdf

20. Basso C, Corrado D, Marcus F, Nava A, Thiene G. Arrhythmogenic right ventricular cardiomyopathy. Lancet. 2009;373(9671): 1289–300.

21. Tester DJ, Ackerman MJ. The role of molecular autopsy in unexplained sudden cardiac death. Curr Opin Cardiol. 2006;21: 166–72.

Embryology of the Heart

6

Michael T. Ashworth

Abstract

The heart is a modified blood vessel, developing from a straight tube that undergoes a complex series of changes, beginning with folding. This folding, termed looping, brings the connecting parts of the heart together in close proximity on its inner curvature. Following this, there is differential outgrowth of the chambers from the heart tube, remodeling of the chamber connections and the formation of septa to separate the systemic and pulmonary blood flow. All the while, the heart provides the blood flow to the developing embryo and builds the capacity to adapt to extrauterine life. Congenital defects of the heart have their origin early in development and can be understood in terms of failure of the normal developmental processes. The illustrations of congenital defects show the consequences.

Keywords

Heart tube • Looping • Septation • Ductus venosus • Foramen ovale • Arterial duct • Postnatal adaptation

Introduction

Modern medical training gives the undergraduate only limited exposure to embryology, and consequently, many medical practitioners find congenital heart disease an impossibly complex field. However, some knowledge of how the heart develops is essential in appreciating normal anatomy and more importantly understanding congenital heart disease [1]. Much of our understanding of the early development of the heart is based on studies in chicken and mouse embryos, supplemented by morphological studies of early human embryos [2]. The heart is at first a simple vessel – the heart tube. By the third week, it shows regular contractions. This heart tube then undergoes looping and septation – a process by which the great vessels, the atria, and the ventricles are delineated. Heart formation is completed with the development of valves, the conduction system, and the formation of coronary arteries.

The Heart Tube

The heart develops from asymmetrical and bilateral plates of cardiac mesoderm that express the cardiac-specific genes NKX2-5 and GATA-4. The heart fields (primary and secondary) are located in the lateral plate mesoderm and give rise to all the lineages present in the differentiated heart – myocardium, endocardium, and smooth muscle [3]. These bilateral plates fuse in the midline to form a primitive heart tube. The blood inflow is caudal and the outflow cranial (Fig. 6.1). The venous inflow is still partly separated; these incompletely fused parts will later fuse and form the atria [4]. The heart tube is lined by endocardium and has a surrounding sleeve of myocardium, both layers separated by abundant extracellular matrix termed the cardiac jelly. Even at the early stages of the heart tube, there is differential expression of genes along its length, a pattern of expression that will determine the fate

M.T. Ashworth, M.D., FRCPath
Department of Histopathology,
Great Ormond Street Hospital for Children,
London WC1N 3JN, UK
e-mail: michael.ashworth@gosh.nhs.uk

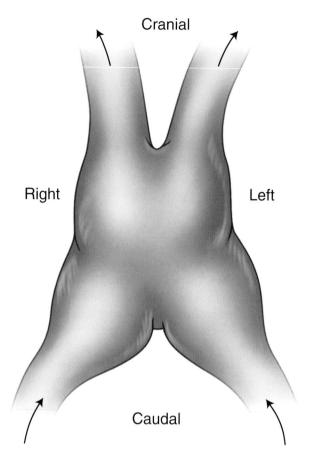

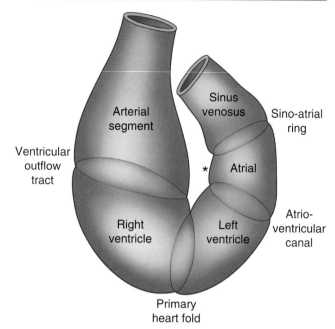

Fig. 6.2 A diagrammatic representation of the looped heart tube. The conventional heart segments are shown together with their transitional zones. Note the close apposition of the transitional zones on the inner curvature of the loop (*asterisk*). These transition zones do not significantly contribute to the formation of the heart chambers; rather they will form the segmental connections

Fig. 6.1 The heart tube. A diagrammatic representation of the heart tube. The inflow is caudal; the two horns of the sinus venosus will later become incorporated into the right atrium. The outflow is cranial – a common arterial trunk

of its various parts [5]. Traditionally, five sequential segments are recognized from caudal to cranial: sinus venosus, atrial, left ventricular, right ventricular, and arterial segments. Between each of the segments lies a transition zone; the sino-atrial ring, the atrioventricular canal, the primary heart fold, and the ventricular outflow tract, respectively. The heart tube is the axis from which cardiac chambers develop as outgrowths. Thus, the original segments contribute more to the connections of the cardiac chambers than to the chambers themselves (Fig. 6.2).

Looping

Looping of the straight heart tube follows activation of a gene cascade that determines right–left symmetry. The genes of this cascade are already expressed in the cardiac mesoderm even before formation of the heart tube. *Pitx2* is considered the controlling gene. Looping of the heart tube is caused because of growth of the tube the ends of which are fixed. This causes the tube to lengthen, and dissolution of the tethering dorsal mesocardium allows the looping of the lengthened tube (Fig. 6.3). Looping is nonrandom and is controlled by genes not yet fully understood. Looping involves both bending of the heart tube ventrally and torsion towards the right [6]. At the same time, the atrial precursors come to lie posterior to the ventricles. The tube normally loops to the right and thereby causes all four transition zones (described above) to be brought into close proximity on the inner curvature of the loop (see Fig. 6.2). This approximation is absolutely essential for correct connection of the chambers [7].

Chamber Development and Septation

Both atria and both ventricles form by ballooning growth from the heart tube, the atria from the dorsal aspect and the ventricles from the ventral aspect [8]. This process is bilateral and in parallel for the atria, but for the ventricles, it is unilateral and in sequence. A consequence of this is that the atria can develop isomerism (Figs. 6.4 and 6.5). Ventricular isomerism is impossible. The endocardial cells of the atrioventricular canal and outflow tracts give rise to cells that populate the cardiac jelly to form cardiac cushions [10] that

Fig. 6.3 Looping of the heart tube. A diagrammatic representation of the looped heart tube. (**a**) is viewed from the ventral surface and (**b**) from the right side. This process of looping results in the atria lying dorsally and the ventricles ventrally. The ventricles come to lie side by side and the arterial trunk ventrally

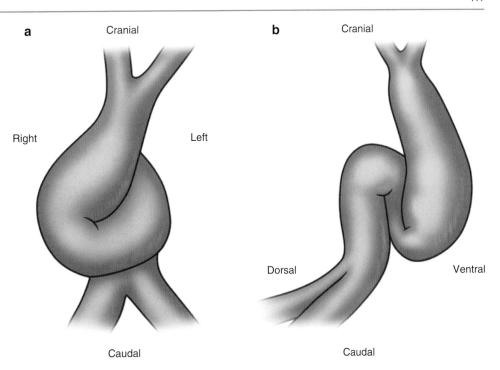

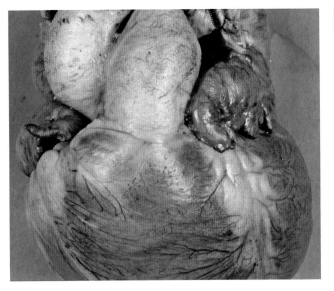

Fig. 6.4 Isomerism of the atrial appendages—left atrial isomerism. A heart showing bilateral atrial appendages of left type. The appendages are long, narrow, and hooked. Hearts with left atrial isomerism often show abnormalities of the systemic venous return and atrioventricular septal defects

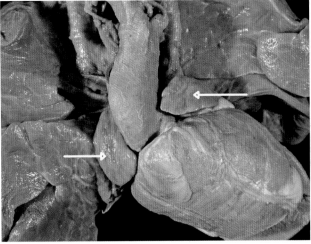

Fig. 6.5 Isomerism of the atrial appendages – right atrial isomerism. There are bilateral atrial appendages of right type with a broad and triangular outline (*arrows*). Such hearts usually exhibit anomalous pulmonary venous return, double inlet ventricle, atrioventricular septal defect, and discordant ventriculoarterial connections with pulmonary stenosis or atresia. In this example, there is pulmonary atresia, the aorta (*asterisk*) being the only vessel arising from the base of the heart (From Ashworth [9]. Reprinted with permission)

contribute to the septation of these areas (Fig. 6.6). At the same time, the atria and ventricles develop trabeculations. The myocardium that forms the chambers acquires specific gene expression (*ANF*, *CX40*, *CX43*) and loses expression of the genes Tbx2 and Tbx3 that are present in the primitive myocardium of the primary heart tube. Tbx5 is expressed in high levels in the prospective left ventricle and low levels in the prospective right ventricle [11]. Reduced dosage of Tbx5 leads to defects in the interventricular septum formation and patterning.

Since the atrial segment is initially connected to the left ventricular segment, there is no direct connection of the atria with the right ventricle [8]. Blood can flow from the atria to the right ventricle via the interventricular

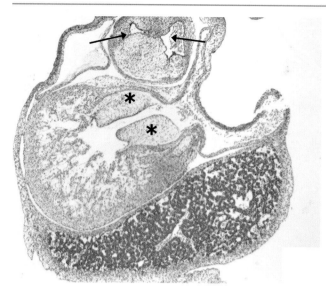

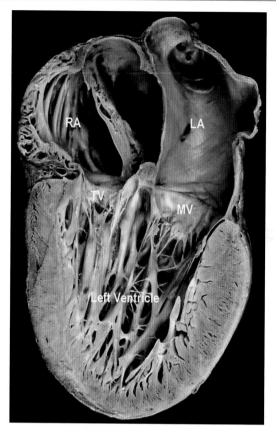

Fig. 6.6 Histological section from an embryo of approximately 37 days gestation/sectioned in the sagittal plane. The right atrium (RA) lies posteriorly and the left ventricle (LV) anteriorly. The liver is present beneath the diaphragm, and the pericardial sac can be seen investing the heart. Note the noncompacted appearance of the left ventricular myocardium. The atrioventricular junction is marked by the presence of upper and lower myxoid swellings (*asterisks*) – the endocardial cushions. They have not yet fused to separate the right and left atrioventricular junctions. The arterial trunk is visible in the upper part of the field, partly surrounded by right and left (LAA) atrial appendages. The trunk also shows myxoid swellings in its intima (*arrows*) that are just fusing to separate the aorta and pulmonary trunk

Fig. 6.7 Double inlet left ventricle. A heart cut in a simulated four-chamber view. The right atrium (*RA*) has a normal tricuspid valve (*TV*), and the left atrium (*LA*) has a normal mitral valve (*MV*). Both valves open into a dominant left ventricle. The right ventricle was small and rudimentary and connected via a ventricular septal defect to the dominant left ventricle. As is usual in these hearts, the aorta takes origin from the right ventricle and the pulmonary trunk from the left ventricle. This feature is not visible in this plane of section (From Ashworth [9]. Reprinted with permission)

foramen. Connection of the atria to the right ventricle develops by growth of the ventricular inlet to the right [7]. Defects in this process result in double inlet left ventricle (Fig. 6.7). Tricuspid atresia (absent right atrioventricular connection) shows a similar morphology (Fig. 6.8). In an analogous manner, the outlet of the heart is connected initially solely to the right ventricle (Fig. 6.9), but by similar differential growth, the outlet comes to overlie both ventricles. Defects in this process will lead to double outlet right ventricle (Fig. 6.10). The interventricular septum grows from the apex of the heart loop between the left and right ventricular segments at the site of the primary heart fold.

The sinus venosus is the venous confluence, which is initially a chamber separate from the atrium that opens into its dorsal wall. It has two horns, left and right, each formed by fusion of the respective right and left vitelline, umbilical and cardinal veins. The left horn becomes the coronary sinus, and the right is incorporated into the wall of the right atrium. A pair of valves develops around the sinus, and fusion of the anterior part of these valves creates the septum spurium which contributes to closure of the atria. The right valve forms the terminal crest (crista terminalis), the prominent muscle bar in the wall of the right atrium that

separates the trabeculated wall of the atrium from the smooth-walled part derived from the sinus venosus (Fig. 6.11). The valve also forms the valve of the inferior caval vein (Eustachian valve) and the valve of the coronary sinus (Thebesian valve). The primary atrial septum develops to the right of sinus venosus. An opening then forms in the primary septum, the ostium secundum, and this is partly closed by growth of the septum secundum – an infolding of the right atrial wall to the right of the primary septum (see Fig. 6.11). The ostium primum is actually beneath the free edge of the septum primum and is obliterated when that edge fuses with the endocardial cushions and the tip of the septum spurium. The pulmonary vein enters the left part of the atrium and is incorporated into it. The exact site of development of the pulmonary vein is still controversial. Incomplete involution of the left horn of the sinus venosus results in persistent left superior caval vein draining to the

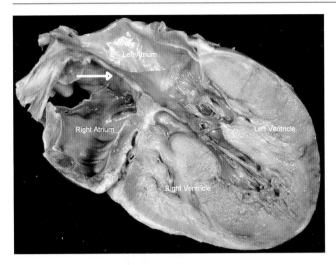

Fig. 6.8 Tricuspid atresia. A heart cut in a simulated four-chamber view. The right atrium is connected to the left atrium by a large atrial septal defect (*arrow*). The left atrium is connected to the left ventricle via a normal mitral valve. The right ventricle is small and connected via a ventricular septal defect to the left ventricle (not visible in this plane of section). There is no connection between the right atrium and the right ventricle

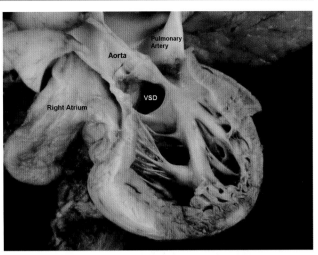

Fig. 6.10 Double outlet right ventricle. The right ventricle has been opened to expose the aorta and pulmonary trunk, both of which arise from the ventricle. A large subarterial ventricular septal defect is present (From Ashworth [9]. Reprinted with permission)

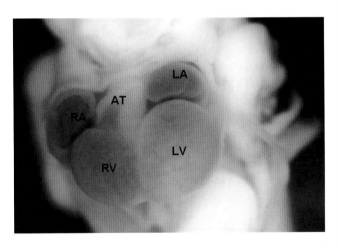

Fig. 6.9 The heart of an embryo at day 36 of gestation from a ruptured ectopic pregnancy. The pericardium has been excised. Note the large size of the heart relative to the thorax. The intracardiac blood is visible through the translucent myocardium. The right (*RA*) and left (*LA*) appendages are visible as are the right (*RV*) and left (*LV*) ventricles and arterial trunk (*AT*). Note the origin of the arterial trunk almost exclusively from the right ventricle at this stage of gestation. Partial septation of the arterial trunk is evident with blood confined to one half of it

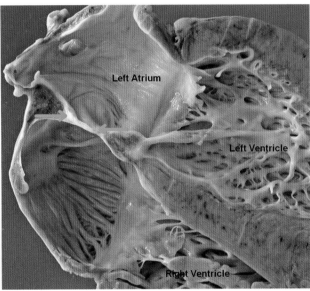

Fig. 6.11 Interatrial septum. A simulated four-chamber view of the heart. The atrial septum has been cut through the oval fossa (*arrows*). The thin flap valve is clearly seen. The infoldings of the atrial wall that will produce the margins of the oval fossa are seen readily. Note the trabeculated wall of the right atrium and the terminal crest (*asterisk*) separating it from the smooth-walled part derived from the sinus venosus

coronary sinus (Fig. 6.12). Deficient atrial septation is among the commoner cardiac defects and is known to be associated with mutations in the genes NKX2-5, GATA-4, TBX20, and MYH6 [1].

During looping, the cardiac jelly is eliminated from much of the heart tube but persists at the site of the endocardial cushions at the atrioventricular junction [10]. These cushions form superiorly and inferiorly and fuse in the midline to create right and left atrioventricular orifices, differential growth of the right atrioventricular canal having brought the right atrium into contact with the right ventricle. Fusion of the cushions with the developing interventricular muscular septum and the atrial primary septum completes septation of the atrial and ventricular chambers, with failure being implicated in ventricular septal defects.

The outflow tracts have a complex origin, partly from the primary heart tube and partly from ingrowth of cells from

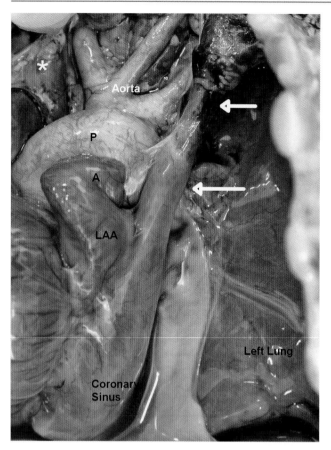

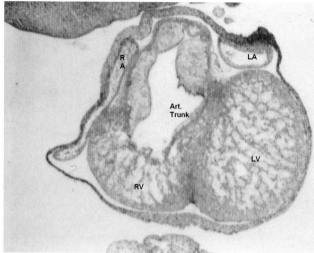

Fig. 6.13 Histological section from an embryo of approximately 37 days of gestation, sectioned in the coronal plane. The right atrial (*RA*) and left atrial (*LA*) appendages lie on either side of the arterial trunk within the pericardial sac. Note the noncompacted appearance of the right (*RV*) and left (*LV*) ventricular myocardium. The arterial trunk arises from the right ventricle and contains myxoid swellings (*asterisks*) – the endocardial cushions. They have not yet fused to separate the aorta and pulmonary trunk

Fig. 6.12 Persistent left superior caval vein draining to the coronary sinus. The thoracic structures viewed from the left with the heart pulled anteriorly and to the right. The persistent left superior caval vein (*arrows*) descends anterior to the left pulmonary (*PA*) artery to enter the coronary sinus on the posterior aspect of the left atrium (*LAA*). Internally the coronary sinus is abnormally large. The right superior caval vein is evident (*asterisk*). There was no brachiocephalic vein, although in some such cases, it may be present

two distinct sources. These two sources are the cardiac neural crest and the secondary heart field, a region of cardiac mesoderm close to, but distinct from, the primary heart plates [1, 12]. The complex interaction of all these tissues gives rise to the ventricular outflow tracts, the arterial valves, and the intrapericardial parts of the aorta and pulmonary trunk (Fig. 6.13).

The pericardium develops as a sac around the developing heart tube. Initially the tube is connected to the posterior mediastinum by the dorsal mesocardium. This later breaks down, permitting the folding of the heart tube on which subsequent development is so critically dependent. The atrioventricular valves develop from the two endocardial cushions at the atrioventricular junction [13]. Defective development leads to atrioventricular septal defects.

The coronary arteries and veins had been thought to develop from cells that grow over the myocardium form the proepicardium. It has recently been shown in the mouse [13]

that their endothelium derives from differentiated venous endothelial cells that sprout onto the developing heart, dedifferentiate, proliferate, and spread to form the coronary plexus [16]. They then redifferentiate and remodel into coronary arteries, capillaries, and coronary veins. There is also a minor contribution from endocardium. Vessel sprouting and outgrowth depend on unknown signals from the epicardium and myocardium.

The conduction tissue develops from the myocardium of the primitive heart tube found in the transitional zones [8]. The formation of an insulating fibrous and fatty tissue plane between atrial and ventricular myocardium occurs only after completion of septation. It begins at 7 weeks and is largely complete by 12 weeks of development.

The Ductus Venosus (Venous Duct) and Foramen Ovale (Oval Foramen)

The fetal blood (in utero) obtains its oxygen and other nutrients via the placenta, returning to the heart through the umbilical vein. The umbilical vein runs to the liver where it enters the portal vein. A shunt between the portal vein and the inferior caval vein termed the ductus venosus (venous duct) bypasses the liver.

The proportion of umbilical venous blood passing through the venous duct varies from 20% to 90%. Blood flow velocity in the venous duct is four to five times that in the inferior caval vein so that as it enters the right atrium, the anterior stream – derived from the abdominal inferior caval – is slow flowing, and the posterior stream originating in the duct venosus is much faster with much higher oxygen saturation. Blood from the venous duct is preferentially directed to the oval foramen by the baffle effect of the Eustachian valve and by nature of its higher velocity. The superior caval blood with that derived from the abdominal vena cava is directed preferentially to the tricuspid valve and right ventricle, only about 5% of it crossing the oval foramen [14].

Arterial Duct, Lungs, and Systemic Circulation

The right ventricle pumps blood into the pulmonary trunk, but over two-thirds of it passes directly via the arterial duct (ductus arteriosus) to the descending aorta. This preferential flow is caused by the high pulmonary resistance. The left atrium receives its blood from across the oval foramen and from the pulmonary veins. This blood flows across the mitral valve and is ejected by the left ventricle into the ascending aorta where it supplies preferentially the head and upper limbs, only about one-quarter of the left ventricular output crossing the aortic isthmus to join the blood flowing through the arterial duct into the descending aorta. The ratio of right to left ventricular output is of the order of 1.2:1 to 1.3:1.

There is mixing of oxygenated and deoxygenated blood at several points in the fetal circulation: in the liver, in the inferior caval vein, and in the left atrium. Streaming of blood partly prevents this mixing by preferentially directing oxygenated blood through the oval foramen to the left heart. This oxygenated blood passes to the head. In addition, by directing inferior and superior caval blood to the right ventricle through the arterial duct to the descending aorta allows deoxygenated blood to return to the placenta.

Postnatal Adaptation

At birth, the function of oxygenation of the blood (hitherto undertaken by the placenta) is assumed by the fetal lungs. The first gasps of the newborn infant expand the lungs with air. This physical expansion, together with the consequent raised local oxygen tension, causes the peripheral pulmonary arterial smooth muscle to relax and the peripheral muscular pulmonary arteries to dilate. This widespread dilatation causes a fall in pulmonary vascular resistance. This reduction continues in the immediate postpartum weeks by remodeling of the pulmonary vascular bed.

The drop in pulmonary vascular resistance has several effects. It causes redistribution of the blood ejected from the right ventricle. The blood, instead of passing preferentially through the arterial duct, now passes to the lungs. This increased volume of blood crossing the lungs increases pulmonary venous return to the left atrium with a subsequent rise in left atrial pressure. This rise in pressure pushes the flap valve of the oval fossa tight against the septum from the left side and seals the interatrial communication. The rise in arterial oxygen saturation brought about by breathing causes the arterial duct to contract and to become functionally closed by 10–15 h after birth. Consolidation of this closure takes place over the following days by fibrosis. The ductus venosus closes about 4 days of age in the term neonate [15].

References

1. Bruneau BG. The developmental genetics of congenital heart disease. Nature. 2008;451:943–8.
2. Tam PPL, Schoenwolf GC. Cardiac fate maps: lineage allocation, morphogenetic movement and cell commitment. In: Harvey RP, Rosenthal N, editors. Heart development. London: Academic; 1999. p. 3–18.
3. Buckingham M, Meilhac S, Zaffran S. Building the mammalian heart from two sources of myocardial cells. Nat Rev Genet. 2005;6:826–35.
4. Moorman A, Webb S, Brown NA, et al. Development of the heart: (1) formation of the cardiac chambers and arterial trunks. Heart. 2003;89:806–14.
5. Kirby ML. Molecular embryogenesis of the heart. Pediatr Dev Pathol. 2002;5:516–43.
6. Taber LA, Voronov DA, Ramasubramanian A. The role of mechanical forces in the torsional component of cardiac looping. Ann N Y Acad Sci. 2010;1188:103–10.
7. Gittenberger de Groot AC, Bartelings MM, Deruiter MC, Poelman RE. Basics of cardiac development for the understanding of congenital heart malformations. Pediatr Res. 2005;57:169–76.
8. Moorman AFM, Christoffels VM. Cardiac chamber formation: development, genes and evolution. Physiol Rev. 2003;83:1223–67.
9. Ashworth MT. The cardiovascular system. In: Keeling JW, Khong TY, editors. Fetal and neonatal pathology. 4th ed. Berlin: Springer; 2007. p. 571–621.
10. Person AD, Klewer SE, Runyan RB. Cell biology of cardiac cushion development. Int Rev Cytol. 2005;243:287–335.
11. Takeuchi JK, et al. Tbx5 specifies the left/right ventricles and ventricular septum position during cardiogenesis. Development. 2003;130:5953–64.
12. Anderson RH, Webb S, Brown NA, et al. Development of the heart: (3) Formation of the ventricular outflow tracts, arterial valves, and intrapericardial arterial trunks. Heart. 2003;89:1110–8.
13. Wessels A, Markman MWM, Vermeulen JLM, et al. The development of the atrioventricular junction in the human heart. Circ Res. 1996;78:10–117.
14. Rudolph AM. The fetal circulation and postnatal adaptation. In: Rudolph AM, editor. Congenital diseases of the heart: clinical-physiological considerations. 2nd ed. Armonk: Futura Publishing Company; 2001. p. 3–44.
15. Kondo M, Itoh S, Kunikata T, et al. Time of closure of ductus venosus in term and preterm neonates. Arch Dis Child Fetal Neonatal Ed. 2001;85:F57–9.
16. Red-Horse K, Ueno H, Weissman IL, Krasnow MA. Coronary arteries form by development al reprogramming of venous cells. Nature. 2010;464:549–53.

Ischemic Heart Disease

7

Katarzyna Michaud

Abstract

Ischemic heart disease as the result of impaired blood supply is currently the leading cause of failure and death. Ischemic heart disease refers to a group of clinicopathological symptoms including angina pectoris, acute myocardial infarction, chronic ischemic heart disease, as well as heart failure and sudden cardiac death. Coronary artery thrombosis is the most common cause of acute myocardial infarction and sudden cardiac death. A thrombotic event is the result of two different processes: plaque disruption and endothelial erosion. The morphology of a "vulnerable plaque" is more clinically indicative than the plaque volume and the degree of luminal stenosis. However, identification of patients with vulnerable plaques remains very challenging and demands the development of new methods of coronary plaque imaging. Sudden death resulting from ventricular fibrillation or AV block frequently complicates coronary thrombosis, accounting for up to 50% of mortality. If a coronary artery is occluded for more than 20 min, irreversible damage to the myocardium occurs. Timely coronary recanalization and myocardial reperfusion limit the extent of myocardial necrosis, but may induce "reperfusion injuries," stunned myocardium, or reperfused myocardial hemorrhagic infarcts, all of which are related to infarct size and coronary occlusion time. Reperfusion injuries have been described after cardiac surgery, percutaneous transluminal coronary angioplasty, and fibrinolysis. A prolonged imbalance between the supply of and demand for myocardial oxygen and nutrition leads to a subacute, acute, or chronic state (aka hibernating myocardium) of myocardial ischemia. Ischemic heart disease is believed to be the underlying cause of heart failure in approximately two-thirds of patients, resulting from acute and/or chronic injury to the heart.

Keywords

Ischemic heart disease • Coronary thrombosis • Sudden cardiac death • Coronary plaque Myocardial infarct • Plaque disruption • Stunned myocardium

Introduction

Cardiovascular disease accounts for nearly one-third of all deaths worldwide [1]. In the United States, cardiovascular disease and stroke cause one death every 33–37 s and cumulatively cause more annual deaths than cancer, respiratory disease, accidents, and diabetes combined [2].

Among cardiovascular diseases, atherosclerotic disease leading to ischemic heart disease continues to be the most frequent cause of death. Ischemic heart disease, resulting

K. Michaud, M.D.
Department of Community Medicine and Public Health, University Hospital of Lausanne, University Center of Legal Medicine of Lausanne and Geneva, Rue du Bugnon 21, 1011 Lausanne, Switzerland
e-mail: katarzyna.michaud@chuv.ch

from an impaired cardiac blood supply, refers to a group of clinicopathological conditions, which can include one, or all, of the following clinical symptoms:

- Angina pectoris (stable or unstable)
- Acute myocardial infarction
- Chronic ischemic heart disease and heart failure
- Sudden cardiac death

Atherosclerosis of coronary arteries is the most frequent cause of impaired myocardial blood supply. Atherosclerosis may be asymptomatic but can be life-threatening in the event of arterial thrombosis. Plaque rupture is the primary underlying cause of luminal thrombosis, responsible for provoking acute coronary syndromes such as myocardial infarction and sudden cardiac death.

The global INTERHEART study of risk factors for acute myocardial infarct demonstrated that nearly 95% of population-attributable risk of myocardial infarction is related to nine potentially modifiable risk factors. These include smoking, altered apolipoprotein B/apolipoprotein A1 ratio, hypertension, diabetes, abdominal obesity, psychosocial factors, daily consumption of fruits and vegetables, regular alcohol intake, and regular physical activity. These risk factors apply to men and women, old and young, and in all regions of the world [3]. Changes in lifestyle and behavior are preventive measures, and the decrease in deaths from coronary artery disease is mostly attributed to risk-factor changes [4].

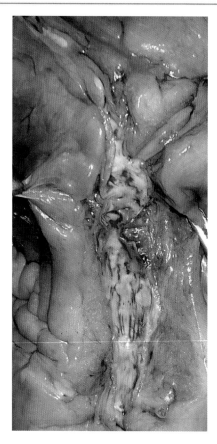

Fig. 7.1 Fatty streaks on the intimal surface of a coronary artery, opened longitudinally, seen as yellow foci on the intimal aspect

Coronary Atheroma

Atherosclerosis is a chronic inflammatory, fibroproliferative disease of large- and medium-sized arteries consisting of the progressive deposition or degenerative accumulation of lipid-containing plaques on the innermost layer of the arterial wall. Endothelial cells, leukocytes, and intimal smooth muscle cells are all major players in the evolution of this disease. Lipid is the essential component of the atherosclerotic disease process. Within each plaque, there are complexes of extracellular lipid, intracellular lipid within foam cells, and collagen with other connective tissue matrix components produced by smooth muscle cells. Endothelial cells, macrophages, and T cells participate in an early and asymptomatic foam-cell lesion, also known as the fatty streak (Fig. 7.1). Atherosclerosis evolves from the subendothelial retention of lipoproteins as a result of a leaky and defective endothelium. The lipoproteins are subsequently modified and rendered cytotoxic, proinflammatory, chemotaxic, and proatherogenic [5].

The "response to injury" hypothesis [6, 7] proposes that the inflammatory process is a central mechanism in early atherogenesis. Arterial wall injury, most often related to aging, diabetes, smoking, dyslipidemia, and hypertension,

triggers an inflammatory response aimed at restoring arterial wall integrity. One of the earliest responses in atherogenesis is the recruitment of circulating monocytes and T lymphocytes. Adhesion molecules and cytokines induce the adhesion of circulating monocytes to the intact endothelial surface and subsequently migration to the intima, where they take up lipid and become foam cells. Atherogenic lipoproteins can also accumulate in the intima without being taken up by foam cells. The atherogenic lipoproteins may be cleared from the intima by scavenging macrophages, resulting in intracellular lipid accumulation.

During the progression of atherosclerosis, endothelial cells, macrophages, and smooth muscle cells die largely by apoptosis. The disintegration of foam cells and loss of smooth muscle cells lead to the formation of a lipid-rich core under a fragile, rupture-prone fibrous cap. The atheromatous core is avascular, hypocellular, and devoid of supporting collagen. The cap is a dynamic connective tissue matrix whose tensile strength is dependent on the constant maintenance by smooth muscle cells.

Plaque inflammation is a pivotal feature of plaque vulnerability. The inflammatory process reduces collagen synthesis and increases apoptosis of smooth muscle cells. Macrophages and T lymphocytes play a major role in the pathophysiology of the fibrous atheroma cap, together being capable of degrading the extracellular matrix by phagocytosis and the secretion of proteolytic enzymes which weaken the thin cap, predisposing it to rupture [8]. Macrophages also contribute to the destruction of the connective tissue matrix through their production of a wide range of metalloproteinases, such as MMP-2 and MMP-9 [9]. These processes are modified by inflammatory cytokines as interferon-γ (gamma), interleukin IL6, CD40 ligand [10]. The immuno-inflammatory response also involves intimal smooth muscle cells, which are responsible for the healing and repair after arterial injury. Smooth muscle cells and collagen stabilize the plaques, protecting them against rupture and thrombosis. If the atherosclerotic stimuli persist over long periods, then the reparative response may dominate and progress to progressively diminish the arterial lumen.

The persistence of risk factor–mediated arterial wall injury leads to ongoing endothelial dysfunction, atheromatous plaque formation, plaque rupture, and thrombotic complications. The concurrent inflammatory process attempts to repair the arterial wall injury with the assistance of endothelial progenitor cells, plaque neovascularization, and cholesterol export. The progression of atherosclerosis from early development to plaque rupture is considered to be a failure of this repair system [11].

Atherosclerotic neovascularization is the process of generating new blood vessels in relevance to the atherosclerotic plaque. It is a response to tissue hypoxia and cholesterol deposition in the vessel wall. In advanced disease, neovascularization may assist in lipid removal from the plaque, leading to plaque regression [12]. Angiogenesis is frequent in advanced atherosclerosis. It is considered as a marker of ongoing disease activity and is a characteristic of high-risk plaques. Coronary neovessels contain endothelial cells of abnormal morphology, leading to an increased permeability that may predispose to intraplaque hemorrhage. The presence of intraplaque bleeding further promotes macrophage recruitment and activation, releasing the proteinases and favoring plaque cap rupture. The coexistence of angiogenesis and inflammation can also mediate rapid plaque progression. Histological studies have shown the highest degree of neovascularization present in ruptured plaques particularly in diabetic patients [8].

Arterial wall remodeling at the site of plaque formation was originally described in a necropsy study [13], demonstrating that the artery responds to plaque growth by increasing the cross-sectional area while retaining normal lumen dimension (positive remodeling). This type of remodeling was later confirmed in vivo with intravascular ultrasound. Plaques that undergo positive remodeling tend to have a large lipid core and a high macrophage content. This may explain the link between compensatory remodeling and plaque rupture. This type of remodeling was higher at target lesions in patients with acute coronary syndromes compared with patients with stable angina. This confirms the histopathological associations between plaque remodeling and vulnerability [14]. The remodeling process has implications for the postmortem measurement of coronary stenosis. When the cross-sectional diameter of the lumen is compared to the dimensions of the vessel at the same point, the degree of stenosis is often overestimated, as the external size of the vessel is larger than normal.

Negative remodeling is defined as local vessel shrinkage and is clinically associated with stable angina. Severe stenosis may even exist months or years before onset of the first symptoms. Furthermore, there is no relationship between the degree of coronary damage and the onset of symptoms, complications, and/or mortality associated with acute coronary syndromes.

Plaque Instability and Vulnerable Plaques

A vulnerable plaque is defined as a nonobstructive, silent coronary lesion that suddenly becomes obstructive and symptomatic [8]. This concept was developed when it was discovered that most lesions leading to acute myocardial infarction were nonobstructive in nature, with a mean diameter of stenosis of 48% [15]. Thus, vulnerable plaques are silent lesions that can give rise to coronary thrombosis.

Thrombosis is the result of two discrete processes: plaque disruption (Fig. 7.2a, b) and endothelial erosion (Fig. 7.2c, d). Plaque disruption (rupture, fissuring) occurs when the plaque cap tears to expose the lipid core to arterial blood (Fig. 7.3). The plaque core is highly thrombogenic, containing tissue factor, fragments of collagen, and a crystalline surface, all of which accelerate the coagulation cascade (Fig. 7.4). The thrombus initially forms within the plaque or at the fissure, but it can expand and diminish the arterial lumen.

Plaque disruption is considered to be an autodestructive phenomenon that is associated with enhanced inflammation. The histological patterns of a ruptured plaque include a thin fibrous cap, a large necrotic core with an increased free esterified cholesterol ratio, increased plaque inflammation, positive vascular remodeling, increased vasa vasorum neovascularization, and intraplaque hemorrhage [8]. Autopsy studies have showed the thickness of the fibrous cap near the rupture site measured 23 ± 19 μm, and 95% of ruptured caps measured 64 μm or less in thickness [16]. Vulnerable plaques also tended to be eccentric.

Progression from an asymptomatic stable plaque, through vulnerable plaque/plaque rupture/thrombus to myocardial infarction, is complex and due to multiple factors. These are incompletely understood due to the inability to accurately detect vulnerable plaques in humans in vivo and in the absence of a good animal model. Heart rate, blood pressure, and pulse pressure are biomechanical factors affecting

Fig. 7.2 Atherosclerotic
vulnerable plaque diagram
showing (**a**) the thin-cap fibrous
atheroma (*arrow*) and necrotic
core (*yellow*), rich in lipids
(*black*). The cap consists of
smooth muscle cells with a
variable number of mac-
rophages and lymphocytes
(*green*). Following plaque
rupture, (**b**) thrombosis occurs,
narrowing the lumen. In cases
of other plaque disease, (**c**)
some lipid may be present deep
in the lesion, but the fibrous cap
is rich in smooth muscle cells
and proteoglycans. There may
be some macrophages, and
lymphocytes may be present,
but there is no necrotic
fibrolipid core. Erosion of the
plaque surface (**d**) allows
thrombosis and lumen
narrowing

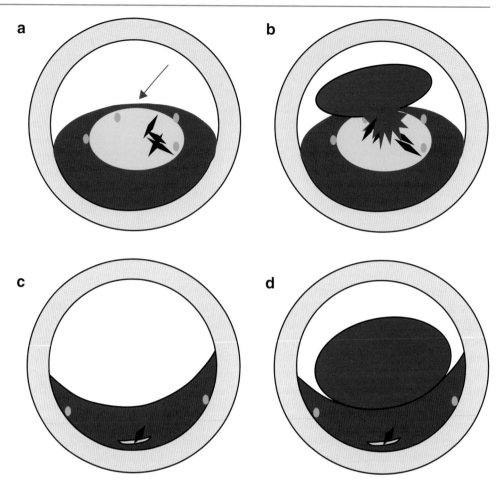

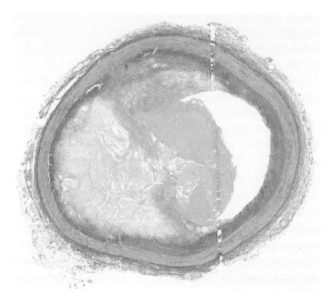

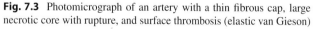

Fig. 7.3 Photomicrograph of an artery with a thin fibrous cap, large
necrotic core with rupture, and surface thrombosis (elastic van Gieson)

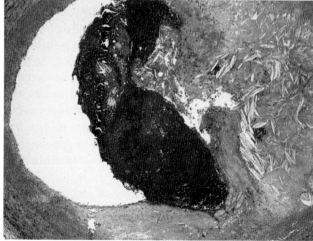

Fig. 7.4 Coronary thrombus over an area of plaque disruption (hematoxylin & eosin)

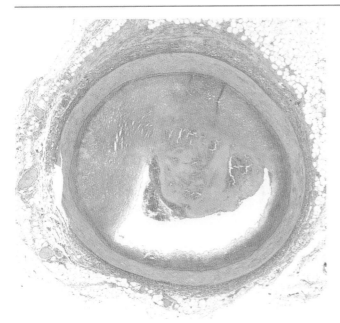

Fig. 7.5 Coronary thrombus over an endothelial erosion of fibrous plaque (elastic van Gieson)

vulnerable arterial fibrous cap, thereby increasing circumferential stress potentially precipitating rupture [9]. Plaque disruption occurs with great frequency; some may result in cardiac infarction or death. Episodes of plaque disruption are associated with the onset or exacerbation of stable angina, caused by a sudden increase in plaque volume and diminution of coronary flow. However, many minor episodes of erosions or disruption are clinically silent and yet contribute to the progression of coronary artery disease. Patients with stable angina usually have segments of chronic high-degree stenosis in one, or more, coronary arteries. Rupture of the plaque surface can be followed by variable amounts of plaque hemorrhage and luminal thrombosis, causing rapid but subclinical progression of the lesion.

The second mechanism favoring thrombus formation is endothelial erosion. This may progress to endothelial denudation which exposes large areas of the subendothelial compartment connective tissue of the plaque, providing an ideal surface for thrombus adherence [17]. Plaques undergoing endothelial erosion contain no specific feature enabling their detection. Histologically, they are characterized by a thick, smooth muscle cell–rich fibrous cap, reduced necrotic core area, and a low degree of inflammation (Fig. 7.5). Plaque erosion is associated with cigarette smoking, suggesting that thrombosis may be related to a systemic, prothrombogenic pathway rather than a local, atherothrombotic mechanism [8].

Focal calcification in atherosclerotic plaques is very common, particularly in older patients. Coronary thrombosis was previously considered to be etiological also related to a calcified nodule with an incidence of 2–6% [18]. However, calcification appears to have no direct causal link to thrombosis with only

one exception. In older individuals, the presence of diffuse intimal calcification coupled with diffuse dilatation of coronary arteries and intimal tears at the margin of calcium plates may cause a thrombotic event [19]. Vascular calcification and inflammation have been shown to rarely coexist, supporting the notion that calcification is a healing response to atherosclerosis [11]. Clinical observations suggest that lesions responsible for acute episodes are generally less calcified than plaques responsible for stable angina.

Imaging of Coronary Atheroma

Atherosclerosis has historically been considered as a segmental disease, but this concept can be challenged as at least 20–30% of patients with an acute coronary syndrome have one or more disrupted plaques present intravascular at ultrasound [20]. Moreover, it is well recognized that the coronary tree of patients with angiographically unseen disease may have plaques at high risk of rupture and thrombosis. Traditional angiography is insensitive for the detection of plaques that do not encroach on the lumen as this technique is intended for the detection of pinpoint stenoses. It allows only an indirect view of the atheroma and is often unable to detect a potentially fatal lesion. Intravascular ultrasound (IVUS) has demonstrated that angiographically normal segments of an artery may contain large plaques, as there is no direct relation between plaque size and the degree of stenosis.

The concept of "vulnerable plaques" indicates that the morphology of plaque is more clinically more important than the plaque volume and/or the degree of luminal stenosis. The identification of patients with vulnerable plaques is difficult and has inspired the development of new methods of in vivo coronary plaque imaging in hopes of providing methods of intervention. Although great progress has been made, invasive and noninvasive methods still provide a limited view of coronary artery disease. The new imaging techniques have yet to provide the resolution necessary for identification of the thin-cap fibroatheroma. The combination of several sophisticated imaging methods (i.e., OCT/backscattered IVUS; IVUS/Raman spectroscopy OCT [optical coherence tomography]; IVUS [intravascular ultrasound]) may provide the most information on the presence or absence of disease [8]. Histology remains the reference method for postmortem examination as it maximizes the understanding of the clinical aspects of acute coronary syndromes.

Acute Coronary Syndromes

Acute coronary syndrome (ACS) refers to a wide spectrum of clinical syndromes including unstable angina (UA), non-ST segment elevation myocardial infarction (NSTEMI), and ST

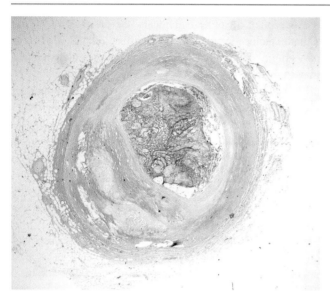

Fig. 7.6 Acute coronary thrombosis seen as the dark red thrombus matter occluding the lumen of the artery. Significant fibrolipid plaque disease is present

segment elevation myocardial infarction (STEMI). Occlusive or mural thrombosis involving a vulnerable plaque represents the main cause of acute coronary syndromes (Fig. 7.6). Such plaque rupture accounts for more than 85% of all thrombi associated with sudden coronary death or acute myocardial infarction in white males with high concentrations of low-density lipoprotein (LDL) [8]. Plaque erosion results in acute myocardial infarction and sudden cardiac death primarily in patients under the age of 50 and represents the majority of acute coronary thrombi in premenopausal women [21].

The pathophysiologic origins and clinical presentations of UA and NSTEMI are similar, but they differ in severity. A diagnosis of NSTEMI can be made when the ischemia is severe enough to cause myocardial damage, resulting in the release of biomarkers of myocardial necrosis into the circulation. The diagnosis of UA is based on the absence of detectable biomarkers hours after the initial onset of ischemic chest pain [22, 23].

The underlining physiopathology of unstable angina, non-ST segment elevation angina, and ST segment elevation myocardial infarction are different. UA and NSTEMI are characterized by partial occlusion of the infarct-related artery. UA is caused by thrombi that project into the arterial lumen without full occlusion. Embolization of platelet/fibrin fragments into the distal vascular bed causes small microscopic foci of necrosis and is thought to be responsible for episodic chest pain. For STEMI, the infarct-related artery is usually rapidly totally occluded. This occlusion is followed soon afterward by the onset of symptoms and/or sudden death (see Fig. 7.6).

Two strategies of coronary reperfusion exist. These include pharmacological (fibrinolysis) and mechanical (primary percutaneous coronary intervention (PCI)). These strategies followed improved appreciation of the role of platelet activation, and aggregation in ongoing ischemic events has led to the use of more effective antiplatelet therapies. In addition, alternative approaches to heparin and antithrombin therapies have been developed in tandem [24].

For patients with STEMI, prompt and complete mechanical restoration of flow in the occluded artery decreased infarct size, preserves left ventricular function, and improves survival rates. Therefore, patients with STEMI require immediate reperfusion therapy with either primary PCI and/or fibrinolysis. Early reopening of the infarct-related artery limits infarct size and also reduces life-threatening complications like transmural extension, ventricular remodeling with aneurysms, cardiogenic shock, and pericarditis.

For patients with UA/NSTEMI, an early invasive strategy involves routine cardiac catheterization followed by PCI. An initial conservative strategy may start with medical management followed by catheterization and revascularization only if ischemia recurs despite vigorous medical therapy.

Antithrombotic therapy is the cornerstone of treatment with two components. Firstly, there is antiplatelet therapy which reduces platelet activation and aggregation. Secondly, there is anticoagulant therapy which targets the clotting cascade to prevent thrombus stabilization [22, 23].

Sudden Coronary Death

Instant death by ventricular fibrillation or atrioventricular (AV) block frequently complicates coronary thrombosis before medical intervention and represents 50% of the mortality of acute myocardial infarction. Intervention in such cases is required within minutes in order to avoid irreversible brain damage [4]. Cardiogenic shock is responsible for the majority of deaths in patients who have reached intensive care. Those with infarcts involving more than 40–50% of the total left ventricular mass rarely survive. These are mostly due to very proximal thrombotic occlusion of the left anterior descending artery [19].

Myocardial Infarction

Coronary artery thrombosis is the most common cause of acute myocardial infarction. If a coronary artery is occluded for more than 20 min, then irreversible damage to the myocardium occurs, but lesser periods of ischemia also cause myocardial tissue dysfunction and tissue loss. Spontaneous reperfusion of the infarcted area can occur, with recanalization of the affected artery (Fig. 7.7), but coronary artery occlusion persists in most patients [25]. Persistent occlusion

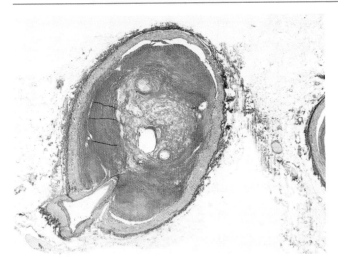

Fig. 7.7 Recanalization of coronary artery in the late stages after thrombosis in which many small capillary-sized channels are noted (elastic van Gieson)

results in a progressive increase of the infarct size with a wave-front transmural extension from the endocardium towards the epicardium [26] reflecting the oxygen/perfusion gradient across the tissue. The infarct size depends on the amount of cardiac muscle perfused by the artery, the magnitude of residual flow based on the degree of occlusion, collateral circulation, and the duration of ischemia [25].

Two coronary arteries arise from the root of the aorta (main left and right), but usually one considers there are functionally three arteries (see Chap. 1). The left anterior descending artery supplies up to 50% of the total left ventricular mass, the whole anterior wall of the left ventricle, and the anterior two-thirds of the interventricular septum. The right coronary artery supplies 30–40% of the left ventricular mass, the right ventricle, and the posterior part of the ventricular septum. The left circumflex coronary artery supplies about 20% of the myocardial mass. There is virtually no overlap between the regions supplied by these three arteries [19]. The coronary arteries are thus considered as "end arteries" since they provide the only source of blood to the varied regions of the myocardium. There is very little redundant blood supply, which explains why blockage of these vessels can be so critical. However, if one artery develops high-grade stenosis, then pressure gradients can enlarge previously existing small vessels and allow collateral flow to a limited extent.

The relationship and outcomes between atherosclerotic stenosis and ischemia are complex (Fig. 7.8). Following an acute coronary occlusion, the infarct size depends mainly on the extent of the territory distal to the culprit coronary plaque, the presence and magnitude of residual flow (subtotal occlusion, collaterals), and the duration of ischemia [25]. The flow reduction depends on many variables as

collateral flow, but also on spasm, increased peripheral resistance by vascular compression, inflammatory nerve irritation, etc. Severe stenosis (Fig. 7.9) may exist months or years before onset of the first symptoms, and there is no relationship between the degree of coronary stenosis and the onset of symptoms, complications, and acute coronary syndrome mortality. A significant proportion of thrombotic occlusions do not develop at sites of preexisting high-grade stenosis or plaque formation. Indeed, up to 75% of the occlusions leading to acute infarction have a previous diameter stenosis less than 50%, and only a minor percentage of occlusions are develop on stenosis with a previous diameter greater than 70% [5].

Histological caution is required in differentiating between a thrombus and coagulum. A thrombus is firmly attached to the vulnerable/damaged plaque and consists of a platelet plug and fibrin deposition of layered growth (Zahn's lines). By contrast, a coagulum is comprised of normal blood components (red blood cells, leukocytes, platelets, and a fine network of fibrin), is not attached to the artery wall, and may occur perimortem. There may be discrepancy between the age of a thrombus and the age of the infarct. Microscopically, fully organized thrombi resulting from previous plaque rupture, known as healed plaque ruptures, have been identified in up to 10% of patients with clinical coronary artery disease [27]. Approximately two-thirds of coronary thrombi in sudden coronary deaths can be seen as well organized, and women have a greater frequency of erosion and late-stage thrombi [28]. In a reperfused infarct, the distal embolization of plaque debris and thrombus into the microvasculature may also be observed.

Acute myocardial infarction presents as two main pathological forms:

- Transmural infarction – full-thickness myocardial necrosis of the ventricular wall, usually precipitated by an occlusive thrombosis of a coronary artery (STEMI)
- Subendocardial myocardial infarction (nontransmural, clinically non-Q-wave infarction) – where the myocardial infarct is confined to the inner subendocardial layers of the ventricular wall, usually resulting from multiple vessel obstructive coronary atherosclerosis without complete luminal occlusion (NSTEMI)

Myocardial infarcts are currently classified by size, location, and duration. Size categories include microscopic (focal necrosis), small (<10% of the left ventricular myocardium), moderate (10–30%), and large (>30%). Temporal categories include evolving (<6 h), acute (6 h to 7 days), healing (7–28 days), and healed (more than 28 days) [29].

The macroscopic and histological changes that result from acute myocardial infarction depend on many factors – most importantly, the time between the onset and completion of coronary occlusion. The presence of a coronary artery thrombus does not necessarily confer a diagnosis of myocardial infarction, particularly in cases without apparent histological

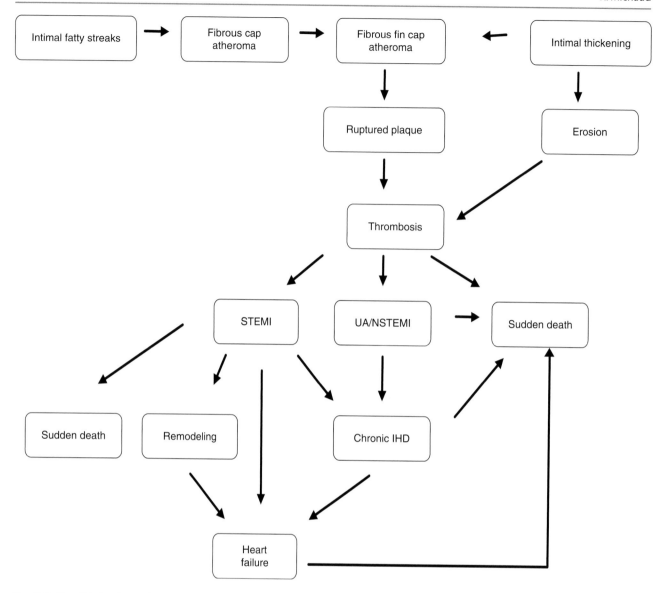

Fig. 7.8 Simplified scheme for ischemic heart disease. Following disruption of a vulnerable plaque or erosion, the flow through the affected epicardial coronary artery will be reduced. In STEMI, the infarct-related artery is usually rapidly totally occluded. This occlusion is followed shortly by the onset of symptoms and/or sudden death. UA and UNSTEMI are characterized by partial occlusion of the infarct-related artery. With unstable angina (UA), thrombi project into the arterial lumen but do not completely occlude it. Cardiac postinfarct remodeling or chronic ischemic heart failure may lead to heart failure/ sudden death

changes, as an occlusive thrombus does not always have time to result in a morphological infarction.

Complications of acute myocardial infarction include ventricular arrhythmias, cardiogenic shock, cardiac rupture (Fig. 7.10), fibrinous pericarditis, aneurysm formation, endocardial thrombosis, and thromboembolism.

Macroscopical Examination

Myocardial changes are difficult to identify on postmortem examination within the first 6 h following complete coronary occlusion. The previous gross histochemical method of immersing a slice of the heart in a solution of nitro blue tetrazolium (NBT), leaving a blue stain due to the enzymes in viable tissue, and not in dead tissue. The historical gross method for identifying infarction involved immersing a slice of the heart in a solution of nitro blue tetrazolium (NBT). This left a blue stain reaction in viable tissue and none in areas of dead tissue. It is no longer used routinely in many laboratories as these chemicals are deemed hazardous/carcinogenic.

However, by naked eye observation, the infarcted region is noted to be paler than normal tissue 6–12 h after vessel occlusion and turns somewhat gray from 18 to 24 h. From 1 to 3 days, the infarcted area becomes centered by a yellow-tan core, which is then surrounded by a hyperemic border

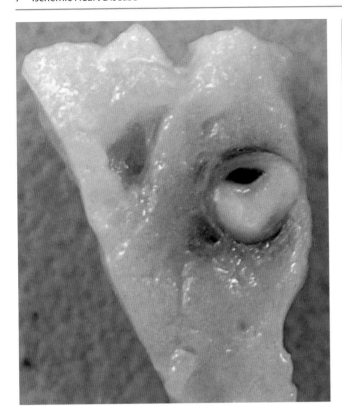

Fig. 7.9 Lipid-rich plaque causing high-grade stenosis, capable of causing angina symptoms or pose a risk for thrombosis and sudden death

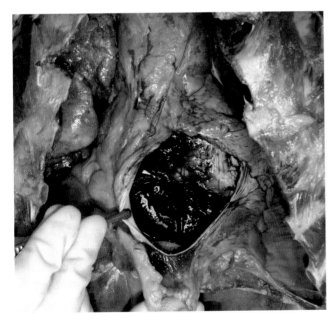

Fig. 7.10 Cardiac tamponade after a myocardial rupture. This is usually 3–6 days after infarction symptoms start

from days 3–7, eventually involving the entire infarct on days 7–10. A fibrous gray scar starts from the periphery and moves to the center of the infarct from the second week. The scar repair process is often complete after the second month (Fig. 7.11) [29].

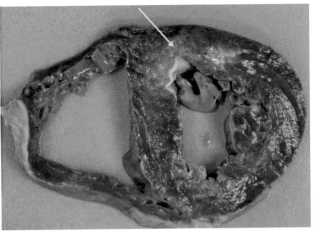

Fig. 7.11 An old myocardial infarction fibrous scar (*arrowed*) following occlusion of the right coronary artery

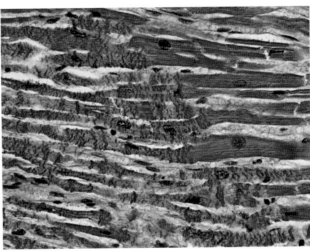

Fig. 7.12 Myocardial infarction showing contraction band necrosis (hematoxylin & eosin)

It must be remembered that virtually no patient currently in a modern hospital setting is left to experience an infarct without some attempted revascularization, antiplatelet, and supportive drug therapy. Consequently, the untreated infarct in evolution is only seen in cases without medical therapy derived from the community.

Histological Patterns of Infarction

In experimental studies, myocardial ischemia results in characteristic metabolic and ultrastructural alterations of myocytes, involving the mitochondria, nuclei, myofilaments, and sarcolemma [30].

The earliest histological signs consist of mild myofibril eosinophilia, elongation of sarcomeres and nuclei [31]. Contraction band necrosis occurs, being seen as irregular

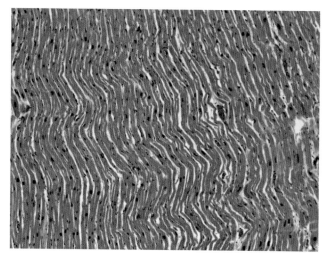

Fig. 7.13 Waviness of myocytes (hematoxylin & eosin)

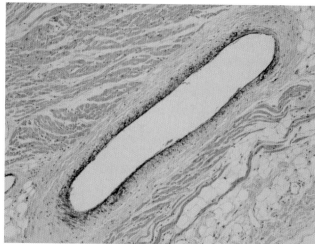

Fig. 7.14 Subendothelial accumulation of c5b9 in early myocardial ischemia (DAB immunohistology)

or pathological bands formed by segments of hypercontracted sarcomeres with scalloped sarcolemmas (Fig. 7.12). Contraction band necrosis is a frequent finding of postmortem examination in sudden death victims of atherosclerotic coronary artery disease. This lesion can also be produced by intravenous infusions of catecholamines and is also known as coagulative myocytolysis, Zenker's necrosis, or catecholamine necrosis. Contraction band necrosis occurs soon after the onset of myocyte death. It is thought to be due to the restoration of calcium ions in the interstitial tissues, which enter the dying myocytes, resulting in intense hypercontraction of the myofibers. Myocyte waviness (Fig. 7.13) of normal cells is visible at the periphery of the infarct [29] but is subjective. Another form of a diffuse pathological contraction band is observed in experimental reperfusion and reflow necrosis studies. In this situation, pathological contraction bands are associated with extensive interstitial hemorrhage.

Current immunohistochemical methods, which utilize plasma (C5b-9, fibronectin) and cellular (myoglobin, cardiac troponin) markers, can improve the ability to detect ischemia when no morphological evidence of necrosis is found (Fig. 7.14). The interpretation of immunohistochemical staining should also consider factors as cardiopulmonary resuscitation and other agonal events that may affect marker expression [32, 33].

Using standard histology staining techniques, the earliest evidence of infarction is visible 6–8 h after the onset of acute ischemia. The infarcted cardiac muscle fibers show a patchy cross striation blurring with increased eosin staining. The capillaries are often engorged, and interstitial edema becomes evident after 8 h.

After 12 h, neutrophilic infiltrates appear, and coagulative necrosis with nuclear pyknosis develops. Coagulative necrosis is characterized by hypereosinophilic changes in the myocytes.

One to 3 days postischemic onset, the infarcted fibers become intensively eosinophilic and lose their nuclei. There

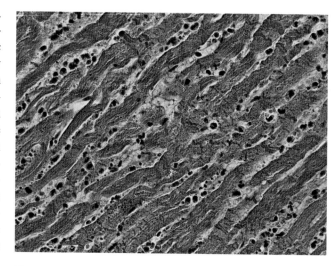

Fig. 7.15 Myocardial infarction with necrosis of myocytes and diffuse infiltration of polymorphonuclear neutrophil cells (hematoxylin & eosin)

is infiltration of neutrophils at the infarct periphery, and these migrate towards the edematous center (Fig. 7.15).

From days 3–7, macrophages remove the necrotic fragments, and a progressive infiltration of lymphocytes and fibroblasts occurs. The necrotic cardiac muscle progressively disappears as a result of the combined phagocytic activity of neutrophils and macrophages, which is replaced by neovascularized granulation tissue (Fig. 7.16). By 14 days, fibrovascular granulation tissue is present at the infarct site, which is progressively replaced by a highly collagenous, virtually acellular scar around 3–6 weeks later (Fig. 7.17). Again, it is emphasized that current medical treatments means that the sequence above is rarely followed verbatim.

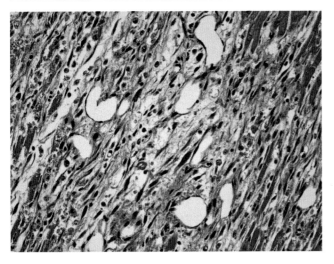

Fig. 7.16 Neovascularized granulation tissue (hematoxylin & eosin)

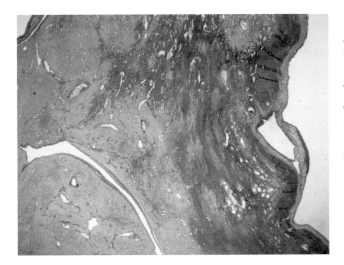

Fig. 7.17 Postinfarct scar showing dense collagen (*red*) with viable myocardial tissue adjacent (elastic van Gieson)

Myocardial Reperfusion

Timely coronary recanalization and myocardial reperfusion limit the extent of myocardial necrosis. However, recanalization techniques have been shown to induce "reperfusion injuries," as described in experimental animals by Klonner [34]. Such injuries include lethal reperfusion injury (myocyte death), "no-reflow" microvascular damage related to the absence of distal myocardial reperfusion after a prolonged period of ischemia, stunned myocardium, and life-threatening reperfusion arrhythmias [4].

A reperfused myocardial hemorrhagic infarct can occur within the area of necrosis, which is significantly related to the infarct size and coronary occlusion time. It has also been described after cardiac surgery, percutaneous transluminal coronary angioplasty, and fibrinolysis therapies.

The infarct following coronary artery recanalization, either pharmacological or interventional, is characterized by frequent subendocardial localization and appears macroscopically red because of interstitial hemorrhage. Hemorrhagic infarcts are thought to be caused by vascular cell damage with leakage of blood from injured vessels [29]. Microscopically, the typical reperfused infarct consists of contraction band necrosis and interstitial hemorrhage. Reperfusion after prolonged coronary occlusion is associated with secondary impairment of microcirculatory flow, which follows endothelial swelling, luminal obstruction, and external compression by edema, hemorrhage, and myocyte swelling. Interventional manipulation may be aggravated by distal embolization of luminal debris. The complications of reperfused myocardial infarcts are related to arrhythmias, increased myocardial stiffness, a propensity to wall rupture, and delayed healing.

Stunned and Hibernating Myocardium

The recognition of noncontracting myocardium (postrevascularization) is a well-known clinical phenomenon. There are two myocardial forms: stunned and hibernating myocardia.

Stunned myocardium is viable myocardium salvaged by coronary reperfusion that exhibits prolonged postischemic dysfunction despite reperfusion [35, 36]. Stunned myocardium has been identified in patients after thrombolysis or percutaneous transluminal angiography, in patients with unstable angina, in exercise-induced angina, after coronary artery spasm, in transient thrombosis of a coronary artery, and immediately after coronary artery bypass surgery. Stunned myocardium returns to normal after a variable period of time (hours to weeks). Normally no treatment is required since there is adequate blood flow, and contractile function recovers spontaneously. If myocardial stunning is severe, involving large parts of the left ventricle impairing its function, inotropic agents and procedures can assist survival and thereby recovery.

Hibernating myocardium reflects a prolonged imbalance between the supply and demand for myocardial oxygen, and nutrition leads to a subacute or chronic state of myocardial ischemia. Hibernating myocardium is supplied by a diminished vasculature. The ischemic cardiac cells remain viable, but contractile function is reduced. Cardiac myocytes adapt to the low-energy supply by reducing their contractile function and metabolic rate, in attempts to conserve resources and preserve myocardial integrity. Hibernating myocardium contains normal myocytes, apoptotic cells, cells with autophagosomes, lysosomes, and vacuoles (Fig. 7.18). Chronic ischemia is also associated with changes in the number, size, and distribution of gap junctions and may give rise to conduction disturbances

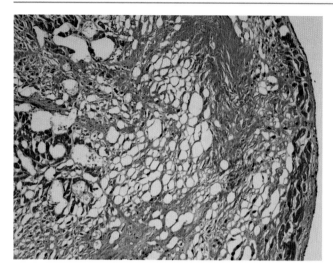

Fig. 7.18 Hibernating myocardium (hematoxylin & eosin)

and arrhythmogenesis. Recent studies suggest that autophagy may play a potential role in myocyte death as a part of the remodeling process in hibernating myocardium and by maintaining the balance between myocyte protein synthesis and degradation in heart failure [37, 38].

The treatment for hibernating myocardium is the restoration of adequate blood flow. Early revascularization may prevent myocyte degradation. The amount of hibernating myocardium and the degree of structural alteration determine the extent of functional recovery after restoration of blood flow. Several new approaches offer promising alternatives, such as vascular endothelial growth factor and fibroblast growth factor-2, which have been shown to be effective for rapid neovascularization. Substances such as statins, resveratrol, some hormones, and omega-3 fatty acids can also enhance recovery in chronically underperfused hearts. For patients with drug-refractory ischemia, intramyocardial transplantation of stem cells into predefined areas of the heart might in the future enhance vascularization and improve cardiac function [39].

The Failing Heart (aka Acute Heart Failure Syndrome) and Remodeling

Heart failure is a complex clinical syndrome that can result from any structural or functional cardiac disorder that impairs the ability of the ventricle to fill and/or eject blood [40]. Most definitions of heart failure are imprecise and include references to typical clinical symptoms and objective assessment of abnormal ventricular function. There are many ways to categorize heart failure. These include the side of the heart involved (left, right, biventricular), whether the abnormality is due to contraction or relaxation of the heart (systolic or diastolic dysfunction), low- or high-output heart states, and

considering the degree of functional impairment conferred by the abnormality (e.g., NYHA functional classification) [40].

Heart failure is usually associated with a structural abnormality of the heart. The pathological causes of heart failure can be put into six major categories [47]:
1. Failure related to myocardial abnormalities, related to any cause of loss of muscle fibers, such as myocardial infarction or inappropriate function, and diminished contractility, such as cardiomyopathies
2. Failure related to overload such as hypertension
3. Failure related to valvular abnormalities
4. Failure related to abnormal rhythm, especially tachyarrhythmia
5. Pericardial abnormalities or pericardial effusion (tamponade)
6. Congenital cardiac lesions

Coronary artery disease is believed to be the underlying cause in approximately two-thirds of patients with heart failure, related to acute or chronic injury to the heart.

Acute heart failure syndrome (AHFS) is defined as gradual or rapid change in heart failure signs and symptoms resulting in a need for urgent care. These symptoms are primarily the result of severe pulmonary congestion due to elevated left ventricular filling pressures. Concurrent cardiovascular conditions such as coronary heart disease, hypertension, valvular heart disease, atrial arrhythmias, and/or noncardiac conditions (including renal dysfunction, diabetes, and anemia) are often present and may precipitate or contribute to the pathophysiology of this syndrome [41]. Approximately 60% of AHFS patients have underlying coronary artery disease and may present with acute coronary syndrome complicated by AHFS or more commonly with AHFS and underlying coronary artery disease [42].

Cardiac remodeling refers to the changes in size, shape, and function of the heart after injury to the ventricles. It represents a series of initially compensatory but subsequently maladapted mechanisms, which can often result in heart failure. The injury is typically due to acute myocardial infarction but may be from any number of causes that result in increased pressure or volume overload on the heart – such as chronic hypertension, congenital heart disease, and valvular heart disease.

The cardiac remodeling that occurs within days to weeks postinfarction is associated with a change in the geometry and structure of the left ventricle. There is radial thinning and circumferential increase of the infarct, such that the chamber becomes dilated and/or hypertrophied and the heart becomes more spherical. This change in chamber size and structure increases the hemodynamic stress on the walls of the failing heart, induces mitral valve incompetence, and reduces cardiac performance. These effects sustain and exacerbate the remodeling process.

Postinfarction remodeling has been divided into two phases: early (<72 h) and late (>72 h). The early phase, which is related to the degradation of the collagen network in the infarcted area, includes expansion of the infarct zone, which can result in early ventricular rupture or aneurysm formation [29]. Early cardiac rupture, leading to tamponade, occurs at the junction of viable and nonviable tissue and is thought to be due to the shearing stress between the noncontractile muscle and contracting viable muscle [43]. Later rupture of the left ventricle is a complication of the expanding infarct. Postinfarction cardiac rupture includes free wall rupture, ventricular septal defects, and papillary muscle rupture. Free wall rupture occurs ten times more frequently than septal or papillary muscle rupture [25]. An ischemic left ventricular aneurysm, resulting from infarct expansion, also has an increased risk of rupture as well as potentially producing systemic emboli. The ischemic aneurysm is also associated with abnormal left ventricular function, with a marked tendency to cause episodic ventricular tachycardia. The aneurysm consists of an aneurysmal sac with a wide neck and a fibrous wall free of residual myocardium. The endocardium is usually fibrous, may contain laminated thrombus, or extend into a large sac. Ventricular septal defects usually arise from expansion of either an anteroseptal or a posteroseptal infarct [19].

Late postinfarction remodeling involves the entire left ventricle and is associated with dilatation and mural compensatory hypertrophy. This is a process lasting several months to years and often precedes the development of chronic heart failure symptoms. Remodeling continues after the appearance of symptoms and substantially contributes to worsening of symptoms despite treatment. The progression of heart failure is also exacerbated by progression of causative diseases and persistence of the risk factors/drivers.

The number of patients surviving with advanced heart failure is increasing rapidly in modern society, and there are multiple guidelines concerning drug therapy choices. Some patients remain symptomatic and have to be managed with surgical therapies such as biventricular pacemakers, ventricular assist devices, and potentially heart transplantation.

Right and Biventricular Heart Failure in Ischemic Heart Disease

Right ventricular involvement in coronary artery disease includes isolated infarcts resulting from right coronary artery occlusion proximal to the right ventricular branches and transmural inferior-posterior left ventricular infarcts. Necropsy studies demonstrate pathologic evidence of right ventricular infarction in 14–60% of patients dying of inferior myocardial infarction typically inscribing a "tripartite" pathologic signature consisting of left ventricle inferior-posterior wall, septal and posterior right ventricular free wall necrosis contiguous with the septum, with less frequent extension into the anterolateral wall. However, the right ventricle appears to be relatively resistant to infarction and has a remarkable ability to recover, even after prolonged occlusion. Right ventricle performance improves spontaneously even in the absence of reperfusion, although recovery of function may be slow and associated with high in-hospital mortality due to a high-grade atrioventricular (AV) block. Bradycardia-hypotension without AV block may complicate inferior myocardial infarction. Reperfusion enhances the recovery of the right ventricular performance and improves the clinical course and survival of patients with ischemic right ventricular dysfunction. Many patients manifest spontaneous clinical improvement within 3–10 days regardless of the patency status of the infarct-related artery. Furthermore, global right ventricular performance typically recovers over several weeks, with subsequent return of right ventricular ejection fraction to near-normal levels within 3–12 months [44, 45].

Nonatherosclerotic Causes of Acute Coronary Syndromes

Not all ischemic events of the heart relate to atheromatous pathology although this is clearly the prime disease process. Other nonatherosclerotic diseases include the following:

Obliterative intimal thickening of the coronary arteries (late stage). This may be found in a variety of pathology such as coarctation of the aorta, transplanted hearts, infectious immune process, polyarteritis nodosa [42], and rheumatic fever.

Coronary artery dissection. In adults, isolated coronary artery dissection may precipitate acute infarction and sudden death (Fig. 7.19). The process often starts as subadventitial hematoma which compresses the vessel lumen from outside.

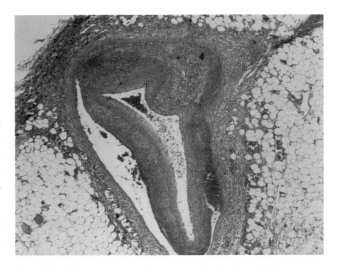

Fig. 7.19 Coronary artery dissection. A subadventitial hematoma between the media and the adventitia in a 42-year-old man

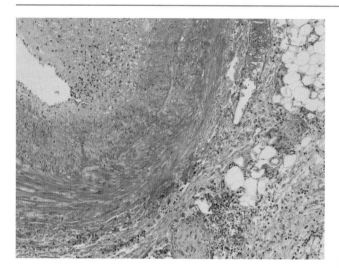

Fig. 7.20 Coronary artery vasculitis in a 36-year-old woman who died suddenly

The pathogenesis is not clear but may follow an eosinophilic inflammatory adventitial process. It can also follow PCI.

Ostial stenosis. This was traditionally related to syphilitic aortitis and is probably more common with Takayasu disease. It may also occur as an isolated phenomenon particularly with other inflammatory arteritis.

Coronary arteritis and aneurysm. This is rare and may be observed in isolated form of vasculitis (Fig. 7.20) or as a manifestation of systematic disease polyarteritis nodosa or Wegener's granulomatosis. Coronary artery aneurysm may be traumatic, congenital, or may follow Kawasaki's disease [19].

Coronary emboli represent a rare finding and may be observed in bacterial endocarditis on the aortic valve carrying emboli beyond the coronary orifices.

Coronary artery spasm is a brief, temporary vessel contraction and can lead to chest pain (angina) and myocardial infarction. The spasm may occur at rest.

Tunneled coronary artery or myocardial bridging defines a congenital coronary abnormality with a segment of a major epicardial coronary artery that burrows intramurally through the myocardium beneath the muscle "bridge." Generally it is seen in the midleft anterior descending artery. The degree of coronary obstruction by the myocardial bridge depends on the location, thickness, length of the bridge, and degree of cardiac contractility. Traditionally, myocardial bridging has been considered a benign condition, but angina, acute coronary syndromes, and sudden death have been reported [46].

References

1. Shah PK. Screening asymptomatic subjects for subclinical atherosclerosis: can we, does it matter, and should we? J Am Coll Cardiol. 2010;56(2):98–105.
2. Gibbons RJ, et al. The American Heart Association's 2008 statement of principles for healthcare reform. Circulation. 2008;118(21):2209–18.
3. Yusuf S, et al. Effect of potentially modifiable risk factors associated with myocardial infarction in 52 countries (the INTERHEART study): case–control study. Lancet. 2004;364(9438):937–52.
4. Thiene G, Basso C. Myocardial infarction: a paradigm of success in modern medicine. Cardiovas Pathol. 2010;19:1–5.
5. Falk E. Pathogenesis of atherosclerosis. J Am Coll Cardiol. 2006;47(8, Supplement 1):C7–12.
6. Ross R, Glomset JA. The pathogenesis of atherosclerosis. N Engl J Med. 1976;295(7):369–77.
7. Ross R. Atherosclerosis – an inflammatory disease. N Engl J Med. 1999;340(2):115–26.
8. Moreno PR. Vulnerable plaque: definition, diagnosis, and treatment. Cardiol Clin. 2010;28(1):1–30.
9. Finn AV, et al. Concept of vulnerable/unstable plaque. Arterioscler Thromb Vasc Biol. 2010;30(7):1282–92.
10. Packard RRS, Libby P. Inflammation in atherosclerosis: from vascular biology to biomarker discovery and risk prediction. Clin Chem. 2008;54(1):24–38.
11. Sanz J, Moreno PR, Fuster V. The year in atherothrombosis. J Am Coll Cardiol. 2010;55(14):1487–98.
12. Moreno PR, Sanz J, Fuster V. Promoting mechanisms of vascular health: circulating progenitor cells, angiogenesis, and reverse cholesterol transport. J Am Coll Cardiol. 2009;53(25):2315–23.
13. Glagov S, et al. Compensatory enlargement of human atherosclerotic coronary arteries. N Engl J Med. 1987;16(22):1371–5.
14. Schoenhagen P, et al. Extent and direction of arterial remodeling in stable versus unstable coronary syndromes: an intravascular ultrasound study. Circulation. 2000;101(6):598–603.
15. Ambrose J, et al. Angiographic progression of coronary artery disease and the development of myocardial infarction. J Am Coll Cardiol. 1988;12(1):56–62.
16. Burke AP, et al. Coronary risk factors and plaque morphology in men with coronary disease who died suddenly. N Engl J Med. 1997;336(18):1276–82.
17. Davies MJ. The pathophysiology of acute coronary syndromes. Heart. 2000;83(3):361–6.
18. Virmani R, et al. Vulnerable plaque: the pathology of unstable coronary lesions. J Interv Cardiol. 2002;15(6):439–46.
19. Sheppard M, Davies MJ. Practical cardiovascular pathology. London: Arnold Publishers, ISBN-10: 034067749X; 1998. p. 17–50.
20. Libby P. Act local, act global: inflammation and the multiplicity of "vulnerable" coronary plaques. J Am Coll Cardiol. 2005;45(10):1600–2.
21. Virmani R, et al. Pathology of the vulnerable plaque. J Am Coll Cardiol. 2006;47(8, Supplement 1):C13–8.
22. Kumar A, Cannon CP. Acute coronary syndromes: diagnosis and management, part II. Mayo Clin Proc. 2009;84(11):1021–36.
23. Kumar A, Cannon CP. Acute coronary syndromes: diagnosis and management, part I. Mayo Clin Proc. 2009;84(10):917–38.
24. White HD, Chew DP. Acute myocardial infarction. Lancet. 2008;372(9638):570–84.
25. Basso C, Thiene G. The pathophysiology of myocardial reperfusion: a pathologist's perspective. Heart. 2006;92(11):1559–62.
26. Reimer KA, Jennings RB. The "wavefront phenomenon" of myocardial ischemic cell death. II. Transmural progression of necrosis within the framework of ischemic bed size (myocardium at risk) and collateral flow. Lab Invest. 1979;40(6):633–44.
27. van der Wal AC. Coronary artery pathology. Heart. 2007;93(11):1484–9.
28. Kramer MCA, et al. Relationship of thrombus healing to underlying plaque morphology in sudden coronary death. J Am Coll Cardiol. 2010;55(2):122–32.
29. Basso C, Rizzo S, Thiene G. The metamorphosis of myocardial infarction following coronary recanalization. Cardiovasc Pathol. 2010;19(1):22–8.
30. Buja LM. Myocardial ischemia and reperfusion injury. Cardiovasc Pathol. 2005;14(4):170–5.

31. Fineschi V, Baroldi G, Silver MD, editors. Pathology of the heart and sudden death in forensic medicine. London/New York: CRC Press/Taylor & Francis; 2006. p. 78–113.

32. Campobasso CP, Dell'Erba AS, Addante A, Zotti F, Marzullo A, Colonna MF. Sudden Cardiac Death and Myocardial Ischemia Indicators: A Comparative Study of Four Immunohistochemical Markers. American Journal of Forensic Medicine & Pathology 2008;29:154–61.

33. Ortmann C, Pfeiffer H, Brinkmann B. A comparative study on the immunohistochemical detection of early myocardial damage. Int J Legal Med. 2000;113(4):215–20.

34. Robert RA, Ganote CE, Jennings RB. The "no-reflow" phenomenon after temporary coronary occlusion in the dog. J Clin Invest. 1974;54(6):1496–508.

35. Kloner RA, Jennings RB. Consequences of brief ischemia: stunning, preconditioning, and their clinical implications: part 2. Circulation. 2001;104(25):3158–67.

36. Kloner RA, Jennings RB. Consequences of brief ischemia: stunning, preconditioning, and their clinical implications: part 1. Circulation. 2001;104(24):2981–9.

37. De Meyer G, De Keulenaer G, Martinet W. Role of autophagy in heart failure associated with aging. Heart Fail Rev. 2010;15:423–30.

38. Kunapuli S, Rosanio S, Schwarz ER. "How do cardiomyocytes die?" Apoptosis and autophagic cell death in cardiac myocytes. J Cardiac Fail. 2006;12(5):381–91.

39. Slezak J, et al. Hibernating myocardium: pathophysiology, diagnosis and treatment. Can J Physiol Pharmacol. 2009;87:252–65.

40. Writing Committee Members, et al. 2009 Focused update incorporated into the ACC/AHA 2005 guidelines for the diagnosis and management of heart failure in adults: A report of the American College of Cardiology Foundation/American Heart Association task force on practice guidelines: developed in collaboration with the International Society for Heart and Lung Transplantation. Circulation. 2009;119(14):e391–479.

41. Gheorghiade M, et al. Acute heart failure syndromes: current state and framework for future research. Circulation. 2005;112(25):3958–68.

42. Pang PS, Komajda M, Gheorghiade M. The current and future management of acute heart failure syndromes. Eur Heart J. 2010;31(7): 784–93.

43. Becker A, van Mantgem J. Cardiac tamponade. A study of 50 hearts. Eur J Cardiol. 1975;3(4):349–58.

44. Rambihar S, Dokainish H. Right ventricular involvement in patients with coronary artery disease. Curr Opin Cardiol. 2010;25(5):456–63. doi:10.1097/HCO.0b013e32833c7bf5.

45. Goldstein JA. Pathophysiology and management of right heart ischemia. J Am Coll Cardiol. 2002;40(5):841–53.

46. Alegria JR, et al. Myocardial bridging. Eur Heart J. 2005;26(12): 1159–68.

47. Butany J. Pathology of cardiac diseases leading to acute and chronic heart failure. Teaching course, Heart failure: causes and modern approach to diagnosis and treatment, Companion Meeting, 25th Anniversary of the Society for Cardiovascular Pathology: an update on endomyocardial biopsy, March 20,2010, 98 th Annual Meeting of the United States & Canadian Academy of Pathology, Washington.

Myocarditis/Inflammatory Cardiomyopathy

8

Ulrik Baandrup

Abstract

Myocarditis/inflammatory cardiomyopathy is defined as inflammatory involvement of heart muscle with leukocytic cell infiltration and nonischemic degeneration/necrosis of myocytes.

The actual incidence of myocarditis is unknown, although the disease process is often related to infections. The commonest driver is primary viral infection, although occasionally reactivation of viral infections may be relevant. Furthermore, bacterial, fungal and protozoal infections may be implicated. Other drivers for myocarditis include autoimmune processes, drugs and toxins. Many cases, however, are ultimately designated idiopathic. The patterns for these myocarditis processes are described and the various pathophysiology is discussed.

In reality, many cases of clinical myocarditis cannot be morphologically verified by endomyocardial biopsy. Clinicians, immunologists, pathologists and those using molecular tests must combine their analyses to explore and redefine myocarditis. At present, whilst considerable progress in the understanding of this disease has been made in the last 50 years, it remains a serious challenge!

Keywords

Myocarditis • Inflammatory cardiomyopathy • Inflammatory heart disease • Dilated cardiomyopathy • Rejection in heart transplantation • Immune disease of the heart Hypersensitivity of the myocardium • Toxic myocarditis • Giant cell myocarditis • Cardiac sarcoidosis Immune-mediated myocarditis • Myocarditis definition • Myocarditis frequency Myocarditis pathogenesis

Introduction

The term myocarditis [1] was first coined by Sobernheim in 1837 but has really only become of interest and concern in the last 50 years. The histological features, subclassification, and varying etiological processes are increasingly being used to determine therapeutic and surgical interventions for this condition.

U. Baandrup, M.D., Ph.D.
Department of Pathology Center for Clinical Research,
Vendsyssel Hospital, Aalborg University,
Bispensgade 37, 9800, Hjørring, Denmark
e-mail: utb@rn.dk

Definition

Myocarditis exists not as one condition but as a group of disorders with the common end point of inflammation within the heart (Figs. 8.1 and 8.2). It is defined as an inflammatory disorder of the heart muscle, characterized by leukocyte infiltration of parenchyma with nonischemic degeneration/ necrosis of cardiac myocytes (Figs. 8.3 and 8.4). This definition does not indicate a specific etiology, other than it being nonischemic in type. The inflammatory infiltrate, in particular, needs analysis and ideally should be quantified, in order to fully appreciate the significance for the individual and the myocardium under assault. Similarly, the consequences of myocarditis need careful consideration as resolution of inflammation can lead to fibrosis and myocytic/

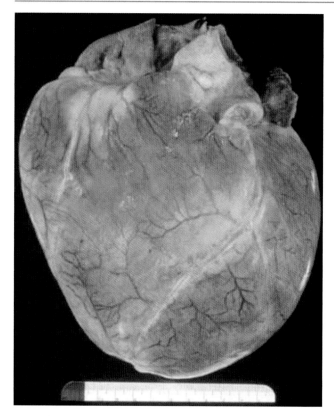

Fig. 8.1 A globally enlarged and dilated heart in a case of acute myocarditis. Note the congested architecture. These cases are often soft on palpation

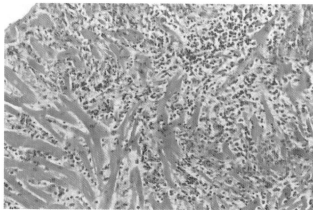

Fig. 8.3 Acute myocarditis of unknown etiology. The infiltrate is granulocytic/lymphocytic. There is obvious eosinophilia with widespread sarcolemmal fraying and myocyte degeneration/necrosis (hematoxylin and eosin)

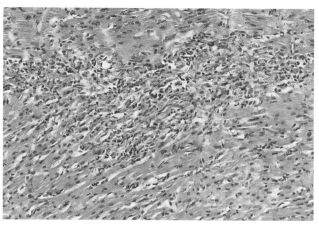

Fig. 8.4 Severe lymphocytic myocarditis with widespread myocyte degeneration. This was a case of a 6-month-old child with adenoviral myocarditis (hematoxylin and eosin)

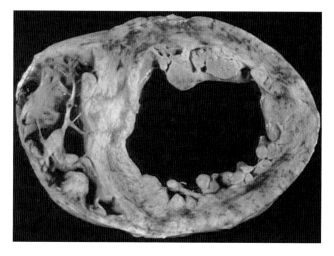

Fig. 8.2 Acute myocarditis, showing the myocardial tissue consistency to be rather soft and congested. Note how it varies in color and tone. There is left ventricle chamber dilatation

myocardial dysfunction. The investigations need to be considered in terms of the disease time line, such that resolving myocarditis and related fibrosis should be considered as the long-term sequelae for any individual.

The term inflammatory cardiomyopathy was reviewed in 1995 by the World Health Organization [2] and is defined as myocarditis in association with cardiac dysfunction, with idiopathic, (auto)immune, and infectious subtypes [3].

The histological criteria for the diagnosis and assessment of myocarditis have been improved following the introduction of standard immunohistochemistry tests and the designation of a cutoff point for infiltrating leukocytes. Specifically, more than 14 lymphocytes/mm^2 and up to 4 macrophages/mm^2 should be required for designation as myocarditis.

Frequency and Incidence

Population analysis to determine the impact of myocarditis has to be accepted as imprecise, at best. The variable symptoms in the acute phase (see below) and the nonspecific features in the chronic/burnt-out phase mean that the full appreciation of the cases of myocarditis is often not

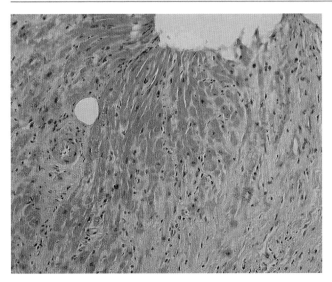

Fig. 8.5 An endomyocardial biopsy from a patient with an earlier diagnosed enteroviral infection. Lymphocytic inflammation and fibrotic scarring are evident, and this may give insight into the possible outcomes for the patient from a clinical perspective, particularly if a series of biopsies are taken over a period of time (hematoxylin and eosin)

recognized.One Swedish general population autopsy study showed a myocarditis rate of 1.06 % [4] although a more focused study of children and young adults showed the incidence from an autopsy cohort to be between 17 and 21 % [5, 6]. Contrastingly, another study of Finnish military service personnel (i.e., the young and fit) showed that acute myocarditis was present at 0.17 per 1,000 man years [7]. In short, it is probably realistic to state that no one actually knows the true prevalence of myocarditis in the general population – unless it is specifically sought by tests as detailed below.

Symptoms

The clinical symptoms [8] of myocarditis range from nil (the asymptomatic cases) through to the rather nonspecific/protean symptoms of malaise and fatigue. More severe cases have significant chest pain, shortness of breath, and advanced symptoms of cardiac failure. Unfortunately, for some individuals, the first symptom is sudden death. Clearly, this wide range of nonspecific symptoms means that diagnosis is often missed, delayed, or completely misinterpreted.

If one survives the acute myocarditis episode (whether there have been symptoms or not), then resolution of the inflammation can lead to a variable degree of fibrosis and myocyte loss (Fig. 8.5). A small degree of myocyte attrition and fibrosis in the walls of the myocardium may have minimal symptomatic or functional effect on cardiac output. However, significant myocardial damage can produce quite severe symptoms of cardiac failure (both left and

Table 8.1 How myocarditis can be sub-typed/grouped

Infectious	Immune-mediated	Toxic	Other/unknown
All types of microorganisms	Post-infectious	Drugs	Sarcoidosis
1. Virus	Systemic disorders	Toxins	Giant cell myocarditis
2. Fungus	Drug hypersensitivity		
3. Bacteria	Transplant rejection		
4. Protozoa			
5. Parasite			

right side) as well as progressive cardiac debility [1, 2, 9] culminating in death.

In many cases, affected individuals present many years after the acute inflammatory process with scarred dysfunctional myocardial parenchyma often in the form of a dilated heart. Indeed, only minor residual nonspecific phenomena may be evident at the point of cardiac transplantation or autopsy investigation [9]. However, any symptoms of potential myocarditis need to be considered with exclusion of coronary artery disease, valvular dysfunction, primary cardiomyopathy, drug-related phenomena, sepsis, and respiratory disease. Just being prepared to consider myocarditis within the differential diagnosis is perhaps the most important aspect in the pathologist: patient interaction.

Etiology and Subtyping of Myocarditis

Myocarditis is classically subdivided according to the pattern of inflammation, the effects on the myocardium, and, if/when identified, the specific etiological pathologies. It is fair to say that the histology can vary to reflect the etiological process, but many common patterns exist in relation to quite diverse pathological insults (Tables 8.1 and 8.2).

Histological review of myocarditis cases reveals a variety of patterns of inflammation which may give insight into the etiology of the inflammation and which may guide treatment. The following discussion is a pragmatic method to subdivide cases – as they present in laboratory practice.

Infections and Myocarditis

Viral Myocarditis

This is perhaps the commonest myocarditic process encountered (Fig. 8.4) and is often diagnosed by endomyocardial biopsy or autopsy techniques when suspected. For subtyping of the precise causative agent, one requires immunohistochemistry, the polymerase chain reaction (PCR), and in-site hybridization(ISH) techniques [10]. The common agents include *coxsackievirus* (A4, A9, and A19 and B1–6

Table 8.2 Some etiological "causes" of myocarditis

Viral, most common	Most common systemic disorders in immune-mediated myocarditis	Toxin and drug-related etiologies
Adenovirus, parvovirus B19, coxsackie B, cytomegalovirus, HHV-6, HIV, influenza A, HSV, respiratory syncytial virus, hepatitis A, vaccinia (smallpox vaccine)[a]	Scleroderma	Amitriptyline, anthracyclines, cefaclor, colchicine, clozapine, furosemide, isoniazid, lidocaine, penicillin, phenytoin, thiazides, tetracycline, trastuzumab.
	Systemic lupus erythematosus	Arsenic, carbon monoxide, copper, ethanol, iron, lead, hymenoptera, snake or scorpion toxins, tetanus toxoid. Hyperpyrexia.
	Polymyositis	
	Wegener's granulomatosis	
	Churg-Strauss syndrome	
	Inflammatory bowel disease (colitis ulcerosa, Crohn's disease, etc.)	

[a]The predominant viral cause of the disease seems to change every decade (Coxsackie virus in 1980s, adenovirus in 1990s, and parvovirus B19 since 2000 [9])

subtypes) *echovirus* (subtypes 4, 9, 16, and 22), and adenovirus infections. These are common causes of lymphocytic myocarditis [1, 5]. Nevertheless, it should be remembered that *measles, mumps, influenza (various subtypes), polio, herpes simplex virus, rubella, respiratory syncytial virus, varicella zoster, Epstein-Barr virus,* and *cytomegalovirus* may also cause a lymphocytic myocarditis.

As indicated, the characteristic format is that of a lymphocytic infiltrate within the interstitial parenchyma with direct myocyte attack causing cellular degeneration. Areas of replaced myocytes can be seen as well as those undergoing active degeneration by the associated lymphoid population. Acute cases often have more than 50 lymphoid cells/mm^2 with associated macrophages. However, it must be remembered that partially resolved or largely quiescent cases can still have some lymphoid cells as indicators of the myocarditis. Rarely, some acute cases have classic viral inclusions. Although uncommonly encountered, inclusions should be sought as part of the investigation protocol. Specialist immunohistochemistry targeting the lymphocyte subtypes, viral epitopes, and molecular techniques for the identification of DNA/RNA sequences may be of benefit. Clearly, those cases with a large degree of myocyte damage and loss will likely have a poor prognosis compared with those with relatively trivial myocyte damage and/or loss.

The detection of viral particles by PCR and in situ hybridization (ISH) techniques has advanced the understanding of myocarditis etiology quite considerably [10]. It is a reality that one ideally needs to suspect/predict the appropriate molecular target and to have a high index of suspicion, if this technique is to yield good quality results. The molecular tests also have to be applied with expertise reflecting the clinical data and compared to other investigation techniques and/or autopsy findings.

Rarely, in cases of immunosuppression, the myocarditic process can reflect reactivation of latent viral infections in the context of diminished immunity. The molecular mechanisms responsible for the reactivation of latent virus infection, the influence of immune activation triggering virus replication, and immune-dependant viral pathogenesis in non-inflamed hearts remain gaps in our current understanding of virus pathogenicity [11].

Bacterial Myocarditis

It is rare for bacteria to directly/diffusely affect the myocardium (opposed to the valves). Nevertheless, generalized bacteremia and showering of embolic material from infected valves can produce a spotty/global myocarditic reaction. In these circumstances (usually autopsy cases), the cause and source is evident and identification of bacteria usually relatively easy by means of standard histochemistry and microbiology culture techniques (see chapter 5). As a general rule, whenever bacterial myocarditis is suspected or encountered, one must think of possible immunosuppression. One specific spirochete infection (*Borrelia burgdorferi*) is recognized to be a rare cause of tick-borne sepsis (*Lyme disease*) with a propensity for myocarditis and later cardiac fibrosis/progressive cardiac failure. There are some cases with fairly specific clinical and pathological features that may provide diagnostic clues [9].

Fungal Myocarditis

In many ways, this is similar to that of bacterial myocarditis. Fungal myocarditis is a relatively rare process and often reflects a localized septic source with vascular dissemination. However, immunosuppression (often chemotherapy induced) can permit a widespread blood-borne fungal infection with colonization of myocardial parenchyma. Often, there are minimal symptoms initially. In cases of fungal myocarditis, the degree of inflammation can also be relatively mild and even fall below the pathological diagnostic

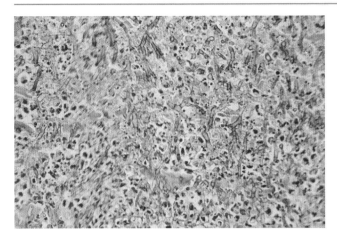

Fig. 8.6 A high magnification photomicrograph of part of an abscess shows *Aspergillus* infection in an immunocompromised patient (periodic acid Schiff)

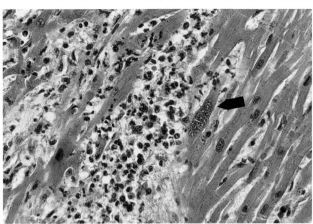

Fig. 8.8 Endomyocardial biopsy from a heart transplant patient with inflammation showing some eosinophilia and an intracellular aggregate (*arrowed*) of *Toxoplasma gondii*. Previously, this was a frequent problem in heart transplant cases, but is rare nowadays (hematoxylin and eosin)

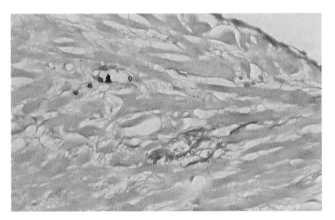

Fig. 8.7 High magnification of an endomyocardial biopsy in a cardiac transplant case stained with *Alcian blue* showing scattered *Cryptococcus* organisms. Such infections can be easily missed if only standard histochemistry is employed. A high degree of suspicion for atypical infective agents in patients with immunosuppressed states is required

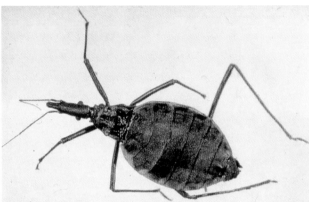

Fig. 8.9 *Triatoma infestans* – a vector of *Trypanosoma cruzi* (like other reduviid bugs)

criteria, in terms of inflammatory cell density. However, fungal myocarditis is clearly an inflammatory process with direct myocyte degeneration in response to the infective agent. The most common organisms involved include *Aspergillus* (Fig. 8.6) and *Candida* species, but others also play a role (Fig. 8.7).

Protozoal Myocarditis

These are relatively rare causes of myocarditis. Aside from those that are directly iatrogenic (immunosuppression during chemotherapy/chronic steroid usage), the possibility of HIV infection and AIDS certainly need to be considered in terms of the differential diagnosis when faced with unusual organisms within myocardial tissue.

Toxoplasma gondii exposure is prevalent in the background population, but rarely causes any clinical effect. However, those with immunosuppression, historically early in the transplant program, were subject to this particular infection reactivation (see cardiac transplantation chapter). Nowadays, better handling of immunosuppression treatments has diminished this risk considerably. The infective agents can be seen within the boundaries of cardiac myocytes as small hematoxyphilic dots (bradyzoites) (Fig. 8.8). There is specific immunohistochemistry available for confirmation. Electron microscopy and serology techniques may also be of value.

In some parts of the world (especially South America), another protozoan, *Trypanosomiasis cruzi* (causing *Chagas disease*) needs to be considered. However, most such cases are chronic and rather indolent, with slow progression toward significant cardiac failure over a period of 10–20 years. Less than 10 % of patients suffer with an acute attack [12, 13] (Figs. 8.9 and 8.10).

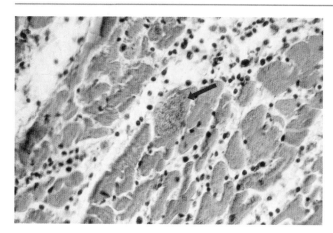

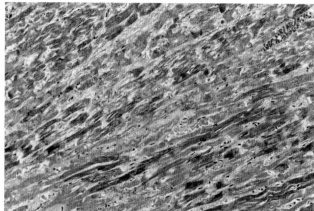

Fig. 8.10 The acute phase of myocarditis in Chagas disease is seen with a myofiber distended by trypanosomes (*red arrow*). There is inflammation and necrosis of individual myofibers (hematoxylin and eosin)

Fig. 8.12 Diphtheria myocarditis. There is severe widespread myocyte degeneration and necrosis. The inflammatory cellular response is relatively sparse (hematoxylin and eosin)

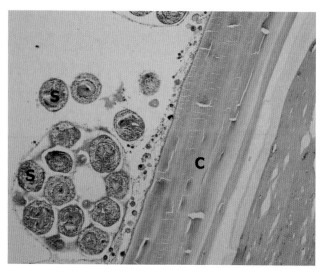

Fig. 8.11 Composite Photomicrograph showing a somewhat hyaline cyst wall of a hydatid cyst (*C*) with scolices (*S*) on the inner lining.

Rarely, amoeba (*Entamoeba histolytica*) infection has been identified as a cause of direct myocardial degeneration and thereby inflammation. Amoebic infection has also been seen as a cause of toxic myocarditis [14], although pericarditis is also recognized [9]. Another rare cause of myocarditis is *hydatid disease*, caused by *Echinococcus granulosus*. This can cause cysts within myocardial tissue [15] or in the pericardial space, but is relatively rare in the Western world. It has a characteristic morphology for the cysts and scolices (Fig. 8.11).

Toxic Myocarditis

As the name implies, this is an inflammatory reaction in relation to a toxic agent. These toxins are commonly drugs, with an associated induced autoimmune cross-reaction or a

direct cytopathic effect on cardiac myocytes, with secondary inflammation. It is debatable whether these should really be classified as true myocarditis. However, since they mostly have some degree of inflammation within the myocardium and thereby exist as a differential diagnosis for infective and other causes of myocarditis, they may be to best considered at this point. Drug reactions associated with myocarditis are usually idiosyncratic (ie: cannot be predicted).

It is often difficult when faced with patients taking multiple drugs to determine which drug or combination was responsible for the myocyte damage and thereby inflammation. Consideration of the drug history may provide some etiological clues, but the side effects of a myocarditic type are often nonspecific. Features seen within the myocardial cells at the ultrastructural level can include myocyte swelling, cytoplasmic vacuolization and fatty change [9]. These can be associated with myocyte degeneration and thereby myocarditis. An index of suspicion for drug-related myocarditis needs to be kept at the forefront of one's mind.

Following the development of potent immunization, *diptheria* is no longer a significant problem in the Western world. Individuals infected with this organism may be inflicted by a toxin created by the infective agent (*Corynebacterium diphtheriae*) and blocking the host cell protein synthesis. The toxin acts directly upon cardiac myocytes which then degenerate and die (Fig. 8.12), causing a degree of inflammation as a consequence.

Immune-Mediated Myocarditis

Autoimmune

Autoimmune systemic disorders have a cause on which we may hypothesize innate, acquired, or adapted autoantibodies.

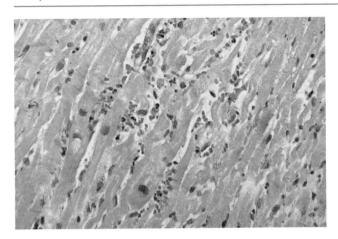

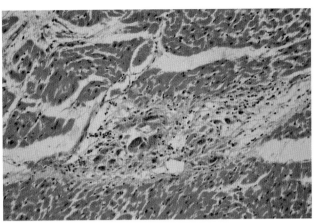

Fig. 8.13 In this section, edema and a slight lymphocytic infiltrate are present together with some sarcolemmal fraying. This was a case of dermatomyositis. Although the features are nonspecific, the biopsy has a distinctly abnormal picture and if left unchecked there will be replacement fibrosis as a consequence (hematoxylin and eosin)

Fig. 8.14 Archive case of an Aschoff nodule in a case of acute rheumatic carditis (hematoxylin and eosin)

There may be lymphocytic and other inflammatory cell activity along with nonspecific degenerative changes of the cardiomyocytes (Fig. 8.13). Often, but not always, some vasculitis is present.

Rheumatic Fever

Rheumatic fever is perhaps the best example of an immune-mediated myocarditic reaction. It is recognized that a *group A beta-hemolytic streptococcus* septic process (often affecting children in the upper respiratory tract/oropharynx) can allow bacterial epitopes to be exposed to the host immune system. These antigens mimic cardiac myosin and other cellular components causing the immunological cross-reaction that is recognized as acute rheumatic fever [8, 16]. The antibody cross-reactivity to various tissues within the heart causes inflammation of the valvular tissue, myocardial parenchyma, and endocardial surfaces. It is rare to see acute cases nowadays, but some global migrants in recent decades have presented unexpectedly in the clinic or autopsy room (Fig. 8.14).

The (acute) inflammatory changes include focal myocyte loss, lymphocytic infiltration, and aggregates of histiocytes, classically described as Aschoff nodules. The individual histiocyte component cells often have a rather bizarre morphology (Anitschkov cells) with some nuclear pleomorphism. Confirmation of the diagnosis requires knowledge of the antecedent history, positive serology, and exclusion of alternate differentials.

With time, the degree of inflammation subsides and one is left with scarring fibrosis and variable myocyte loss. It should be remembered that it is the valvular tissue component [8, 9] which usually causes the progressive

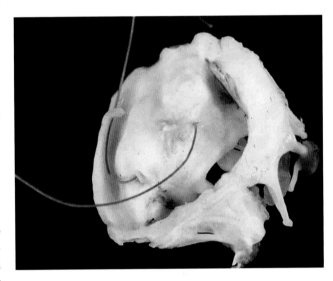

Fig. 8.15 Macroscopic view of a mitral valve involved previously by rheumatic fever. The valve leaflets are fibrotic, stiff, and the commissures are fused. Mechanical stenosis of the valve is the result

cardiac dysfunction over many decades, rather than myocyte replacement (Fig. 8.15). The differential diagnosis of the acute cases includes giant cell reactions in response to vasculitis (Wegener's, giant cell arteritis), sarcoid, drugs, mycobacterial infection, idiopathic giant cell myocarditis, etc. [9].

Cellular Rejection

The most common myocarditis type diagnosed in the current era reflects cellular rejection in heart-transplanted patients (see chapter 10). While cellular rejection is well described and can be diagnosed rather precisely (Fig. 8.16), there are still problems related to antibody-mediated (humoral) rejection [17].

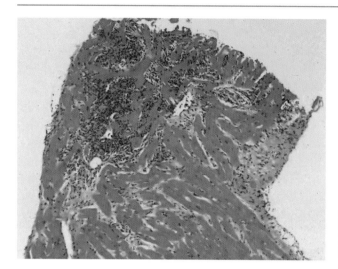

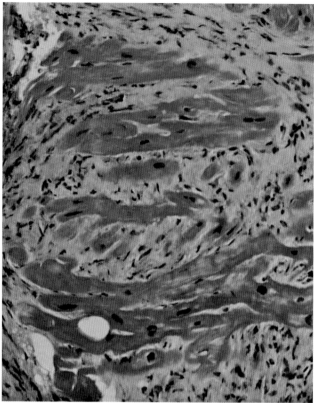

Fig. 8.16 Grade 3R (severe, high grade, acute cellular rejection) in a cardiac transplant case. The R suffix denotes the revised grade to avoid confusion with the 1990 scheme. There is a pronounced inflammatory infiltrate with many lymphocytes and some macrophages associated with myocyte damage (hematoxylin and eosin)

Eosinophilic Myocarditis

Eosinophilic myocarditis is a rare form of myocarditis with a notable/profound infiltration of the interstitial compartment by eosinophils [18]. The density of eosinophils can vary. The degranulation of eosinophilic cytoplasmic components causes direct local damage to cardiac myocytes with subsequent myocyte degeneration/loss and replacement fibrosis (Figs. 8.17 and 8.18). It is likely that this probably exists as part of the inflammatory vasculitic disorder spectrum (e.g., Churg-Strauss), Loeffler's endomyocardial inflammation, hypersensitivity reactions (often drug induced), and atypical parasitic infections. The possibility of drug reactions needs to be carefully scrutinized even when there is focal vascular reactivity and involvement.

Giant Cells in Myocarditis

Giant cells are often seen as part of a myocarditic process. They may be the key feature of the inflammatory process [19], or they may just be part of the background pathology. They may occur singly or may be diffuse in type. Diffuse infiltration cases with degeneration of cardiac myocytes are usually designated idiopathic giant cell myocarditis (see below) [19]. However, giant cells are often seen in association with macrophage aggregates or granulomatous inflammatory process and may lead one toward more the diagnosis of infective agents and autoimmune processes [1, 9]. If one has excluded atypical infective agents (tuberculo-

Fig. 8.17 A case of Churg-Strauss is seen with a high magnification view of myocardial tissue. There is inflammation and eosinophilia together with interstitial fibrosis and myocyte degeneration. The patient had characteristic lung pathology. The release of eosinophil granules is recognized to be damaging to local myocytes (hematoxylin and eosin)

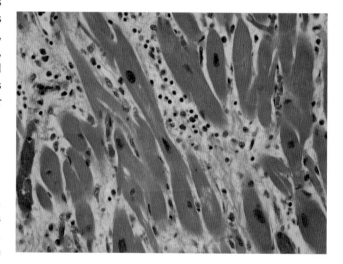

Fig. 8.18 A case of eosinophilic myocarditis. One requires to consider hypersensitivity and drug reactions as well as parasitic infections (hematoxylin and eosin)

sis, fungal organisms), then a granulomatous myocarditis with giant cells is more likely to point towards sarcoid and sarcoid-like processes (Fig. 8.19).

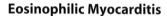

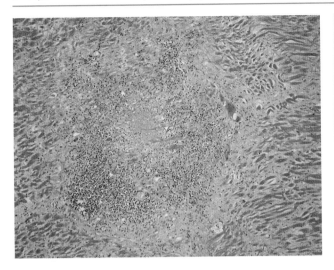

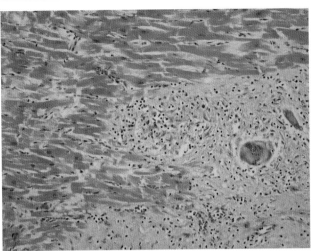

Fig. 8.19 A zone of necrobiosis with a granulomatous reaction with moderate numbers of lymphocytes. A giant cell is seen peripherally (hematoxylin and eosin)

Fig. 8.21 Sarcoidosis involving the left ventricle produces significant fibrous replacement myocytes with scattered lymphocytes and characteristic giant cells (hematoxylin and eosin)

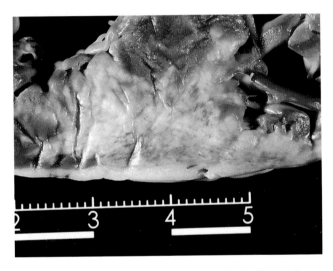

Fig. 8.20 Autopsy sample of a case of sudden death with the left ventricle showing previous sarcoidosis-related fibrosis (Courtesy of Dr. PJ Gallagher)

Sarcoid Myocarditis

Sarcoidosis commonly affects the myocardium, perhaps more commonly that might be expected clinically, but rarely causes significant myocardial debility. The characteristic systemic features of sarcoid are well recognized, and one may identify granulomatous foci within the myocardium in cases of patients who present with cardiac dysrhythmias, or, indeed, sudden death (Figs. 8.20 and 8.21). Exclusion of atypical infective agents is important in this diagnosis, but there is no specific confirmatory test available. Sudden death in cases of sarcoid is relatively rare, but those dying in this format often have granulomatous foci of inflammation and replacement fibrosis at key points within the cardiac conduction system. These areas of scarring are liable to produce reentrant tachyarrhythmias and thereby potentially sudden death [20].

Idiopathic Giant Cell Myocarditis

The etiology of this condition is unclear, but it is recognized that this diffuse inflammatory and degenerative process with abundant associated giant cells is a potent cause of rapidly progressive cardiac failure and sudden death [19] (Figs. 8.22 and 8.23). Even when transplanted, the disease may recur in the allograft [21].

Tissue Handling and Practical Aspects of Case Handling/Diagnosis

Since myocarditis is considered to be a global (rather than focal) myocardial disorder, it is reasonable to sample the myocardium by the endovascular bioptome approach for in vivo studies. Despite being diffuse, the intensity of inflammation can vary significantly within the myocardial tissue and consequently ideally five endomyocardial tissue biopsies should be taken, with biopsy sample number consideration being required if additional special investigations are being contemplated [22, 23]. The size of each biopsy should be between 0.5 and 2 mm and should include endomyocardial tissue rather than scarred tissue. The precise number of samples and staining reactions used will usually reflect individual case considerations.

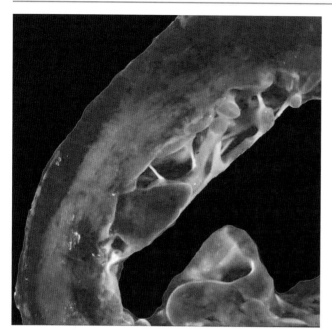

Fig. 8.22 Autopsy macroscopic view of part of the left ventricle showing acute infarction-like features of the anterior wall in a case of idiopathic giant cell myocarditis

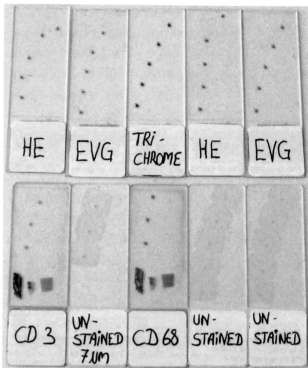

Fig. 8.24 Ideal handling of endomyocardial tissue samples shows a run of sections taken on to many glass slides with different histochemical and immunohistochemical stains. Some unstained sections are often kept back for additional stains, as required/suggested by the initial review

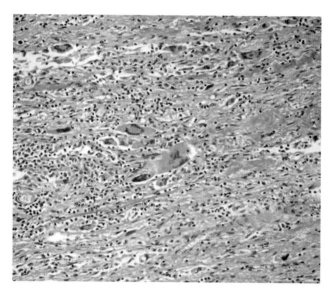

Fig. 8.23 High magnification view of idiopathic giant cell myocarditis with abundant pleomorphic giant cells, edema, an inflammatory infiltrate with histiocytes, and lymphocytes and myocyte loss (hematoxylin and eosin)

Endomyocardial Biopsy

Ideal practice requires the samples of endomyocardial tissue for routine light microscopy analysis to be examined with serial/level sections being cut. The sections should include stains for hematoxylin and eosin, elastic van Gieson (for elastic and connective tissue), Masson's trichrome (for muscle and connective tissue), and eventually Congo Red histochemistry for amyloid

(this section shall be about 7 μm thick when only 3-4 μm thick the reation is sometimes so weak that it cannot be assessed correctly). Spare sections can be cut for immunohistochemistry, with particular emphasis on CD3 and CD68 antigens (Fig. 8.24). Other inflammatory cell antisera can be of use, although this tends to be more in a research setting (Table 8.3).

One piece of tissue may be reserved for microbiology sampling, either by direct culture or molecular assay. Common viral culprits can be assessed by PCR analysis. Alternatively, this sample may be reserved for later investigation by being snap frozen/stored in liquid nitrogen. A sample can be reserved for electron microscopy, although the diagnostic yield from this investigation tends not to be high. Clearly, not every test needs to be employed in every case, but the choices made must reflect the individual case specifics.

The routine light microscopy assessment of the samples will normally document the number of endomyocardial fragments and the status of the cardiac myocytes, with particular emphasis upon myocytolysis, apoptosis, sarcolemmal fraying, infective agent/viral inclusions, etc. The interstitial compartment will be of particular interest of in terms of edema and the quantitation of the degree of fibrosis. Furthermore, inflammatory cell components need to be quantitated in number per unit area (mm²). The role of immunohistochemistry cannot be underestimated in this regard.

Table 8.3 Some usual staining and immunohistochemical reactions performed on endomyocardial biopsy material

Staining reactions	Immunohistochemical reactions
Hematoxylin–eosin	CD 3
Elastic van Gieson	CD 4
Masson's trichrome	CD 20
PAS	CD 45
Perl (iron)	CD 65
Congo red (amyloid)	Antihuman amyloid A
	Prealbumin (transthyretin)
	Specific viral antibodies (e.g., CMV)
	HLA-ABC
	HLA-DR
	C4d

Of course this list is endless. One has to be guided by morphology with a levelheaded and sensible mind

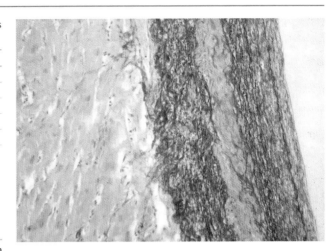

Fig. 8.25 A section from a case of fibroelastosis, dilated type. It is noted that there is a continuous rim of smooth muscle cells within the fibroelastotically thickened endomyocardium (elastic van Gieson)

On the endocardial aspect, one looks for inflammatory cells and increase of smooth muscle cells, the latter denoting cavity dilatation (Fig. 8.25). Especially in the initial stages of an inflammatory condition of the myocardium, there may be morphological clues to a specific diagnosis: the acute phase of the Aschoff granuloma in rheumatic fever, myocytic cysts in toxoplasmosis, eosinophilia (not specific, but pointing in certain diagnostic directions), and so on.

Subacute cases and those cases wherein the inflammation has largely subsided may simply show myocyte loss, the occasional lymphocyte and well-defined established fibrosis. The role of molecular techniques in particular, ISH and the PCR, have advanced the diagnosis quite dramatically in the last 10–20 years. Molecular analysis for viral detection, particularly amplification methods like PCR or nested PCR, allows the detection of a low number of copy viral genomes even from an extremely small amount of tissue such as endomyocardial biopsies [11, 24]. It is very important to use a molecular technique as a diagnostic tool and ancillary to other mandatory investigations (clinical and morphological) and apply it with skilled expertise. Different cardiotropic viruses (already earlier mentioned), other than enterovirus, should always be considered.

Autopsy

The autopsy handling of a cardiac specimen follows similar patterns of investigation and tissue investigation, but by being a much larger tissue resource can have full tissue sampling for the different tests required, as above.

The macroscopic appearances at autopsy can be blatant on occasion (Figs. 8.1 and 8.21), but are mostly quite subtle or nonspecific, and it is only after considering myocarditis as a potential differential that one may be prompted to take appropriate samples (see also Chap. 5, 14). Florid cases show considerable myocyte damage and degeneration with edematous, hemorrhagic, and softened parenchyma macroscopically.

Histological changes of hemorrhagic foci, edema, and myocyte loss/cytoplasmic degeneration are clear pointers to the diagnosis. By contrast, the presence of a dilated cardiomyopathy (as an end point) should not stop one from sampling for subacute myocarditis.

It is often also important to collect some peripheral blood (5–10 ml) EDTA and sodium citrate tubes for other molecular investigations as an adjunction to those performed directly upon the myocardial tissue itself.

Aspects of pathogenesis

Chronic cases can be particularly difficult to diagnose. Many lack the significant inflammatory cell infiltrates and show only nonspecific myocyte loss and fibrosis. Many cases are seen in the format of a dilated cardiomyopathy (Fig. 8.26). However, proving this is often not possible without other cross-correlation data in the form of prior serology, clinical history, or radiology data.

Molecular analysis for viral detection, introduction of new molecular techniques, particularly amplification methods like Polymerase Chain Reaction (PCR) or nested – PCR, allow the detection of a low number of copy viral genomes even from an extremely small amount of tissue such as endomyocardial biopsy [11]. It is very important to use a molecular technique as a diagnostic tool and ancillary to other mandatory investigations (clinical and morphological) and apply it with expertise. Different cardiotropic viruses (already mentioned) other than enterovirus should be sought.

Specifically, the pathogenesis of viral myocarditis is generally felt to involve three phases. The initial phase involves viral infection and then viral replication. The second stage reflects the inflammatory response that can be both innate

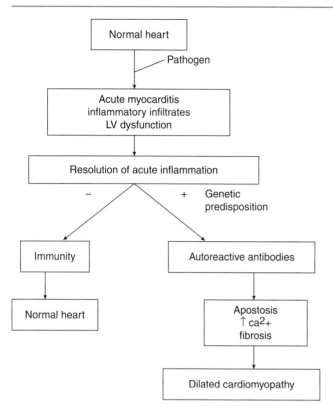

Fig. 8.26 Pathogenesis. Based on Fig. 2 from [25]

Table 8.4 Efficacy of various diagnostic modalities for myocarditis

Diagnostic modality	Sensitivity range (%)	Specificity range (%)
Troponin (lower threshold of >0.1 mg/ml)	34–53	89–94
Antibodies to virus or myosin	25–32	40
Indium-111 antimyosin scintigraphy	85–91	34–53
Cardiac magnetic resonance imaging	86	95
Myocardial biopsy (Dallas criteria of pathology)	35–50	78–89
Myocardial biopsy (viral genome by PCR)	38–65	80–100

Based on Table 66.3 from Libby et al. [30]
AV atrioventricular, *ECG* electrocardiogram, *PCR* polymerase chain reaction

that myocardial inflammation in some patients can trigger and manifest ARVC – an inherited myocardial disease with a complex genetic background.

Prognostic Information from the Endomyocardial Biopsy

The histological assessment and subclassification of biopsy-proven myocarditis by means of endomyocardial biopsy has been shown to predict patient outcome [19, 26]. However, the prognostic significance of identification of the viral agents remains controversial/contradictory in terms of patient prognosis/outcome [27–29]. Nevertheless, it remains vital for a full understanding of viral myocarditis that appropriate consideration is made for the identification of potential viral triggers. A comparison of efficacy of various diagnostic modalities for myocarditis has been shown (see Table 8.4), but caution should be exercised when reading this table. However, ultimately, the molecular techniques allied to histology have led to some better understanding of disease evolution.

and acquired/adaptive in quality. The third and final phase revolves around cardiac remodelling as a consequence of myocyte damage/loss and resultant fibrosis.

Mimics of Myocarditis

It is well recognized that many cardiovascular disorders have an element of myocardial inflammatory cell infiltrate, and the issue will be to separate the innocent "bystander cell" from a truly pathological reaction. Certainly, a few mast cells and very occasional lymphoid cells may be seen routinely in myocardial tissues from autopsies in which the individuals have no cardiovascular disease.

In atherosclerosis of the coronary arteries, there may be considerable adventitial aggregates of lymphocytes observed. This response to vascular atheroma can spill a short way into myocardial tissues. It is important not to over-interpret such phenomena, particularly on small samples. Similar issues can be seen in a limited tissue sampling of systemic or localized vasculitis cases.

In arrhythmogenic right ventricular cardiomyopathy (ARVC), lymphocytic infiltrates and myocytic degenerative changes have been described in some cases of ARVC [9]. This may reflect a response to myocyte loss from degenerative processes, although one idea previously put forward was

Treatments for Myocarditis

Myocarditis is often underdiagnosed with only basic treatment really being available for those presenting to clinicians with acute symptoms [8, 16, 31]. Treatment in these cases mostly involves immunosuppression with little being available for specific conditions. Other treatments are directed to address the cardiac function consequences of the myocarditis process (e.g., anti-failure therapy).

However, for most patients, significant myocarditis results in chronic damage. Treatment for those with chronic effects is usually aimed at ameliorating any dysrhythmias and cardiac failure. These supportive treatments progress from standard oral drug therapy regimens, include provision

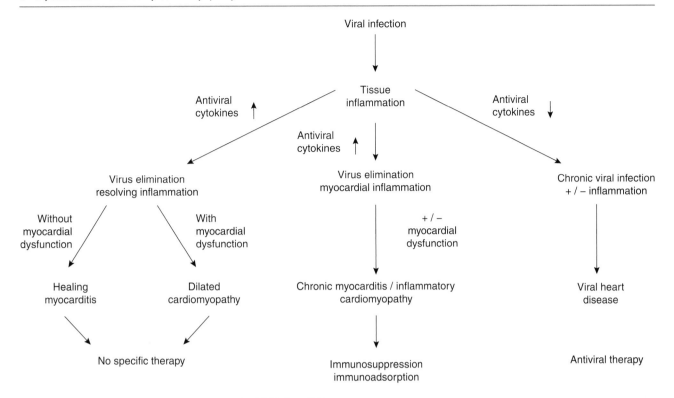

Fig. 8.27 Crude treatment algorithm. Based on Fig. 18.29 from [32]

of pacemakers (various types), and may progress through to heart transplantation for end-stage cardiac failure.

The role of immunosuppression for myocarditis remains a complex reality, and it needs appropriate confirmation/understanding of the causative agent/process as well as the understanding of the consequences of immunosuppression itself. Clearly, potentiation of an infective process (in an immune-suppressed state) could lead to further myocyte damage and a significant deleterious effect on the individual (Fig. 8.27).

Concluding Remarks

It is clear that myocarditis is underdiagnosed, underappreciated, and a complex mixture of different conditions with a common theme (myocardial inflammation, myocyte damage and loss). A high index of clinical and pathological suspicion, appropriate tissue sampling, and targeted specific pathological investigations can yield information on affected cases [33]. Nevertheless, it is likely that myocarditis will remain a serious challenge for the foreseeable future for clinicians, pathologists, and society.

Acknowledgment   I am grateful for a long-lasting cooperation with Dr. Sabine Pankuweit, Universitätsklinikum Giessen & Marburg, Germany, who has been very educational and always kind. Sabine has once again been of great help when preparing this chapter.

References

1. Aretz HAT, Billingham ME, Edwards WD, et al. Myocarditis: a histopathologic definition and classification. Am J Cardiovasc Pathol. 1987;1:3–14.
2. Richardson P, Mckenna W, Bristow M, et al. Report of the 1995 World Health Organization/International Society and Federation of Cardiology Task Force on the Definition and Classification of cardiomyopathies. Circulation. 1996;93(5):841–2.
3. Maisch B, Bültman B, Factor S, et al. World Heart Federation consensus conferences' definition of inflammatory cardiomyopathy (myocarditis): report from two expert committees on histology and viral cardiomyopathy. Heartbeat. 1999;4:3–4.
4. Gravanis MG, Sternby NH. Incidence of myocarditis. Arch Pathol Lab Med. 1991;15:390–2.
5. Woodruff JF. Viral myocarditis: a review. J Infect. 1998;37: 424–79.
6. Eckart RE, Scoville SL, Campell Cl, et al. Sudden death in young adults: a 25-year review of autopsies in military recruits. Ann Intern Med. 2004;141:829–34.
7. Karjalainen J, Heikkilä J. Incidence of three presentations of the acute myocarditis in young men in military service: a 20-year experience. Eur Heart J. 1999;20:1020–5.
8. Bloomfield P, Bradbury A, Grubb NR, Newby DE. Cardiovascular disease. In: Davidson's principles and practice of medicine. 20th ed. Edinburgh: Churchill Livingstone; 2005. p. 519–646.
9. Winters GL, McManus BM. Myocarditis. In: Silver MD, Gotlieb AI, Schoen FJ, editors. Cardiovascular pathology. 3rd ed. New York: Churchill Livingstone; 2001. p. 256–84.
10. Bowles NE, Bowles KR, Towbin JA. Viral genomic detection and outcome in myocarditis. Heart Fail Clin. 2005;3:407–17.
11. Lotze U, Egerer R, Glück B, Zell R, Sigusch H, Erhardt C, Heim A, Kandolf R, Bock T, Wutzler P, Figulla HR. Low level myocardial

parvovirus B19 persistence is a frequent finding in patients with heart disease but unrelated to ongoing myocardial injury. J Med Virol. 2010;82(8):1449–57.

12. Rassi Jr A, Rassi A, Marin-Neto JA. Chagas disease. Lancet. 2010;37(9723):1388–402.

13. Carod-Artal FJ. Trypanosomiasis, cardiomyopathy and the risk of ischemic stroke. Expert Rev Cardiovasc Ther. 2010;815(5):717–28.

14. Manoji Muditha Pathirage LP, Kularante SAM, Wijesinghe S, Ratnatunga NVI, Gaarammana IB. Fulminant colitis and toxic myocarditis: a unifying cause? Lancet. 2009;374:2026.

15. Tejada JG, Saavedra J, Molina L, Forteza A, Gomez C. Hydatid disease of the interventricular septum causing pericardial effusion. Ann Thorac Surg. 2000;71:2034–5.

16. Hess OM, McKenna W, Schultheiss H-P. Myocardial disease. In: Camm AJ, Lüscher TF, Serruys PW, editors. Cardiovascular medicine. 2nd ed. Oxford: Oxford University Press; 2009. p. 665–716.

17. Boon NA, Colledge NR, Walker BB, Hunter JAA. Diseases of the heart valves. In: Davidson's principles and practice of medicine. 20th ed. London: Churchill Livingstone; 2006. p. 616–8; Stewart S, Winters GL, Fishbein MC, et al. Revision of 1990 working formulation for the standardization of nomenclature in the diagnosis of heart rejection. J Heart Lung Transplant. 2005;24:1710–20.

18. Sheppard MNS. Myocarditis, in practical cardiovascular pathology. 2nd ed. London: Hodder Arnold; 2011. p. 193–219.

19. Cooper LT, Berry GJ, Shabetai R. Idiopathic giant cell myocarditis – natural history and treatment. N Engl J Med. 1997;336:1860–6.

20. Silverman KJ, Hutchins GM, Bulkley BM. Cardiac sarcoid. A clinicopathological evaluation of 84 unselected cases with systemic sarcoidosis. Circulation. 1978;58:1204–11.

21. Das BB, Recto M, Johnsrude C, Klein L, Orman K, Shoemaker L, Mitchell M, Austin EH. Cardiac transplantation for pediatric giant cell myocarditis. J Heart Lung Transplant. 2006;25:474–8.

22. Konno S, Sakakibara S. Endomyocardial biopsy. Dis Chest. 1963;44:345–50.

23. Baandrup U, Florio RA, Olsen EGJ. Do endomyocardial biopsies represent the morphology of the rest of the myocardium? Eur Heart J. 1982;1:171–8.

24. Bock C-T, Klingel K, Kandolf R. Human parvovirus B19-associated myocarditis. N Engl J Med. 2010;362(13):1248–9.

25. MacLellan WR, Lusis AJ. Dilated cardiomyopathy: learning to live with yourself. Nat Med. 2003;9:1455–6.

26. Magnani JW, Danik HJS, Dec GW, DiSalvo TG. Survival in biopsy-proven myocarditis: a long-term retrospective analysis of the histopathologic, clinical, and hemodynamic predictors. Am Heart J. 2006;151:463–70.

27. Kuhl U, Pauschinger M, Seeberg B, Lassner D, Noutsias M, Poller W, Schultheiss HP. Viral persistence in the myocardium is associated with progressive cardiac dysfunction. Circulation. 2005;112:1965–70.

28. Caforio ALP, Calabrese F, Angelini A, Tona F, Vinci A, Bottaro S, Ramondo A, Carturan E, Iliceto S, Thiene G, Daliento L. A prospective study of biopsy-proven myocarditis: prognostic relevance of clinical and aetiopathogenetic features at diagnosis. Eur Heart J. 2007;28:1326–33.

29. Kuethe F, Sigusch HH, Hilbig K, Tresselt C, Gluck B, Egerer R, Figulla HR. Detection of viral genome in the myocardium: lack of prognostic and functional relevance in patients with acute dilated cardiomyopathy. Am Heart J. 2007;153:850–8.

30. Libby P, et al. Braunwald's heart disease. 8th ed. Philadelphia: Saunders, Elsevier; 2008.

31. Liu PP, Schultheiss H-P. Myocarditis. In: Libby P, Bonow RO, Mann DL, Zipes DP, Braunwald E, editors. Heart disease. 8th ed. Philadelphia: Saunders/Elsevier; 2008. p. 1775–92.

32. Camm JA, Lüscher TF, Serruys PW, editors. The ESC textbook of cardiovascular medicine. 2nd ed. Oxford: Oxford University Press; 2009.

33. Baughman KL. Diagnosis of myocarditis – death of Dallas criteria. Circulation. 2006;113:593–5.

Valvular Heart Disease

9

Siân Hughes

Abstract

This chapter deals with current topics in valvular heart disease, focusing on the most common types of diseased valve encountered in routine surgical practice including floppy mitral valves, senile tricuspid aortic valves, and congenital bicuspid aortic valves. The pathology of infective endocarditis and rheumatic valvular heart disease is also discussed. Macroscopic and microscopic images of the different valve pathologies are provided as well as a detailed description of valve pathophysiology, and scientific data underlying the pathogenesis of the different forms of valvular heart disease is provided.

Keywords

Stenosis • Regurgitation • Vegetation • Calcification • Rheumatic fever • Congenital bicuspid valve • Infective endocarditis • Myxomatous degeneration • Aortic dilatation

Introduction

The spectrum of valvular heart disease has changed significantly over the last half century reflecting the decline in rheumatic fever, advances in interventional cardiology, and cardiothoracic surgical techniques, albeit balanced against disorders in an increasing elderly population. With the advent of the antibiotic era and improved living conditions, rheumatic fever, the principal cause of valvular heart disease worldwide, has declined and is seen infrequently in industrialized nations. Advanced cardiothoracic surgery including the development of cardiopulmonary bypass, effective cardioplegic solutions, and modern heart valve prostheses means the pathologist is more likely to receive excised floppy mitral valves, congenital bicuspid aortic valves, and senile tricuspid aortic valves as part of their

S. Hughes, MBBS, M.Sc., Ph.D., FRCPath
Department of Histopathology,
University College Hospital London,
21 University St., Rockefeller Building,
London WC1E 6JJ, UK
e-mail: sian.hughes@ucl.ac.uk, rmkdshu@ucl.ac.uk

routine surgical practice. This chapter will focus primarily on the pathology of excised cardiac valves in the adult seen most frequently (Table 9.1) in surgical pathology practice and will describe the underlying valvular disease processes and the diagnostic macroscopic and histological features.

Normal Structure and Function of the Valves

The aortic and pulmonary valves are comprised of three semilunar cusps. The aortic valve cusps are designated as the right coronary, left coronary, and noncoronary cusp, which are inserted within their curved outer edges within a connective tissue sleeve. The cusps are apposed at three commissures at which they are equally spaced and firmly attached to the supra-aortic ridge. The ventricular surfaces of each aortic cusp have a small nodule in the center of its free edge called the nodulus of Arantii. Two ridges extend down from the nodulus of Arantii, representing the closure line where the cusps abut one another, when the valve is closed. The portion of the cusp above the closure lines is known as the lunula. Fenestrations are common at this site in normal valves, but these are not usually functionally significant. The structure and function of the pulmonary valve is similar to that of the

S.K. Suvarna (ed.), *Cardiac Pathology*,
DOI 10.1007/978-1-4471-2407-8_9, © Springer-Verlag London 2013

Table 9.1 The common causes of cardiac valvular dysfunction

Mitral regurgitation

Chronic rheumatic valvular heart disease

Floppy mitral valve

Chordal rupture (pregnancy, closed chest trauma)

Ischemic papillary muscle damage

Infective endocarditis

Aortic regurgitation

Chronic rheumatic valvular heart disease

Congenital bicuspid aortic valve

Infective endocarditis

Aortic root abnormalities (e.g., inflammatory aortitis, syphilis)

Age-related degenerative change

Marfan's syndrome

Idiopathic dilatation of the ascending aorta

Aortic dissection

Aortic stenosis

Congenital bicuspid aortic valve

Chronic rheumatic valvular heart disease

Senile tricuspid calcific aortic stenosis

Mitral stenosis

Chronic rheumatic valvular heart disease

Severe annular calcification

Tricuspid stenosis

Chronic rheumatic valvular heart disease

Tricuspid regurgitation

Tricuspid ring dilatation (Marfan's syndrome, right ventricular failure, chronic rheumatic valvular heart disease)

Carcinoid heart disease

Ebstein's anomaly

Infective endocarditis (may reflect cusp destruction, but ring dilatation also must occur to cause functional disturbances)

Pulmonary valve stenosis

Congenital pulmonary stenosis

Carcinoid heart disease

Pulmonary regurgitation

Carcinoid heart disease

Note: Many of these different diseases affecting valves may produce overlapping functional abnormalities. This broad summary does not provide an exhaustive list but outlines the most common causes of functional valvular abnormalities

aortic valve, and the cusps are named as right, left, and anterior. The structure of both valves is similar in that they have a dense collagen core (fibrosa) and are covered by endothelium. Between these are loose structures myxoid tissue (spongiosa), which may often contain adipose tissue, a delicate layer of collagen, and elastic fibers on the ventricular side of the valve (ventricularis).

The mitral and tricuspid valves are comprised of two and three cusps, respectively. They differ in structure and function to the semilunar valves. Both mitral and tricuspid valves are inserted into a fibrous ring or annulus, which serves to separate the atria and ventricles. Chordae tendineae are attached to the edges and undersurface of the cusps and prevent prolapse of the valves into the atria during systole. Chordal

tension is regulated by the papillary muscles. The mitral valve is comprised of a large triangular anterior cusp, whereas the posterior cusp is crescentic, narrower and comprised of three scallops lateral, medial, and central. In the Carpentier surgical classification system, the three scallops of the posterior leaflets are designated as P1 (anterolateral), P2 (middle), and P3 (posteromedial). The corresponding portions of the anterior cusp are labeled A1, A2, and A3 [1]. Each leaflet has a rough zone near the free edge and a central clear zone at the base of the cusp [2]. The two cusps appose one another at the medial and lateral commissures, which can be identified by fan-shaped commissural chordae. The tricuspid valve shows wide anatomic variation but is essentially comprised of a septal cusp, which is attached to the ventricular septum, and a large anterior cusp, which overlies most of the ventricular cavity, and a smaller posterior cusp. Both types of have a dense inner core (fibrosa), which is comprised of collagen over which there is abundant myxomatous connective tissue (spongiosa). These valves are avascular structures with sparse fibroblasts within the fibrosa. The atrial and ventricular aspects of the valves are composed of a thin layer of collagen and elastic tissue, being known as the atrialis and ventricularis, respectively [3]. There is a standard monolayer endothelial surface (see also chapter 1).

Infective Endocarditis

Infective endocarditis is a disorder wherein microorganisms or fungi grow within a platelet thrombus (vegetation) on the endocardial surface of a heart valve. This disease damages valve tissues and is a serious illness with considerable morbidity and mortality. The types of valves most at risk of endocardial damage are regurgitant rather than stenotic valves, where turbulent flow plays a significant role in causing damage to the endothelial/valve surface. In the preantibiotic era, the most common underlying cardiac abnormality was rheumatic valvular heart disease [4, 5]. Today, infective endocarditis is most commonly seen in young adult patients with a regurgitant congenital bicuspid aortic valve (BAV). Furthermore, it is observed four times more commonly in patients with a floppy mitral valve [6–11], where there is a mitral regurgitant murmur and redundant thickened leaflets, when compared with normals [9, 11–13] In several surgical series, it has been observed that infected BAVs occur in a significant proportion of all cases [14, 15]. *Viridans streptococci* and *staphylococci* accounted for 72% of cases in one study, where there was also strong male predominance [16]. Infective endocarditis may also be observed in the elderly with degenerative calcific valvular heart disease [9, 17].

Traditionally, infective endocarditis was classified as either acute or subacute depending on the virulence of the causative organism. The clinical features of this disease are wide-ranging, and a multitude of different microorganisms may cause infective endocarditis. It is now better classified as infective endocarditis, according to the offending microorganism. Infective endocarditis classically presents clinically with a heart murmur, fever, anemia, raised white cell count, splenomegaly, and hematuria. Other features, which may variably be present, include petechia, Osler's nodes, Janeway lesions, Roth spots, and splinter hemorrhages in nails. The diagnosis is usually confirmed by positive blood cultures and the characteristic echocardiographic finding of a vegetation on a heart valve [18].

The pathogenesis of infective endocarditis has been studied using animal models, which provide an accurate picture of the disease seen in humans [19, 20]. The principal risk factors for developing this disease reflect endocardial damage to the valve surface in association with bacteremia. Small platelet and fibrin thrombi form on the valve surface and serve as a focal point (nidus) in which an infection can settle and grow. The ability of a particular microorganism to cause infection is partially mediated by the presence of cell surface specific receptors, which enable it to bind to tissue components of platelets and/or the damaged valve. It is also facilitated by the difficulty for neutrophil polymorphs to penetrate a mass of infected thrombotic material.

A broad range of microorganisms can cause infective endocarditis including *Staphylococcus aureus*, *Staphylococcus epidermidis*, *Streptococcus viridans*, *Aspergillus* species, *Candida* species, and various *enterococci*. Atypical infections may also occur. Several series have been reported detailing the incidence of a comprehensive range of organisms [4, 9, 17, 20, 21]. However, the majority of cases of infective endocarditis are due to *staphylococcal* and *streptococcal* organisms. It is recognized that most cases of tricuspid valve endocarditis in intravenous drug abusers are due to either *Staphylococcus aureus* or *Candida* species. Although endocardial damage is regarded as a prerequisite for developing infective endocarditis, highly virulent organisms such as *Staphylococcus aureus* are capable of infecting normal native valves.

The principal causes of bacteremia include routine dental treatment and/or dental sepsis. Other invasive procedures such as urogenital and gastrointestinal instrumentation may also provide a source of infection, and these procedures are the leading cause of *enterococcal* endocarditis. Infective endocarditis may also occur due to sepsis at other organ sites. Thus, skin infections, pneumonia, and meningitis are all significant risk factors for the development of this disease.

Macroscopically, the vegetation is pathognomonic of infective endocarditis (Fig. 9.1). Vegetations may vary considerably in size and number ranging from small sessile lesions to large polypoid masses. Factors influencing size include the valve site, hemodynamic pressures within the heart, and type of microorganism. The vegetation is a mass of thrombus, comprising platelets, fibrin, and microorganism colonies – often walled off from neutrophil polymorphs (Fig. 9.2). The vegetations typically spread along the closure

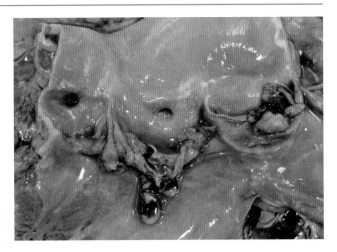

Fig. 9.1 Bacterial endocarditis in an intravenous drug abuser affecting the aortic valve. Irregular *yellow* vegetations are present on the closure line of the cusps of the aortic valve. *Staphylococcus aureus* was isolated

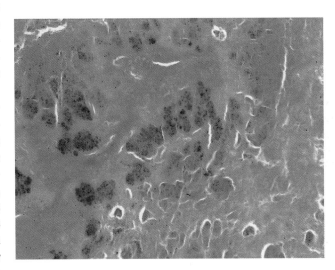

Fig. 9.2 Photomicrograph of the histology of a vegetation caused by bacterial endocarditis. The valve cusp is covered by a mass of eosinophilic thrombus containing basophilic colonies of bacteria. The colonies occur within the deeper layers of the thrombus, where it is difficult for neutrophil polymorphs to penetrate (hematoxylin & eosin)

line of the valves and are friable and craggy. Some vegetations, containing *Staphylococcus aureus* or fungal species (Fig. 9.3), tend to be large and locally destructive. Those due to less virulent organisms may be smaller and flatter – causing less damage to the valve.

Floppy mitral valve autopsy studies have shown that the primary site of infection is the valve leaflet. Spread of the infection in these valves may occur with spread to the left atrial wall at the site of jet lesions [22] or friction lesions in the left ventricular wall [23]. Secondary involvement of the chordae has also been observed [3].

The complications of infective endocarditis depend very much on the virulence of the organism and may include cusp perforation, chordal rupture, aneurysmal bulging of the valve, and perivalvular abscess formation. This may lead to

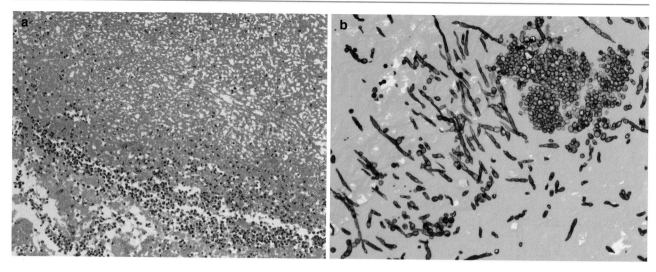

Fig. 9.3 Photomicrograph of the histology of a vegetation caused by fungal endocarditis (hematoxylin & eosin). The vegetation (**a**) comprises of a dense eosinophilic mass of thrombus, containing spores and hyphae confirmed by Grocott staining (**b**). The underlying valve cusp was heavily inflamed, and neutrophil polymorphs were present at the periphery of the vegetation. *Candida* was isolated from the vegetation

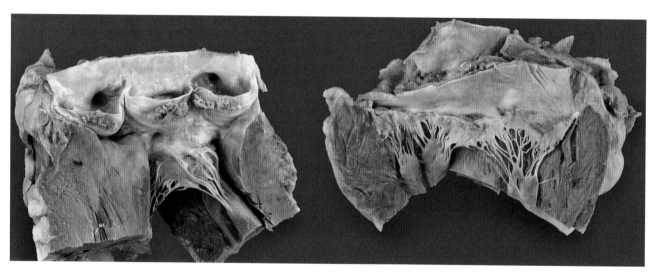

Fig. 9.4 Nonbacterial thrombotic endocarditis involving the aortic and mitral valves, respectively. On the aortic valve, there are small, pink, friable vegetations attached to the noduli Arantii of the cusps. On the mitral valve, the vegetations are yellow/gray and are arranged evenly along the closure line of the cusps. Both patients had underlying terminal malignancies

catastrophic aortic or mitral regurgitation with congestive heart failure. Systemic embolic events may also occur, and the risk of this complication increases according to the size of the vegetation, especially in those more than 10 mm in diameter [18]. Surgery is indicated in patients with infective endocarditis who have heart failure and either a stenotic or regurgitant valve [24].

In recent years, there have been radical changes in the recommendations for antibiotic prophylaxis to prevent infective endocarditis in patients with valvular heart disease or other risk factors. Discussion of these recommendations is beyond the scope of this chapter. However, they have been reviewed in detail for the management of patients with valvular heart disease [24].

Nonbacterial Thrombotic Endocarditis

Noninfective thrombotic endocarditis (NBTE) is characterized by large masses of thrombus, which often develop on the aortic and mitral valves. They are also known as marantic vegetations. They occur on the atrial surface of the mitral and tricuspid valves and the ventricular surface of the pulmonic and aortic valves. The most commonly affected valves are the aortic and/or mitral valve (Fig. 9.4) [25]. Histologically, these vegetations are comprised of fibrin and platelets with only occasional inflammatory cells [26]. They do not destroy the underlying valvular tissue, which shows only edema with minimal inflammatory change. The vegetations of NBTE typically occur in patients with terminal malignancy, such as adenocarcinomas, chronic infection, or acute disseminated intravascular coagulation – reflecting a prothrombotic state [25, 27]. The vegetations are not infected or destructive. However, they are of clinical importance as they may give rise to systemic emboli and are easily dislodged due to the lack of inflammatory reaction at the site of attachment [25, 28].

Libman–Sacks endocarditis is a type of NBTE and occurs in the setting of the antiphospholipid syndrome. This can be either primary or secondary to an underlying condition, usually systemic lupus erythematosus. Libman–Sacks endocarditis predominantly affects the ventricular aspects of the aortic and mitral valves and is characterized by small, sterile verrucous vegetations on the valve cusps comprised of thrombotic material. NBTE is usually associated with regurgitation as a consequence of valvulitis and healing due to fibrous thickening of the valve as well as thromboembolic complications [29].

Rheumatic Valvular Heart Disease

Rheumatic valvular heart disease may potentially affect any of the heart valves, but most commonly the mitral and aortic valves are affected. This disease occurs after an episode of acute valvulitis following acute rheumatic fever. Acute rheumatic fever is a disease of childhood caused by group A β(beta)-hemolytic *streptococci*. Initially causing a pharyngitis, the *Streptococcal* infection manifests as a febrile illness with a rash, polyarthritis, and involvement of the heart in the form of a pancarditis.

In the acute stage of the illness, pancarditis occurs and involves all three layers of the heart (pericardium, myocardium, and endocardium). Chronic rheumatic valvular disease is a long-term complication of immunologically mediated injury to the valve cusps. There are currently no medical treatments to prevent or delay disease progression [24].

Those with rheumatic mitral stenosis are prone to develop pulmonary hypertension and atrial fibrillation, which is associated with left atrial dilatation [30]. Indeed, a systemic embolic event from an atrial thrombus may be the first manifestation of this disease [31].

Although the incidence of rheumatic fever has steadily declined in the industrialized world since the 1970s [24], its incidence remains high in developing countries. In these areas, rheumatic valvular heart disease is commonly observed in the elderly population or immigrants from less developed nations.

Acute Rheumatic Valvulitis and Carditis

In the acute phase, rheumatic fever is characterized by pancarditis. Initially, a fibrinous pericarditis occurs with no specific histological features and may be associated with

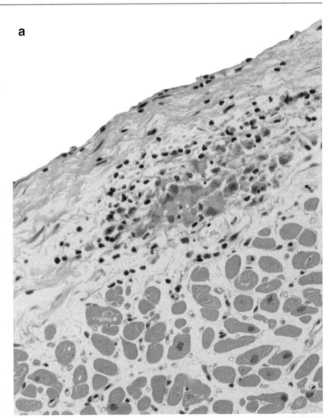

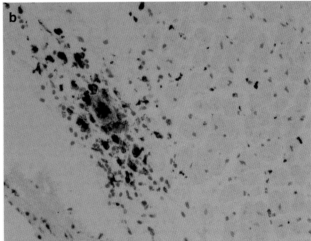

Fig. 9.5 (a) Photomicrograph of an Aschoff body in rheumatic fever. In the subendocardium, there is a rounded collection of giant cells and histiocytes surrounded by lymphocytes (hematoxylin & eosin). This was an incidental finding in the papillary muscle of an elderly patient with chronic rheumatic valvular heart disease. (b) Immunostains for CD68 confirm the presence of cells of macrophage origin in the Aschoff body

pericardial effusion. In contrast, the myocarditis is associated with microscopic granulomas in the cardiac interstitium – termed Aschoff bodies (Fig. 9.5). These are characterized by a central core of collagen surrounded by epithelioid histiocytes. The granulomas are comprised of a combination of Anitschkow cells, which have a central rod of chromatin and Aschoff giant cells, which are formed from the coalescence of multinucleated histiocytes. The Aschoff bodies are usually associated with a lymphocytic chronic inflammatory cell infiltrate. They are most commonly found in a subendocardial location but rarely occur in the valves themselves.

Myocarditis remains a rare but life-threatening complication of acute rheumatic fever and is characterized by congestive cardiac failure, arrhythmias, and heart block. Although long-term myocardial dysfunction is generally not observed, the Aschoff bodies disappear over time and are replaced by fibrous scars. However, the Aschoff bodies may persist for over a decade after the initial illness. They are not indicative of active disease. In the acute phase of the disease, the valvulitis is associated with small translucent nodules along the line of closure of the valve, sometimes involving the chordae.

Chronic Rheumatic Valvulitis and Carditis

Chronic rheumatic valvular heart disease may often present after a latent period of between 20 and 40 years after the initial infection. It runs a slow, stable course followed by accelerated progression later in life [30]. Clinically, it may present with stenosis and/or regurgitation, often affecting the aortic and mitral valves. Macroscopically, rheumatic aortic and mitral valves have a variable appearance depending on the underlying functional abnormality. The valve often becomes hyalinized, fibrotic, and there is commissural fusion.

Microscopically, the hallmarks of chronic rheumatic valvular heart disease include the triad of fibrosis, calcification, and thick-walled blood vessels with, or without, chronic inflammation (Fig. 9.6). The normal valvular architecture is effaced by dense fibrosis, and thick-walled blood vessels can be seen permeating the valve. The presence of thick-walled blood vessels is not pathognomonic of rheumatic valvular heart disease and may occur in healed infective endocarditis. These vessels serve as an indicator of a severe inflammatory insult to the valve in the past. However, the diagnosis can usually be confidently made, given the characteristic macroscopic features of rheumatic valves coupled with the mixed functional abnormalities observed echocardiographically.

Early studies have shown that the mitral valve is involved in 85% of cases, the aortic in 44%, the tricuspid in 10–16%, and the pulmonary valve in 1–2% of cases [32]. Isolated mitral stenosis occurs in 40% of patients with rheumatic fever and is more commonly observed in women [33–35].

For example, in stenotic rheumatic mitral valves, there is commissural fusion, nodular calcification, as well as thickening, shortening, and fusion of the chordae [36]. The valve orifice is reduced to a narrow opening, and stenotic mitral valves have a so-called "fish-mouth" appearance with an oval aperture (Fig. 9.7). The area of the normal mitral valve is often reduced by 50% [37]. In rheumatic mitral valves, the chordae tendineae are typically fused and thickened causing outflow tract obstruction. This is a helpful clue to the macroscopic diagnosis of stenotic valves. By contrast, regurgitant valves are fibrotic, lack commissural fusion, and have a reduced surface area. Other features include the presence of atrial dilatation combined with the presence of "jet" lesions.

The valve in association with mitral regurgitation from rheumatic valves is often thickened, shortened, and has fused chordae, anchoring the posterior cusp of the mitral valve to the wall of the left ventricle. This is more commonly observed in children [38]. Complications associated with regurgitant mitral valves include the formation of thrombus in the atria

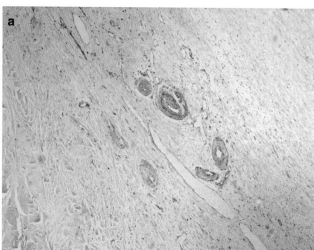
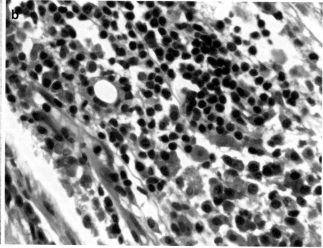

Fig. 9.6 (**a**) Photomicrograph of *thick-walled* blood vessels accompanied by fibrosis in a mitral valve affected by chronic rheumatic valvular heart disease. These vessels are not pathognomonic of rheumatic valvular heart disease but may serve as an indicator of a severe inflammatory insult to the valve in the past. (**b**) Photomicrograph of a dense lymphoplasmacytic inflammatory cell infiltrate in a rheumatic mitral valve (hematoxylin & eosin)

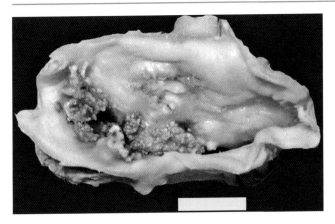

Fig. 9.7 Surgically excised stenotic rheumatic mitral valve viewed from the atrial aspect. The orifice is narrowed due to commissural fusion and has a characteristic "fish-mouth" appearance with an oval aperture. Nodular calcification and fibrotic thickening of the cusps are evident. In rheumatic mitral valves, the chordae tendineae are typically fused and thickened causing outflow tract obstruction (*bar marker* 1 cm)

or atrial appendages, leading to systemic emboli, infective endocarditis, and pulmonary hypertension.

The surgical treatment of choice for rheumatic mitral stenosis is either commissurotomy or percutaneous mitral valvotomy, whereby one or more large endovascular balloons are inflated across the valve orifice. Mitral valve replacement with, or without, chordal reconstruction is reserved for patients with significant calcification and deformity of the chordal apparatus [24].

Senile Tricuspid Calcific Aortic Stenosis

Senile tricuspid calcific aortic stenosis is the commonest cause of aortic stenosis requiring valve replacement surgery in the elderly population of the industrialized world, with an estimated prevalence of 2.9% in the 75–86-year age group [39]. Symptoms are rare in patients less than 70 years of age. In contrast to BAV, senile tricuspid calcific valves are also associated with aortic root dilatation and dissection albeit at a much later age [40, 41].

Senile calcific aortic stenosis is not a passive degenerative condition but is an active disease process characterized by inflammation, dystrophic calcification, and osseous metaplasia with risk factors similar to those observed for the development of atherosclerosis [42]. Macroscopically, it is characterized by the three cusps having relatively equal size, being studded with nodules of calcification over the aortic aspect of the cusp without commissural fusion (Fig. 9.8). The calcification progresses from the base of the cusp to the leaflet causing loss of valve area and reduced cusp motion. Thrombosis and ulceration can occur over the calcific nodules. Microscopically, calcification starts within the valve fibrosa towards the free edge of the cusps, and

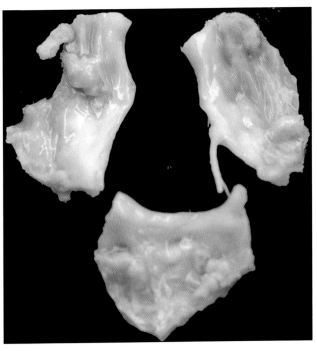

Fig. 9.8 Surgically excised senile tricuspid calcific aortic stenosis. The lack of commissural fusion enables the surgeon to remove the cusps individually. The cusps are of roughly equal size and studded by nodules of calcification. No vegetations are seen

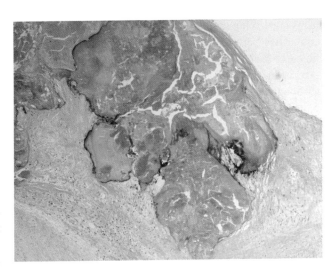

Fig. 9.9 Photomicrograph of senile tricuspid calcific aortic stenosis. The valve architecture is largely effaced by nodular calcific deposits. The calcification elicits neovascularization of the cusp. A mild chronic inflammatory cell infiltrate comprised of lymphocytes and/or plasma cells is often evident (hematoxylin & eosin)

there is associated fibrosis (Fig. 9.9). The calcium elicits a neovascular response, and thin-walled capillary-sized blood vessels are a common feature. A mild chronic inflammatory cell infiltrate comprised of lymphocytes and/or plasma cells may also be evident. The cusps may often be submitted piecemeal, making the diagnostic distinction from other calcific processes affecting the valve (e.g., rheumatic valvular disease) difficult. However, thick-walled blood vessels are rarely apparent, being a common feature of postinflammatory valves. Another feature, also frequently seen in end-stage senile tricuspid calcific valves, is heterotopic ossification sometimes with hematopoietic elements. This has been ascribed to tissue remodeling and pathological microfracture repair and is accompanied by the expression of the bone matrix morphogenetic proteins, BMP 2 and BMP 4 [43]. Indeed, it has been postulated that a calcifying osteoblast phenotype is the final common pathway for the development of valve calcification [42].

The risk factors for developing senile tricuspid calcific aortic stenosis are similar to those for atheroma and include male gender, abnormal lipid profiles, hypertension, diabetes mellitus, chronic renal disease, and cigarette smoking [43–50]. It has been recently shown that paraoxonase-1 (PON-1) activity is reduced in patients with severe calcific aortic stenosis. PON-1 is a high-density lipoprotein-bound enzyme with antiatherogenic properties preventing oxidative modification of LDL. Indeed, PON-1 activity appears inversely correlated with the severity of aortic stenosis and is significantly lower in patients with severe aortic stenosis compared with patients with only mild and moderate disease [51].

There has been significant progress over the past decade in our understanding of the molecular and cellular mechanisms underlying senile calcific aortic stenosis [42, 52]. The similarities between the pathology of atherosclerosis and the early lesions of senile tricuspid calcific aortic stenosis have been shown histologically by the demonstration of apolipoproteins, foamy macrophages, and T lymphocytes in the valve and the expression of cell adhesion proteins [44, 45, 53]. Furthermore, experimental animal models have confirmed that experimental hypercholesterolemia causes both atherosclerosis and aortic valve calcification [42, 54]. Valvular calcification appears to be actively regulated in tricuspid calcific aortic valves, as shown by the expression in macrophages and at mineralization zones of osteopontin – a protein involved in the regulation of both normal and dystrophic calcification [55, 56]. The presence of myofibroblastic cells with an osteoblastic phenotype within the valve appears to regulate calcification and bone formation via bone morphogenetic proteins 2 and 4 [43, 57, 58]. It has also been shown that stenotic aortic valves have increased activity of matrix metalloproteinases [59–61] and elastolytic cathepsins S, K, and V and their inhibitor cystatin C [62, 63]. The latter appear to participate in degeneration of the aortic valvular extracellular matrix and the promotion of neovascularization, as well as bone formation and remodeling, thereby promoting aortic stenosis. Furthermore, the increased production of proinflammatory cytokines, such as tumor necrosis factor-alpha (TNF-α(alpha)) and interleukin-1 (IL1) by inflammatory cells within the valve, mediates the upregulation of cathepsins and matrix metalloproteinases [62–64],

as well as promoting an osteoblast-like phenotype in human aortic valve myofibroblasts [63]. Other cytokines, such as tissue growth factor beta-1 (TGFβ(beta)-1), are present in calcified human aortic valve leaflets and have been shown to mediate calcification of sheep aortic valve interstitial cells in culture by mechanisms involving apoptosis [65]. Recent studies have shown that the activator of nuclear factor kappa-B ligand (RANKL) and osteoprotegerin (OPG) cytokine system is also involved in bone turnover and vascular calcification and is differentially expressed in human aortic calcified stenotic valves. RANKL also promotes matrix calcification, induces an osteoblastic phenotype in vitro in cultured human aortic valve myofibroblasts, and promotes matrix metalloproteinase expression. This suggests further novel pathways are involved in calcific aortic stenosis [64, 66]. The presence of angiogenic growth factors, such as vascular endothelial growth factor (VEGF) in stenotic aortic valves, implies that angiogenesis may influence disease progression [67]. Clearly, there appears to be a complex interplay between mediators of inflammation, angiogenesis, osteoblastic differentiation, cathepsin, and matrix metalloproteinase activity in senile calcific aortic stenosis, which may represent future potential therapeutic targets [58, 59, 63–65, 68].

Several genetic studies have shed light on the risk factors determining the genetic predisposition to the development of aortic valve calcification. These include the finding that the B allele of the vitamin D receptor is more common in patients with senile tricuspid calcific aortic stenosis [69]. Another study showed that estrogen receptor alpha gene polymorphisms are related to lipid levels in adolescent females and the development of aortic stenosis in postmenopausal women. Consequently, this polymorphism may influence the risk of developing disease by affecting lipid metabolism [70].

The natural history of senile tricuspid calcific aortic stenosis consists of a prolonged latent period explaining how it is a disease of the elderly [71]. Later symptoms of heart failure, angina, and syncope supervene. There is a significant increase in morbidity, and patients are at risk of sudden cardiac death [72]. Appropriate surgical intervention in the form of aortic valve replacement is essential [73], and it may be performed at any age.

Some studies have shown that statins appear to slow the progression of aortic stenosis [56, 74, 75], whereas others have yielded lesser results [76, 77]. Indeed, statins per se may actually induce bone formation [78]. Other therapeutic strategies are aimed at reversing the effects of atherosclerosis. ACE inhibitors may provide an alternative medical therapy in elderly patients, as shown by the presence of ACE, angiotensin II, and the AT-1 receptor in stenotic calcified aortic valves [79]. Certainly, standard medical therapies for cardiac failure and angina may bridge the gap before valve surgery/intervention.

Congenital Bicuspid Aortic Valves

Congenital bicuspid aortic valves (BAVs) are the most common form of congenital heart disease and a leading cause of aortic stenosis and aortic regurgitation. They typically affect 1–2% of the population [80, 81] and present at a younger age than those with senile tricuspid calcification. There is strong male (3:1) predominance [82]. BAVs may also occur in patients with Turner's syndrome [83], William's syndrome [80, 84] and are associated with other forms of congenital heart disease including coarctation of the aorta [85], patent ductus arteriosus [86], and ventricular septal defects [87] and Shone's anomaly [88]. BAV is inherited as an autosomal dominant trait with low penetrance [89, 90]. Thus, screening of first-degree relatives of patients with a BAV is now recommended [90–92].

Typically, BAVs are comprised of one large cusp together with a smaller cusp, although a very small percentage may be unicuspid (Fig. 9.10) [93]. Classically, the larger valve leaflet has a central prominent central raphe or ridge, which lacks valve tissue, and a V-shaped notch along the free edge of the cusp. The cusp margins are smooth and straighter than that observed in normal valves. Commissural fusion is evident by the position of the raphe. Different anatomical patterns of the bileaflet valve are evident according to which cusps have fused. Fusion of the left and right coronary cusps is often observed with coarctation of the aorta and fusion of the right, and noncoronary cusp is associated with more severe valve dysfunction in children [82, 94]. There are various classifications describing the orientation of the leaflets and presence or absence of a raphe in BAVs [93, 95–97]. In stenotic BAVs, the superior surfaces of the cusp are studded with varying amounts of nodular calcification predominantly affecting the base of the cusp and the raphe [93]. The main principal differential diagnosis when the pathologist is confronted with two heavily calcified valve cusps is between aortic stenosis due to chronic rheumatic valvular heart disease and a heavily calcified BAV. The presence of a raphe in a stenotic valve is a feature more commonly seen in a BAV. Alternatively, this can usually be resolved by correlation with echocardiography (prior to surgery) and microscopy. In most cases of rheumatic valvular heart disease, there will often be concomitant disease involvement of the mitral valve. Furthermore, plump thick-walled blood vessels, in general, are not a prominent feature of BAVs but are germane to rheumatic valves. Their presence within a valve indicates that the valve has been subjected to a severe inflammatory insult in the past. It is not uncommon for calcification to elicit some neovascularization of the valve, but the presence of large caliber vessels is less common in the BAV. Calcification occurs at a much younger age in patients with BAV and is accelerated with symptomatic valvular disease occurring at 50–60 years of age [98]. The pathogenesis and propensity of BAVs to undergo calcification appear to be partly regulated

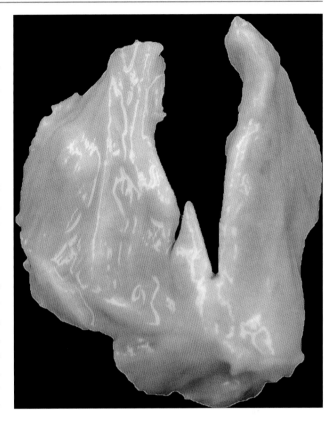

Fig. 9.10 Surgically excised unicommissural congenital aortic valve with an oval orifice. A prominent raphe indicating commissural fusion is evident

by the modulation calcification-related genes [99]. The development of calcification in valve cusps appears to be similar to that observed in patients with senile tricuspid calcific stenosis [100], and BAV patients often have hypercholesterolemia [101] and high C-reactive protein levels [102], both of which appear to accelerate the process of calcification. Calcification in BAV also appears to be inversely linked to endothelial nitric oxide synthase (eNOS).

Congenital BAVs may also present with aortic regurgitation. This typically necessitates valve replacement and is commonly seen in a younger age group. A complication of these valves is infective endocarditis [103]. Regurgitant BAVs are translucent, and one cusp is commonly larger in area than the other. These cusps are unable to support each other during valve apposition, and the free edge of the valve cusps has a tendency to slide under one another. Macroscopically, congenital BAVs that are regurgitant are soft, translucent, and lack calcification. The free edge of the cusp has a rolled appearance due to regurgitant blood flow. Microscopically, bicuspid regurgitant valves have a characteristic "tadpole" appearance where there is nodular fibrosis of the free edge of the cusp in association with myxomatous degeneration of the valve spongiosa.

Both regurgitant, stenotic, and hemodynamically normal BAVs are associated with aortic root dilatation, aortic dissection, and aneurysm formation [104–107]. Thus, aortic root dilatation begins at an early age in BAV patients and is

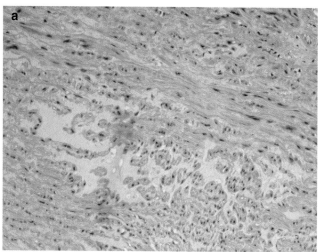 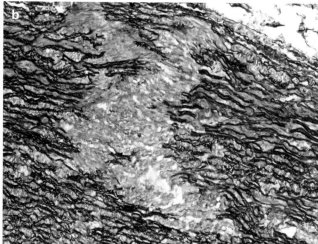

Fig. 9.11 Photomicrograph of a dilated aortic root from a Turner's syndrome patient with a congenital bicuspid aortic valve. (**a**) There is prominent cystic medial necrosis with smooth muscle cell loss, accumulation of basophilic ground substance (hematoxylin & eosin). (**b**) Fragmentation of elastic fibers confirmed (elastic van Gieson)

associated with midascending-type dilatation [108] and can occur in patients with normally functioning valves [109]. The risk of aortic dissection in patients with a BAV is considerably higher than those with a tricuspid valve [41]. Frequently the pathologist is sent aortic wall due to aortic root dilatation following reconstruction of the aortic root. Indeed, BAVs should be considered as a disease of the entire aortic root and aorta, and it has been suggested that replacement of the aortic root and valve (rather than isolated valve replacement) should be performed in these patients [110, 111].

Individuals with regurgitant BAV have defects in the fibrillin-1 gene and altered matrix metalloproteinase activity leading to loss of structural stability, root dilatation, and a risk of proximal thoracic aneurysms. Histologically, there is prominent Erdheim-type "cystic medial necrosis" [112] with fragmentation of elastic fibers and noninflammatory smooth muscle cell loss and accumulation of basophilic ground substance (Fig. 9.11) [113, 114]. Indeed, the aortic pathology is indistinguishable from that observed in patients with Marfan's syndrome or Ehlers–Danlos syndrome. Although some of the dilatation observed can be ascribed to haemodynamic abnormalities, it has become increasingly apparent that there are structural changes at the cellular level rendering the aorta prone to dilatation and aneurysm formation [104, 105, 113, 114].

Noncalcific Age-Related Degenerative Change of the Aortic Valve

Aortic regurgitation may also occur due to age-related degenerative change. This is characterized by myxomatous degeneration of the valve spongiosa and is analogous to the macroscopic and microscopic phenomena observed in floppy mitral valves. Fenestrations with fine cord-like structures are often observed at the free edges of the expanded cusps. Aortic root dilatation, the so-called "annuloaortic ectasia," may also feature.

Floppy Mitral Valve (Mitral Valve Prolapse)

Floppy mitral valves are now the leading cause of isolated mitral regurgitation in the industrialized world and represent a large subset of patients requiring surgery, often presenting in the fifth and sixth decade [115–117]. Floppy mitral valves are due to billowing and prolapse of one or more mitral valve leaflets during systole into the left atrium. The entity was first described by Read in 1965, and a wide range of terms have since been used in the literature to describe these valves, including Barlow disease [118]. The prevalence is considered to be 1–2.5% of the general population [119], being both familial and sporadic. The familial forms are transmitted as an autosomal dominant trait with incomplete penetrance [7] and are associated with several different chromosomal loci, including chromosomes 13, 11, 16, and the X chromosome [117, 120–122]. However, no specific gene has been identified. Inherited floppy mitral valves are observed more commonly in patients with connective tissue disorders, such as Marfan's syndrome, pseudoxanthoma elasticum, osteogenesis imperfecta, and Ehlers–Danlos syndrome [3]. It has been postulated that they may occur as a consequence of a generalized disorder of connective tissue.

Floppy mitral valves are characterized by an increase in cusp area with attenuation and elongation of the chordae tendineae, which have a propensity to rupture. The valve loses its elasticity and resistance and becomes redundant

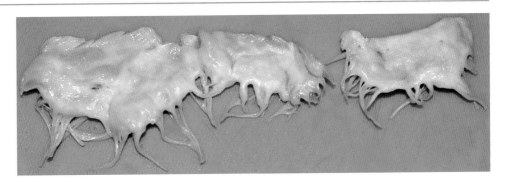

Fig. 9.12 Surgically excised floppy mitral valve. There is *dome-shaped* billowing of the valve cusps, less marked than when the valve is under pressure in vivo. The chordae tendineae are elongated and thinned with a propensity to rupture

hence the designation – i.e., floppy. During systole, the valve prolapses into the atria, leading to regurgitation. The posterior cusp is most commonly affected. There is also dilatation of the mitral annulus [123]. Macroscopically, the valve appears ballooned or hooded, being translucent and soft to touch. In contrast to chronic rheumatic valvular heart disease, there is no commissural fusion (Fig. 9.12). Microscopically, there is no calcification or neovascularization of the valve. Instead, there is prominent myxomatous degeneration with connective tissue degradation and accumulation of proteoglycans in the spongiosa, which encroaches on the fibrosa, leading to loss of normal structure. It is accompanied by surface fibrosis over the atrial aspect of the valves (Fig. 9.13) [3, 124–127].

Echocardiography is the method of choice for assessing significant prolapse, but some 80% of asymptomatic and healthy individuals will show a minor degree of cusp prolapse – clearly of no significance. The natural history of the floppy valve can vary from a benign course with normal life expectancy to severe mitral regurgitation, which is associated with significant morbidity and early mortality [128].

Floppy mitral valves are subject to several complications, including chordal rupture, leading to acute, severe mitral regurgitation [128] and a risk of infective endocarditis. The elongated chordae may also interact on the endocardium, leading to endocardial fibrosis and so-called "friction lesions" on the left ventricular wall, which may entrap the chordae and/or promote mitral regurgitation. Atrial fibrillation due to left atrial enlargement is a well-recognized complication in patients with floppy mitral valves. This is associated with an increased risk of sudden cardiac death or heart failure [129]. There is also a rare but increased risk of sudden cardiac death in patients with floppy mitral valves due to malignant ventricular arrhythmias [123, 130].

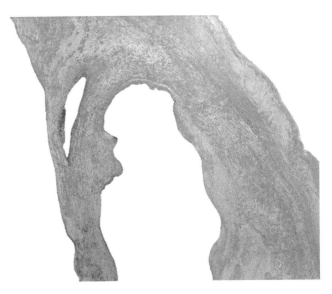

Fig. 9.13 Photomicrograph of a floppy mitral valve showing myxomatous degeneration and accumulation of proteoglycans with loss of collagen in the valve spongiosa, which impinges on the fibrosa. This leads to loss of normal structure. It is accompanied by surface fibrosis (Alcian blue and elastic van Gieson)

causing acute and severe mitral regurgitation. Of the two ventricular papillary muscles, the posteromedial muscle has a lesser blood supply, and lesions are more frequently observed in this muscle compared to the anterolateral muscle [38]. Papillary muscle dysfunction can also be observed in a wide range of cardiac diseases including endomyocardial fibrosis, anomalous coronary arteries, and various infiltrative disease of the myocardium. Congenital malformations of the papillary muscles themselves have also been described and include a single muscle in the left ventricle – the so-called "parachute" mitral valve [38].

Mitral Regurgitation Due to Papillary Muscle Rupture

Mitral regurgitation can also occur in the setting of ischemic heart disease, where damage and rupture of ischemic papillary muscles secondary to acute myocardial infarction occur,

Tricuspid Valve Disease

Disease of the tricuspid valve is much rarer than the other forms of valvular heart disease. The most common causes of tricuspid regurgitation include rheumatic heart disease, infective endocarditis, carcinoid heart disease, radiation damage, Marfan's syndrome, and Ebstein's anomaly.

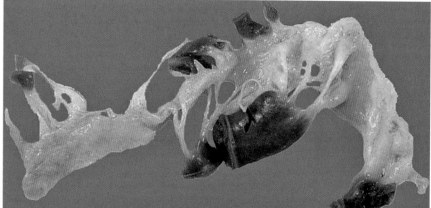
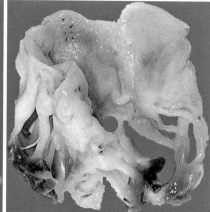
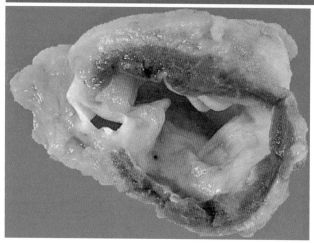

Fig. 9.14 A surgical resection sample set from a case of carcinoid syndrome. The valves were all thickened, opaque, reduced in cross-sectional area and irregular in morphology. No vegetations were present. Tricuspid valve (*top left*), mitral valve (*top right*), pulmonary valve (viewed from the conus, *bottom*)

Ebstein's anomaly is a congenital heart disorder that may present in adulthood. It is characterized by inferior displacement of the septal and posterior cusps of the tricuspid valve into the right ventricle and leads to variable tricuspid regurgitation. Carcinoid heart disease occurs in approximately half of patients with a functionally and significantly active carcinoid tumor. The tricuspid leaflets become opaque, thickened, and reduced in area (Fig. 9.14). Histologically, there is cellular fibroblast-rich tissue on the surfaces of the cusps. The proliferation occurs in response to vasoactive amines including serotonin and 5-hydroxytryptamine released from the tumor.

Tricuspid stenosis occurs in most frequently in the setting of rheumatic heart disease, and there is usually a concomitant degree of regurgitation, as well as aortic and mitral valve involvement. In rheumatic disease, there is commonly commissural fusion, and the valve may appear as a fibrous diaphragm with a central aperture. Other rare causes of tricuspid stenosis include infective endocarditis with large vegetations, Fabry's disease, Whipple's disease, treatment with methysergide (for refractory migraine), and giant blood cysts [131–133].

Pulmonary Valve Disease

The pulmonary valve is rarely involved in adult life (as acquired valvular heart disease) compared with the other valves and is operated on the least. The most commonly observed diseases of this valve include carcinoid heart disease and pulmonary valve stenosis, which is usually part of congenital heart disease [134, 135]. In carcinoid heart disease, the pulmonary valve cusps appear white, fibrotic, and shrunken causing either pulmonary stenosis or insufficiency. It may be part of congenital heart disease.

Conclusion

Over the last half century, significant progress has been made in our understanding and treatment of valvular heart disease. With the decline in rheumatic heart disease, the pathologist is most likely to encounter floppy mitral valves, senile tricuspid aortic valves, and congenital BAVs as part of routine practice.

In the future, advances in our understanding of the cellular and molecular mechanisms underlying valvular heart disease will hopefully lead to the emergence of new therapeutic modalities to prevent disease progression. This will invariably reduce the need for open surgical intervention, which remains a significant economic burden in the industrialized world.

References

1. Carpentier A. Cardiac valve surgery – the "French correction". J Thorac Cardiovasc Surg. 1983;86:323–37.

2. Ranganathan N, Lam JHC, Wigle ED, et al. Morphology of the human mitral valve: II. The valve leaflets. Circulation. 1970;41:459–67.

3. Lucas Jr RV, Edwards JE. The floppy mitral valve. Curr Probl Cardiol. 1982;7:1–48.

4. Cherubin CE, Neu HC. Infective endocarditis at the Presbyterian Hospital in New York City. Am J Med. 1971;51:83–95.

5. Rabinovich S, Evans J, Smith IM, et al. A long-term view of bacterial endocarditis. Ann Intern Med. 1965;63:185–98.

6. Devereux RB, Frary CJ, Kramer-Fox R, et al. Cost-effectiveness of infective endocarditis prophylaxis for mitral valve prolapse with or without a mitral regurgitant murmur. Am J Cardiol. 1994;74:1024–9.

7. Devereux RB, Brown WT, Kramer-Fox R, et al. Inheritance of mitral valve prolapse: effect of age and sex on gene expression. Ann Intern Med. 1982;97:826–32.

8. Clemens JD, Horwitz RI, Jaffe CC, et al. A controlled evaluation of the risk of bacterial endocarditis in persons with mitral valve prolapse. N Engl J Med. 1982;307:776–81.

9. McKinsey DS, Ratts TE, Bisno AL. Underlying cardiac lesions in adults with infective endocarditis. The changing spectrum. Am J Med. 1987;82:681–8.

10. Hickey AJ, MacMahon SW, Wilcken DEL. Mitral valve prolapse and bacterial endocarditis: when is antibiotic prophylaxis necessary? Am Heart J. 1985;109:421–35.

11. Danchin N, Voiriot P, Briancon S, et al. Mitral valve prolapse as a risk factor for infective endocarditis. Lancet. 1989;1:743–5.

12. MacMahon SW, Hickey AJ, Wilcken DE, et al. Risk of infective endocarditis in mitral valve prolapse with and without precordial murmurs. Am J Cardiol. 1987;59:105–8.

13. Marks AR, Choong CY, Sanfilippo AJ, et al. Identification of high-risk and low-risk subgroups of patients with mitral-valve prolapse. N Engl J Med. 1989;320:1031–6.

14. Varstela E, Verkkala K, Pohjola-Sintonen S, et al. Surgical treatment of infective aortic valve endocarditis. Scand J Thorac Cardiovasc Surg. 1991;25:167–74.

15. Janatuinen MJ, Vanttinen EA, Nikoskelainen J, et al. Surgical treatment of active native endocarditis. Scand J Thorac Cardiovasc Surg. 1990;24:181–5.

16. Lamas CC, Ekyn SJ. Bicuspid aortic valve – a silent danger: analysis of 50 cases of infective endocarditis. Clin Infect Dis. 2000;30:336–41.

17. Moulsdale MT, Eykyn SJ, Phillips I. Infective endocarditis 1970–1979. A study of culture-positive cases in St. Thomas Hospital. Q J Med. 1980;49:315–28.

18. Mugge A, Daniel WG, Frank G, et al. Echocardiography in infective endocarditis: reassessment of prognostic implications of vegetation size determined by the transthoracic and the transesophageal approach. J Am Coll Cardiol. 1989;14:631–8.

19. Freedman LR, Valone Jr J. Experimental infective endocarditis. Prog Cardiovasc Dis. 1979;22:169–80.

20. Petersdorf RG, Pelletier LL, Durack DT. The 1976 Paul B. Beeson lecture. Some observations on experimental endocarditis. Yale J Biol Med. 1977;50:67–75.

21. Von Reyn CF, Levy BS, Arbeit RD, et al. Infective endocarditis: an analysis based on strict case definitions. Ann Intern Med. 1981;94:505–18.

22. Ringer M, Feen DJ, Drapkin M. Mitral valve prolapse: jet stream causing mural endocarditis. Am J Cardiol. 1980;45:383–5.

23. Kuhn III C, Weber N. Mural bacterial endocarditis of a ventricular friction lesion. Arch Pathol. 1973;95:92–3.

24. Bonow RO, Carabello BA, Chatterjee K, et al. 2008 focused update incorporated into the ACC/AHA 2006 guidelines for the management of patients with valvular heart disease: a report of the American College of Cardiology/American Heart Association Task Force on Practice Guidelines (Writing Committee to revise the 1998 guidelines for the management of patients with valvular heart disease). Endorsed by the Society of Cardiovascular Anesthesiologists, Society for Cardiovascular Angiography and Interventions, and Society of Thoracic Surgeons. J Am Coll Cardiol. 2008;52:e1–142.

25. El-Shami K, Griffiths E, Streiff M. Nonbacterial thrombotic endocarditis in cancer patients; pathogenesis, diagnosis and treatment. The Oncologist. 2007;12:518–23.

26. Eiken PW, Edwards WD, Tazelaar HD, et al. Surgical pathology of nonbacterial thrombotic endocarditis in 30 patients, 1985–2000. Mayo Clin Proc. 2001;76:1204–12.

27. Kim H, Suzuki M, Lie J, et al. Non-bacterial thrombotic endocarditis (NBTE) and disseminated intravascular coagulation (DIC). Arch Pathol Lab Med. 1977;101:65–8.

28. Olney B, Schattenberg T, Campbell J, et al. The consequences of the inconsequential: marantic (non-bacterial thrombotic) endocarditis. Am Heart J. 1979;98:513–22.

29. Hojnik M, George J, Ziporen L, et al. Heart valve involvement (Libman-Sacks Endocarditis) in the antiphospholipid syndrome. Circulation. 1996;93:1579–87.

30. Selzer A, Kohn KE. Natural history of mitral stenosis: a review. Circulation. 1972;45:878–90.

31. Abernathy WS, Willis III PW. Thromboembolic complications of rheumatic heart disease. Cardiovasc Clin. 1973;5:131–75.

32. Cabot RC. Facts on the heart. Philadelphia: W. B. Saunders; 1926.

33. Wood P. An appreciation of mitral stenosis, I: clinical features. Br Med J. 1954;4870:1051–63.

34. Rowe JC, Bland EF, Sprague HB, et al. The course of mitral stenosis without surgery: ten- and twenty-year perspectives. Ann Intern Med. 1960;52:741–9.

35. Olesen KH. The natural history of 271 patients with mitral stenosis under medical treatment. Br Heart J. 1962;24:349–57.

36. Rusted IE, Schiefley CH, Edwards JE. Studies of the mitral valve, II: certain anatomic features of the mitral valve and associated structures in mitral stenosis. Circulation. 1956;14:398–406.

37. Gorlin R, Gorlin SG. Hydraulic formula for calcification of the area of the stenotic mitral valve, other cardiac valves, and central circulatory shunts. Am Heart J. 1951;41:1–29.

38. Roberts WC. Morphologic features of the normal and abnormal mitral valve. Am J Cardiol. 1983;51:1005–28.

39. Lindroos M, Kupari M, Heikkila J, et al. Prevalence of aortic valve abnormalities in the elderly: an echocardiographic study of a random population sample. J Am Coll Cardiol. 1993;91:1220–5.

40. Yuan S-M, Jing H, Lavee J. The bicuspid aortic valve and its relation to aortic dilation. Clinics. 2010;65:497–505.

41. Larson EW, Edwards WD. Risk factors for aortic dissection: a necropsy study of 161 cases. Am J Cardiol. 1984;53:849–55.

42. Rajamannan NM. Calcific aortic stenosis: lessons learned from experimental and clinical studies. Arterioscler Thromb Vasc Biol. 2009;29:162–8.

43. Mohler III ER, Gannon F, Reynolds C, et al. Bone formation and inflammation in cardiac valves. Circulation. 2001;103:1522–8.

44. O'Brien KD, Reichenbach DD, Marcovina SM, et al. Apolipoproteins B (a), and E accumulate in the morphologically early lesion of "degenerative" valvular aortic stenosis. Arterioscler Thromb Vasc Biol. 1996;16:523–32.

45. Olsson M, Dalsgaard CJ, Haegerstrand A, et al. Accumulation of T lymphocytes and expression of interleukin-2 receptors in nonrheumatic stenotic aortic valves. J Am Coll Cardiol. 1994;23:1162–70.

46. Aronow WS, Schwartz KS, Koenigsberg M. Correlation of serum lipids, calcium, and phosphorus, diabetes mellitus and history of systemic hypertension with presence or absence of calcified or thickened aortic cusps or root in elderly patients. Am J Cardiol. 1987;59:998–9.

47. Mohler ER, Sheridan MJ, Nichols R, et al. Development and progression of aortic valve stenosis: atherosclerotic risk factors – a causal relationship? A clinical morphologic study. Clin Cardiol. 1991;14:995–9.

48. Stewart BF, Siscovick D, Lind BK, et al. Clinical factors associated with calcific aortic valve disease. J Am Coll Cardiol. 1997;29:630–4.

49. Palta S, Pai AM, Gill KS, et al. New insights into the progression of aortic stenosis. Implications for secondary prevention. Circulation. 2000;101:2497–502.

50. Nassimiha D, Aronow WS, Ahn C. Association of coronary risk factors with progression of valvular aortic stenosis. Am J Cardiol. 2001;87:1313–4.

51. Cagirci G, Cay S, Karakurt O, et al. Paraoxonase activity might be predictive of the severity of aortic valve stenosis. J Heart Valve Disease. 2010;19:453–8.

52. Yetkin E, Waltenberger J. Molecular and cellular mechanisms of aortic stenosis. Int J Cardiol. 2009;35:4–13.

53. Ghaisas NK, Foley JB, O'Brien DS, et al. Adhesion molecules in nonrheumatic aortic valve disease: endothelial expression, serum levels and effects of valve replacement. J Am Coll Cardiol. 2000;36:2257–62.

54. Sider KL, Blaser MC, Simmons CA. Animal models of calcific aortic valve disease. Article ID 364310, doi: 10.4061/2011/364310. Int J Inflamm 2011;2011:1–18.

55. O'Brien KD, Kuusisto J, Reichenbach M, et al. Osteopontin is expressed in human aortic valvular lesions. Circulation. 1995;92:2163–8.

56. Rajamannan NM, Subramaniam M, Springett M, et al. Atorvastatin inhibits hypercholesterolaemia-induced cellular proliferation and bone matrix production in the rabbit aortic valve. Circulation. 2002;105:2260–5.

57. Rajamannan NM, Subramaniam M, Rickard D, et al. Human aortic valve calcification is associated with an osteoblast phenotype. Circulation. 2003;107:2181–4.

58. Mohler III ER, Chawla MK, Chang AW, et al. Identification and characterization of calcifying valve cells from human and canine aortic valves. J Heart Valve Dis. 1999;8:254–60.

59. Kaden JJ, Bickelhaupt S, Grobholz R, et al. Receptor activator of nuclear factor kappaB ligand and osteoprotegerin regulate aortic valve calcification. J Mol Cell Cardiol. 2004;36:57–66.

60. Fondard O, Detaint D, Iung B, et al. Extracellular matrix remodelling in human aortic valve disease: the role of matrix metalloproteinases and their tissue inhibitors. Eur Heart J. 2005;26:1333–41.

61. Satta J, Oiva J, Salo T, et al. Evidence for an altered balance between matrix metalloproteinase-9 and its inhibitors in calcific aortic stenosis. Ann Thorac Surg. 2003;76:681–8.

62. Helske S, Syvaranta S, Lindstedt KA, et al. Increased expression of elastolytic cathepsins S, K, and V and their inhibitor cystatin C in aortic stenotic valves. Arterioscler Thromb Vasc Biol. 2006;26:1791–8.

63. Kaden JJ, Dempfle CE, Grobholz R, et al. Inflammatory regulation of extracellular matrix remodelling in calcific aortic valve stenosis. Cardiovasc Pathol. 2005;14:80–7.

64. Kaden JJ, Dempfle CE, Grobholz R, et al. Interleukin-1 beta promotes matrix metalloproteinase expression and cell proliferation in calcific aortic valve stenosis. Atherosclerosis. 2003;170:205–11.

65. Jian B, Narula N, Li QY, et al. Progression of aortic valve stenosis: TGF-beta 1 is present in calcified aortic valve cusps and promotes aortic valve interstitial cell calcification via apoptosis. Ann Thorac Surg. 2003;75:457–65.

66. Kaden JJ, Dempfle C-E, Kilic R, et al. Influence of receptor activator nuclear factor kappa B on human aortic valve myofibroblasts. Exp Mol Pathol. 2005;78:36–40.

67. Soini Y, Salo T, Satta J. Angiogenesis is involved in the pathogenesis of nonrheumatic aortic valve stenosis. Hum Pathol. 2003;34:756–63.

68. Yang X, Fullerton DA, Su X, et al. Pro-osteogenic phenotype of human aortic valve interstitial cells is associated with higher levels of Toll-like receptors 2 and 4 and enhanced expression of bone morphogenetic protein 2. J Am Coll Cardiol. 2009;53:491–500.

69. Ortlepp JR, Hoffmann R, Ohme F, et al. The vitamin D receptor genotype predisposes to the development of calcific aortic valve stenosis. Heart. 2001;85:635–8.

70. Nordstrom P, Glader CA, Dahlen G, et al. Oestrogen receptor alpha gene polymorphism is related to aortic valve sclerosis in postmenopausal women. J Intern Med. 2003;254:140–6.

71. Sprigings DC, Forfar JC. How should we manage symptomatic aortic stenosis in the patient who is 80 or older? Br Heart J. 1995;74:481–4.

72. Horstkotte D, Loogen F. The natural history of aortic valve stenosis. Eur Heart J. 1988;9(Suppl E):57–64.

73. Schwarz F, Baumann P, Manthey J, et al. The effect of aortic valve replacement on survival. Circulation. 1982;66:1105–10.

74. Novaro GM, Tiong IY, Pearce GL, et al. Effect of hydroxymethyl-glutaryl coenzyme a reductase inhibitors on the progression of calcific aortic stenosis. Circulation. 2001;104:2205–9.

75. Aronow WS, Ahn C, Kronzon I, et al. Association of coronary risk factors and use of statins with progression of mild valvular aortic stenosis in older persons. Am J Cardiol. 2001;88:309–15.

76. Cowell SJ, Newby DE, Prescott RJ, et al. A randomized trial of intensive lipid-lowering therapy in calcific aortic stenosis. N Engl J Med. 2005;352:2389–97.

77. Rossebo AB, Pedersen TR, Boman K, et al. Intensive lipid lowering with simvastatin and ezetimibe in aortic stenosis. N Engl J Med. 2008;359:1343–56.

78. Mundy G, Garret R, Harris S, et al. Stimulation of bone formation in vitro and in rodents by statins. Science. 1999;286:1946–9.

79. O'Brien KD, Shavelle DM, Caulfield MT, et al. Association of angiotensin-converting enzyme with low-density lipoprotein in aortic valvular lesions and in human plasma. Circulation. 2002;106:2224–30.

80. Braverman AC, Guven H, Beardslee MA, et al. The bicuspid aortic valve. Curr Probl Cardiol. 2005;30:470–522.

81. Hoffman JI, Kaplan S. The incidence of congenital heart disease. J Am Coll Cardiol. 2002;39:1890–900.

82. Siu SC, Silversides CK. Bicuspid aortic valve disease. J Am Coll Cardiol. 2010;55:2789–800.

83. Sybert VP. Cardiovascular malformations and complications in Turner syndrome. Pediatrics. 1998;101:E11.

84. Lopez-Rangel E, Maurice M, McGillivray B, et al. William's syndrome in adults. Am J Med Genet. 1992;44:720–9.

85. Roos-Hesselink JW, Scholzel BE, et al. Aortic valve and aortic arch pathology after coarctation repair. Heart. 2003;89:1074–7.

86. Deshpande J, Kinare SG. The bicuspid aortic valve – an autopsy study. Indian J Pathol Microbiol. 1991;34:112–8.

87. Suzuki T, Nagai R, Kurihara H, et al. Stenotic bicuspid aortic valve associated with a ventricular septal defect in an adult presenting with congestive heart failure: a rare observation. Eur Heart J. 1994;15:402–3.

88. Bolling SF, Iannattoni MD, Dick 2nd M, et al. Shone's anomaly: operative results and late outcome. Ann Thorac Surg. 1990;49:887–93.

89. Garg V, Muth AN, Ransom JF, et al. Mutations in NOTCH1 cause aortic valve disease. Nature. 2005;437:270–4.

90. Huntington K, Hunter AG, Chan KL. A prospective study to assess the frequency of familial clustering of congenital bicuspid aortic valve. J Am Coll Cardiol. 1997;30:1809–12.

91. Cripe L, Andelfinger G, Martin J, et al. Bicuspid aortic valve is heritable. J Am Coll Cardiol. 2004;44:138–43.

92. Warnes CA, Williams RG, Bashore TM, et al. ACC/AHA 2008 guidelines for the management of adults with congenital heart disease: a report of the American College of Cardiology/American Heart Association Task Force on Practice Guidelines (Writing Committee to Develop Guidelines on the Management of Adults With Congenital Heart Disease). J Am Coll Cardiol. 2008;52:e1–121.

93. Roberts WC. The congenitally bicuspid aortic valve. A study of 85 autopsy cases. Am J Cardiol. 1970;26:72–83.

94. Fernandes SM, Khairy P, Sanders SP, et al. Bicuspid aortic valve morphology and interventions in the young. J Am Coll Cardiol. 2007;49:2211–4.

95. Sievers HH, Schmidtke C. A classification system for the bicuspid aortic valve from 304 surgical specimens. J Thorac Cardiovasc Surg. 2007;133:1226–33.

96. Sabet HY, Edwards WD, Tazelaar HD, et al. Congenitally bicuspid aortic valves: a surgical pathology study of 542 cases (1991 through 1996) and a literature review of 2,715 additional cases. Mayo Clin Proc. 1999;74:14–26.

97. Angelini A, Ho SY, Anderson RH, et al. The morphology of the normal aortic valve as compared with the aortic valve having two cusps. J Thorac Cardiovasc Surg. 1989;89:362–7.

98. Beppu S, Suzuki S, Matsuda H, et al. Rapidity of progression of aortic stenosis in patients with congenital bicuspid aortic valves. Am J Cardiol. 1993;71:322–7.

99. Nigam V, Sievers HH, Jensen BC, Simpson PC, Srivastava D, Mohamed SA. Altered microRNAs in bicuspid aortic valve: a comparison between stenotic and insufficient valves. J Heart Valve Dis. 2010;19:459–65.

100. Rajamannan NM. Bicuspid aortic valve disease: the role of oxidative stress in Lrp5 bone formation. Cardiovasc Pathol. 2011;20:168–76.

101. Rabus MB, Kayalar N, Sareyyupoglu B, et al. Hypercholesterolaemia association with aortic stenosis of various etiologies. J Card Surg. 2009;24:146–50.

102. Yagubyan M, Sarkar G, Nishimura RA, et al. C-reactive protein as a marker of severe calcification among patients with bicuspid aortic valve disease. Journal of Surgical Research. 2004;121:281.

103. Fedak PW, Verma S, David TE, et al. Clinical and pathophysiological implications of a bicuspid aortic valve. Circulation. 2002;106:900–4.

104. Pachulski RT, Weinberg AL, Chan KL. Aortic aneurysm in patients with functionally normal or minimally stenotic bicuspid aortic valve. Am J Cardiol. 1991;67:781–2.

105. Hahn RT, Roman MJ, Mogtader AH, et al. Association of aortic dilation with regurgitant, stenotic and functionally normal bicuspid aortic valves. J Am Coll Cardiol. 1992;19:283–8.

106. Edwards WD, Leaf DS, Edwards JE. Dissecting aortic aneurysm associated with congenital bicuspid aortic valve. Circulation. 1978;57:1022–5.

107. Roberts CS, Roberts WC. Dissection of the aorta associated with congenital malformation of the aortic valve. J Am Coll Cardiol. 1991;17:712–6.

108. Della Corte A, Bancone C, Quarto C, et al. Predictors of ascending aortic dilatation with bicuspid valve: a wide spectrum of disease expression. Eur J Cardiothrac Surg. 2007;31:397–405.

109. Nistri S, Sorbo MD, Marin M, et al. Aortic root dilatation in young men with normally functioning bicuspid aortic valves. Heart. 1999;82:19–22.

110. Ergin MA, Spielvogel D, Apaydin A, et al. Surgical treatment of the descending dilated aorta: when and how? Ann Thorac Surg. 1999;67:1834–9.

111. Morgan-Hughes GJ, Roobottom CA, Owens PE, et al. Dilatation of the aorta in pure, severe, bicuspid aortic valve stenosis. Am Heart J. 2004;147:736–40.

112. McKusick VA. Association of congenital bicuspid aortic valve and Erdheim's cystic medial necrosis. Lancet. 1972;1:1026–7.

113. Niwa K, Perfloff JK, Bhuta SM, et al. Structural abnormalities of great arterial walls in congenital heart disease: light and electron microscopic analyses. Circulation. 2001;103:393–400.

114. Bonderman D, Gharehbaghi-Schnell E, Wollenek G, et al. Mechanisms underlying aortic dilatation in congenital aortic valve malformation. Circulation. 1999;99:2138–43.

115. Olson LJ, Subramanian R, Ackermann DM, et al. Surgical pathology of the mitral valve: a study of 712 cases spanning 21 years. Mayo Clin Proc. 1987;62:22–34.

116. Waller BF, Morrow AG, Maron BJ, et al. Etiology of clinically isolated, severe, chronic, pure mitral regurgitation: analysis of 97 patients over 30 years of age having mitral valve replacement. Am Heart J. 1982;104:276–88.

117. Freed LA, Acierno Jr JS, Dai D, et al. A locus for autosomal dominant mitral valve prolapse on chromosome 11p15.4. Am J Hum Genet. 2003;72:1551–9.

118. Read RC, Thal AP, Wendt VE. Symptomatic valvular myxomatous transformation (the floppy valve syndrome). A possible forme fruste of the Marfan syndrome. Circulation. 1965;32:897–910.

119. Freed LA, Levy D, Levine RA, et al. Prevalence and clinical outcome of mitral valve prolapse. N Engl J Med. 1999;341:1–7.

120. Disse S, Abergel E, Berrebi A, et al. Mapping of a first locus for autosomal dominant myxomatous mitral-valve prolapse to chromosome 16p11.2-p12.1. Am J Hum Genet. 1999;65:1242–51.

121. Nesta F, Leyne M, Yosefy C, et al. New locus for autosomal dominant mitral valve prolapse on chromosome 13: clinical insights from genetic studies. Circulation. 2005;112:2022–30.

122. Kyndt F, Schott JJ, Trochu JN, et al. Mapping of X-linked myxomatous valvular dystrophy to chromosome Xq28. Am J Hum Genet. 1998;62:627–32.

123. Virmani R, Atkinson JB, Forman MB. The pathology of mitral valve prolapse. Herz. 1988;13:215–26.

124. Cole WG, Chan D, Hickey AJ, et al. Collagen composition of normal and myxomatous human mitral heart valves. Biochem J. 1984;219:451–60.

125. Tamura K, Fukuda Y, Ishizaki M, et al. Abnormalities in elastic fibres and other connective-tissue components of floppy mitral valve. Am Heart J. 1995;129:1149–58.

126. Olsen EG, Al-Rufaie HK. The floppy mitral valve: study on pathogenesis. Br Heart J. 1980;44:674–83.

127. Prunotto M, Primo Caimmi P, Bongiovanni M. Cellular pathology of mitral valve prolapse. Cardiovasc Pathol. 2010;19:e113–7.

128. Fontana ME, Sparks EA, Boudoulas H, et al. Mitral valve prolapse and the mitral valve prolapse syndrome. Curr Probl Cardiol. 1991;16:309–75.

129. Grigioni F, Averinos JF, Ling LH, et al. Atrial fibrillation complicating the course of degenerative mitral regurgitation: determinants and long-term outcome. J Am Coll Cardiol. 2002;40:84–92.

130. Vohra J, Sathe S, Warren R, et al. Malignant ventricular arrhythmias in patients with mitral valve prolapse and mild mitral regurgitation. Pacing Clin Electrophysiol. 1993;16:387–93.

131. Waller BF, Howard J, Fess S. Pathology of tricuspid valve stenosis and pure tricuspid regurgitation – part III. Clin Cardiol. 1995;18:225–30.

132. Waller BF, Howard J, Fess S. Pathology of tricuspid valve stenosis and pure tricuspid regurgitation – part I. Clin Cardiol. 1995;19:97–102.

133. Waller BF, Howard J, Fess S. Pathology of tricuspid valve stenosis and pure tricuspid regurgitation – part II. Clin Cardiol. 1995;18:167–74.

134. Waller BF, Howard J, Fess S. Pathology of pulmonic valve stenosis and pure regurgitation. Clin Cardiol. 1995;18:45–50.

135. Altrichter PM, Olson LJ, Edwards WD, et al. Surgical pathology of the pulmonary valve: a study of 116 cases spanning 15 years. Mayo Clin Proc. 1989;64:1352–60.

Transplant Pathology

10

Desley A.H. Neil

Abstract

This chapter provides a general overview of the diagnosis of acute cellular rejection, antibody-mediated rejection, and chronic vascular rejection (graft vasculopathy) and how to differentiate from the mimics of rejection. Also described are other entities encountered in cardiac transplant recipients including peritransplant injury both in endomyocardial biopsies and failed allografts, infections, and post-transplant lymphoproliferative disorders. The examination of a failed allograft is discussed.

Keywords

Heart transplant • Rejection • Quilty • Antibody-mediated rejection • Allograft vasculopathy Chronic vascular rejection • Post-transplant lymphoproliferative disorder • Infection Allograft • Previous biopsy site

Introduction

Cardiac transplantation is the gold standard therapy for advanced heart failure, and the outcome is independent of preoperative severity of the heart failure with 1- and 10-year survival rates reaching nearly 80% and over 60%, respectively [1, 2]. Early mortality within the first month remains unchanged with time, at around 15%, but accounting for around 40% of deaths, with 55% of these due to primary graft failure [1]. Acute cellular rejection is becoming less common with improvements in immunosuppression with an associated decrease in mortality related to acute cellular rejection, accounting for 12–15% of transplant failures [1]. However, almost 30% of deaths between 1 month and 1 year are due to rejection [1]. Data for antibody-mediated rejection is incomplete as reliable methods of detecting it have only been developed recently. Death after the first year is largely due to malignancy in around 33% and the development of chronic vascular rejection (coronary allograft vasculopathy) in about 25% [1].

In adults, non-ischemic cardiomyopathy is now the most common indication for cardiac transplantation accounting for over 50% of cases, with ischemic heart disease the next most common indication. Together they account for 90% of cardiac transplants [2]. Prior to 2006, non-ischemic and ischemic cardiomyopathy accounted for roughly equal numbers of cases [3]. In the pediatric group, congenital heart disease is the most common disease group requiring transplantation in the under 1-year-olds with cardiomyopathy and congenital heart disease being the two main indications in older children [3].

Cardiac transplant recipients are routinely monitored for rejection by endomyocardial biopsies (EMB) of the right ventricle. Rejection can be either cell mediated or antibody mediated. EMBs are the mainstay for diagnosis. They are initially performed weekly with decreasing frequency post-transplantation, with some centers stopping biopsies at 1 year post-transplant [2]. Early post-transplant EMBs may be complicated by perforation and tamponade. Fibrous obliteration of the pericardial space, eliminating further such risk, occurs as a healing response to pericardial blood accumulation.

D.A.H. Neil, BMedSc, MBBS, Ph.D., FRCPath
Department of Cellular Pathology, Level – 1,
Queen Elizabeth Hospital Birmingham,
Edgbaston, Birmingham B15 2WB, UK

Department of Histopathology, Queen Elizabeth Hospital
Birmingham, Birmingham, UK
e-mail: desley.neil@uhb.nhs.uk

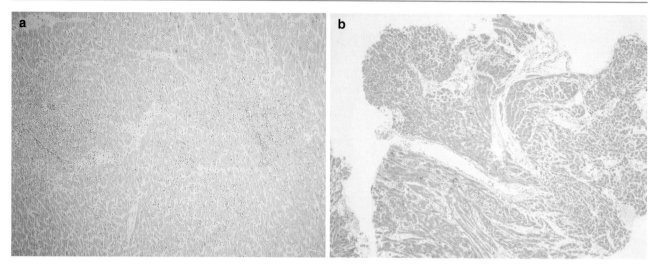

Fig. 10.1 (**a**) Hematoxylin & eosin-stained section showing several foci of inflammation. This is the ISHLT 1990 "A" pattern of rejection. (**b**) Hematoxylin & eosin-stained section showing a diffuse inflammatory cell infiltrate. This is the ISHLT 1990 "B" pattern of rejection

Prior to 1990, many "homegrown" grading schemes for cardiac rejection were developed and used, many being modifications of the Billingham grading system [4]. This resulted in an inability to accurately compare results between centers or assess the impact of immunosuppressive agents. In 1990, under the direction of the International Society of Heart and Lung Transplantation (ISHLT), a standardized grading system was agreed by pathologists from large transplant centers [5]. They also standardized minimum numbers of biopsies and minimum numbers of sections for each biopsy in an attempt to reduce missing rejection due to sampling error. This was further modified in a revision in 2005 [6]. The 1990 grading system split histological patterns resulting in six grades, not necessarily meant to be indicative of a sequential increase in severity but to allow subsequent assessment of the clinical significance of the different patterns.

Specimen Adequacy and Number of Slides

As the infiltrate for rejection is often patchy, ISHLT requires a minimum of three fragments, preferably four, of myocardium. Each should have at least 50% of the muscle free from previous biopsy sites or Quilty lesions (see below) for the biopsy to be considered adequate to exclude rejection [6]. For similar reasons, at least three levels should be cut with a least three sections/slide and stained with hematoxylin and eosin [6]. With three biopsies, there is 5% chance of missing a mild rejection, but negligible risk of missing moderate or severe rejection [7], and if there are four biopsies, the rate of missing mild rejection falls to 2%. The more pieces containing a mild rejection infiltrate increases the risk of missing a higher-grade rejection [8]. One piece may also be frozen for immunofluorescence or other studies. No tissue is normally required for electron microscopy. The recent consensus group working for ISHLT concluded that immunostaining with an anti-C4d antisera is also performed at 2 weeks and 1, 3, 6, and 12 months to aid in the detection of antibody-mediated rejection [9, 10].

Rejection

The 1990 ISHLT grading scheme was designed for the assessment of cell-mediated rejection (acute cellular rejection (ACR)) involving an infiltrate of lymphocytes and macrophages, with injury to the myocytes [5]. While antibody-mediated rejection (AMR) was recognized as an entity, diagnostic criteria were unreliable and could not be reproduced in every center, and this "diagnosis" was a diagnosis of exclusion in cases of biopsy-negative graft dysfunction, when other causes were ruled out clinically. The development of an antibody to the complement fragment C4d [11, 12] has allowed the detection of AMR in tissue sections. C4d is formed during activation of the classical pathway of complement activation, primarily by antigen-antibody reactions. It binds covalently to tissues and remains for several weeks allowing detection of AMR in biopsies.

Donor-specific antibodies (DSAs) can be present in the recipient prior to transplantation (preformed) resulting in early AMR and hyperacute rejection. They also may develop post-transplant causing AMR in both the early and late post-transplant periods [9, 13, 14]. ACR and AMR can occur simultaneously or alone. ACR alone is the most common pattern of rejection. After that, combined ACR and ACR is next most frequent with AMR alone as the least common, although exact prevalences are unreliable at the moment [10].

Cell-Mediated Rejection (Acute Cellular Rejection)

Old "1990" ISHLT Grading System [5]

This is divided into focal (Fig. 10.1a) and diffuse (Fig. 10.1b) infiltrates with and without muscle damage (Fig. 10.2) (see Table 10.1). This unified grading system allowed all units across the world to be able to compare results. Subsequent

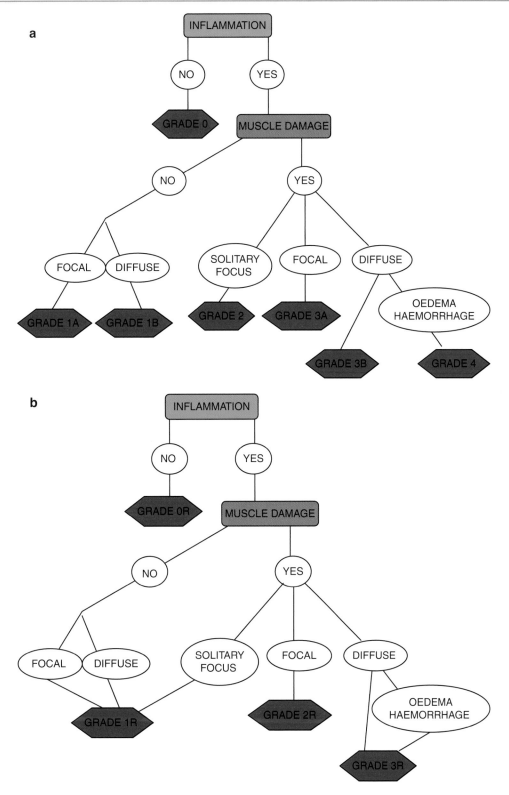

Fig. 10.2 (a) Flow chart outlining the steps involved in arriving at the "old" ISHLT 1990 cell-mediated rejection grade. (b) Flow chart outlining the steps involved in arriving at the "new" ISHLT 2005 cell-mediated rejection grade

Table 10.1 ISHLT grading schemes for cellular rejection

ISHLT 1990		ISHLT 2005	
Grade 0	No/minimal inflammation	Grade 0R	No/minimal inflammation
Grade 1a	Multifocal infiltrate without muscle damage	Grade1R	Inflammation with no muscle damage or a single focus of muscle damage
Grade 1b	Diffuse infiltrate without muscle damage		
Grade 2	Single focus of inflammation with muscle damage		
Grade 3a	Multifocal infiltrate with muscle damage	Grade 2R	Multifocal infiltrate with muscle damage
Grade 3b	Diffuse infiltrate with muscle damage	Grade 3R	Diffuse infiltrate with muscle damage +/− edema and hemorrhage
Grade 4	Severe diffuse inflammation, often mixed with muscle damage, edema, and hemorrhage		

studies however showed that there was very poor reproducibility of grades between centers using this complicated scoring system [3, 6]. Grades 1A, 1B, and 2 behaved in a similar manner, having no clinical signs or symptom [15], with only a 10–15% risk of progressing to high-grade rejection [6]. One single-center study showed inconsistent grading of grade 2 rejection and indicated that it usually represented a Quilty lesion and the removal of the grade did not result in an increase in higher-grade rejection [16]. All transplant units treated grades 3b and 4 aggressively such that subdifferentiation was unnecessary [6]. The grading system was simplified to the current four-grade system [6] by the merging of several grades, although in many centers, both the "old" 1990 and "new" 2005 grading systems are being used simultaneously [17].

New 2005 ISHLT Grading System [6]

An R is put after the grade to indicate that it is the new revised grading system. Grade 0R remains the same, while grade 1R amalgamates grades 1a, 1b, and 2. Grade 2R replaces the old grade 3a, and grade 3R amalgamates grades 3b and 4 (see Table 10.1).

Myocyte Injury

The grade of rejection relies on the identification of myocyte injury, which is difficult to define. It is best assessed by looking for changes across all levels of the biopsy and taking into account a combination of subtle features. On low power, distortion of the normal architecture with apparent loss of myocytes (Fig. 10.3a) and, at higher magnification, an inflammatory encroachment on myocytes with irregular cytoplasmic borders (Fig. 10.3b, c), lymphocytes within myocytes, fragments of myocytes (Fig. 10.3b), and evidence of myocytolysis with clearing/vacuolization of the cytoplasm (Fig. 10.3b) can be seen. A perinuclear halo (Fig. 10.3c),

nuclear enlargement, and occasionally prominent nucleoli [3, 6] may also be seen. Hypereosinophilia, nuclear pyknosis, and loss of nuclei are features of coagulative necrosis (Fig. 10.4) and are not features of acute cellular rejection [18] occurring in relation to previous biopsy sites, peritransplant injury, and later ischemic injury in the form of microinfarcts or zonal infarcts. Coagulative necrosis stains with complement 9 (C9) [19–21] (Fig. 10.5) and to lesser extents with C3d and C4d antisera. Myocyte injury related to acute cellular rejection and contraction band necrosis in the early stages does not stain with complement.

Antibody-Mediated Rejection

Until recently, antibody-mediated rejection (AMR), also known as vascular rejection by the surgeons, was a diagnosis of exclusion considered to occur with biopsy-negative unexplained hemodynamic compromise [22]. A few centers were able to make a tissue diagnosis of AMR by demonstrating the deposition of immunoglobulins and complement within capillaries on frozen sections [23–25], but this technique could not be reproduced reliably in other centers [26]. In the early 1990s, capillary deposition of a polyclonal antibody to complement fragment C4d was shown to correlate with worse renal transplant outcome [12]. This was subsequently shown to correlate with the presence of donor-specific antibodies, most commonly against human leucocyte antigens (HLA) [27], and was also shown to correlate with poor outcome in heart transplants [11].

C4d is produced via activation of the classical pathway (usually antigen-antibody-mediated activation) and becomes covalently bound to tissues, allowing detection for up to 7–10 days after the event. C4d staining is considered positive when there is multifocal or diffuse strong capillary immunoperoxidase (IP) staining and 2–3+ (moderate to marked) diffuse staining of capillaries using immunofluorescence (IF) (Fig. 10.6) [9, 13]. Staining of venules and particularly arterioles occurs normally so can be used as an inbuilt positive

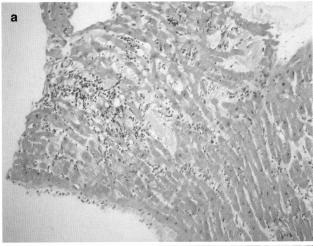

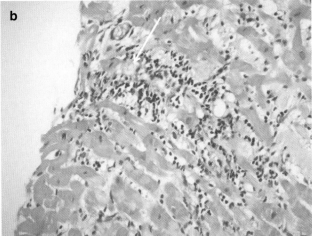

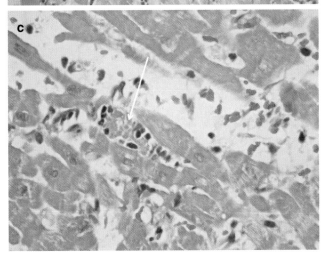

Fig. 10.3 (**a**) Muscle damage is suggested at low power when distortion to the normal architecture of the myocytes is identified (Hematoxylin & eosin). (**b**) Muscle damage is identified when myocytes show myocytolysis with clearing of the cytoplasm (*arrow*), and there is encroachment of lymphocytes on the myocyte with irregular cell borders. Fragments of myocyte cytoplasm are seen within the area of inflammation (Hematoxylin & eosin). (**c**) Lymphocyte encroachment on a myocyte producing irregular cell borders and cytoskeletal disruption (*arrow*). Several surrounding myocytes demonstrate a perinuclear halo (Hematoxylin & eosin)

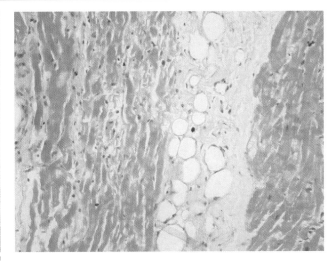

Fig. 10.4 Coagulative necrosis is present on the *left* with hypereosinophilic wavy myocytes with loss of nuclei. Normal muscle is present on the *right* for comparison. An area of fat necrosis separates the two areas (Hematoxylin & eosin)

control [9]. There is good correlation between immunoperoxidase and immunofluorescence staining for C4d [9, 28, 29]. An international study, as part of Banff 2009, showed good reproducibility between centers on a formalin-fixed paraffin-embedded tissue microarray of controls and positive samples [9].

With the introduction of the C4d immunostain, the hematoxylin and eosin appearances of AMR could be clarified. The histological features suggestive of AMR (Fig. 10.7) are inflammatory cells within capillaries, in particular macrophages, and prominent/swollen endothelial cells. This latter feature is indicative of injury/activation [6, 9, 10, 30, 31], and interstitial edema and hemorrhage may be apparent, particularly in the more severe cases [9, 10]. Since this infiltrate is within vessels, it is usually diffuse in an "old 1B" pattern, and the myocardium appears "busy" at low power (Fig. 10.8).

There are four stages of AMR recognized:

1. Latent humoral response – circulating DSA only
2. Silent humoral reaction – circulating DSA + C4d deposition without histological features of AMR and no graft dysfunction
3. Subclinical AMR – circulating DSA + C4d deposition + histological features of AMR without clinical dysfunction
4. AMR – circulating DSA + C4d deposition + histological features of AMR + graft dysfunction [32]

Stages 2 and 3 have been linked with poor outcome [33–35]. For these reasons, the original ISHLT recommendation for the diagnosis of AMR that included the presence of graft dysfunction [6, 14] has been changed to a purely pathological diagnosis [9, 10]. In the 2005 ISHLT recommendations for the diagnosis of AMR, the histological features of AMR

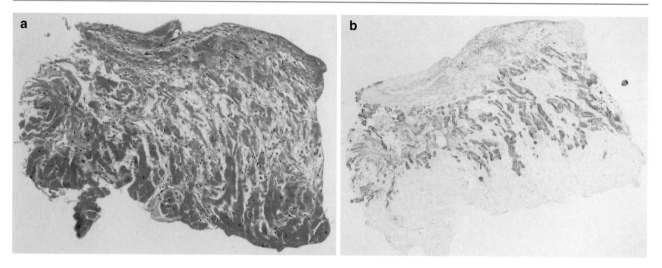

Fig. 10.5 (**a**) Hematoxylin & eosin-stained biopsy of heart showing extensive coagulative necrosis. (**b**) Complement 9 immunostain on the same biopsy as in Fig. 10.5a. The coagulative necrosis stains *brown*

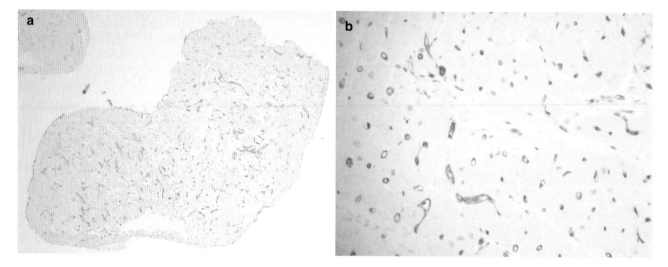

Fig. 10.6 (**a**) Low power of C4d immunoperoxidase stain showing strong diffuse C4d staining of capillaries. (**b**) High power of C4d immunoperoxidase stain showing circumferential capillary staining

should be looked for in each biopsy. If present, either an IF panel (comprising IgG, IgM, and/or IgA + C3d, C4d, and/or C1q to assess capillary staining) or an immunoperoxidase (IP) panel (of C4d to assess capillary staining and CD68 to identify intravascular macrophages) should be performed. The biopsy would be graded as AMR0 (no histological features of AMR or histological features, but negative IF/IP) or AMR1 (histological features + positive IF/IP). This grading scheme will be replaced in the near term with one encompassing the other stages of AMR including C4d staining without histological features and histological features without C4d. In addition, the requirement for immunoglobulins in IF has been removed [9, 10]. The new AMR grading system will be designated with a "p" prior to the grade to indicate that it is "pathologically" defined AMR. The proposed grades are shown in Table 10.2 [9, 10]. If C4d staining of capillaries and/or histological features of AMR are present, testing for DSA should be suggested to the clinician.

The recommendations for timing of assessment of biopsies for AMR is that all biopsies should be assessed for the histological features and their presence triggers IF/IP staining. Additionally IF/IP should be routinely performed at 2 weeks, 1, 3, 6, and 12 months post-transplant. Similarly DSAs should be assessed at the same time points as well as annually thereafter. After a C4d-positive biopsy, all subsequent biopsies greater than 2 weeks after the positive biopsy should be assessed for C4d. The 2-week time gap is because C4d can remain positive prior to this without ongoing complement activation [9].

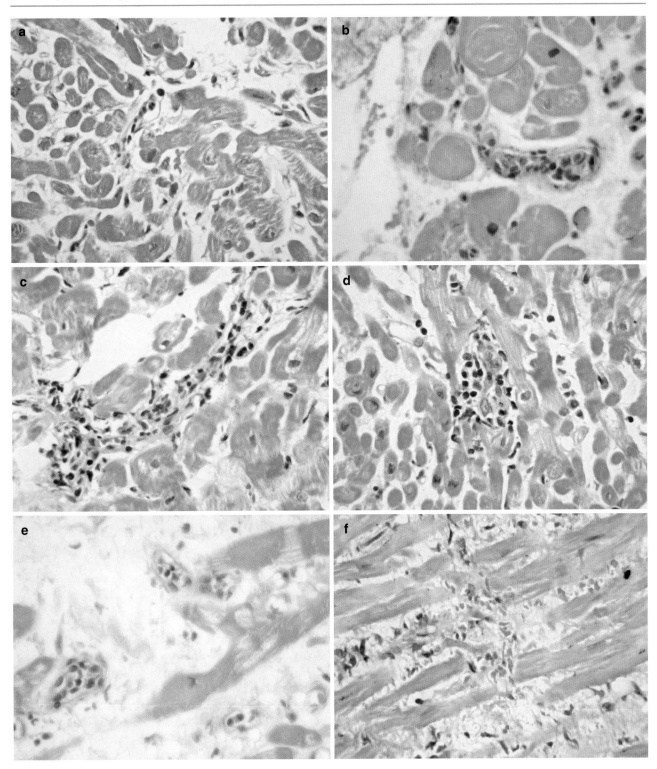

Fig. 10.7 (**a**) A few inflammatory cells, including a neutrophil within a small vessel. A relatively subtle finding requiring high-power assessment (Hematoxylin & eosin). (**b**) A vessel stuffed with inflammatory cells (Hematoxylin & eosin). (**c**) The inflammatory infiltrate also extends around vessels in AMR (Hematoxylin & eosin). (**d**) Swollen endothelial cells are evident in this section as well as inflammatory cells within the vessel (Hematoxylin & eosin). (**e**) Edema and inflammatory cells within vessels (Hematoxylin & eosin). (**f**) Hemorrhage + interstitial inflammation (Hematoxylin & eosin)

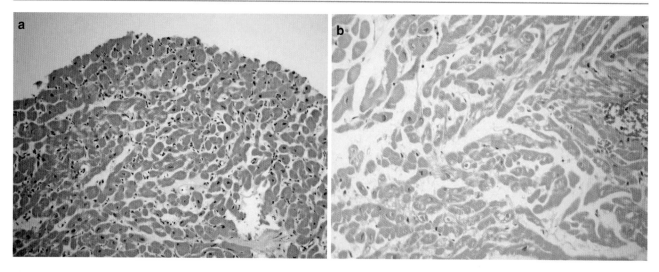

Fig. 10.8 The low-power clue for AMR is a busy myocardium (**a**) with a normal uninflamed myocardium for comparison (**b**) (both Hematoxylin & eosin stains)

Table 10.2 ISHLT grading scheme for antibody-mediated rejection

pAMR0		Negative for AMR	No evidence of AMR histologically and C4d negative
pAMR1	pAMR1H+	Suspicious of AMR	EITHER histological features of AMR (H+)
	pAMR1I+		OR C4d positive (I+)
pAMR2		AMR	BOTH histological features of AMR and C4d+
pAMR3		Severe AMR	C4d+ and histological features of AMR + marked edema, interstitial hemorrhage, capillary fragmentation, mixed inflammatory infiltrate, endothelial cell pyknosis, and/or karyorrhexis

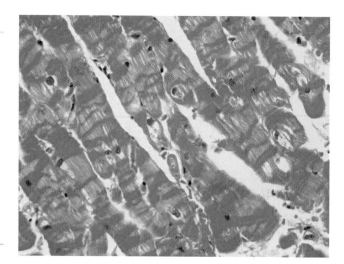

Fig. 10.9 Thick and thin transverse contraction bands are seen across the myocytes (Hematoxylin & eosin)

Contraction Band Artifact

Contraction bands (Fig. 10.9) are readily identified in cardiac transplant biopsies and are not an indicator of contraction band necrosis. They occur as a result of the procedure and placing in the cold fixative [3].

Quilty Lesion

This lesion, named after the first patient, is a mononuclear cell infiltrate (Fig. 10.10), which can be limited to the endocardium (Quilty A lesion) or involve the underlying myocardium, generally with quite conspicuous muscle damage (Quilty B lesion). These first became recognized with the introduction of cyclosporine, not being present in the azathioprine and prednisolone era [36], and there has been some change in the balance between A and B lesions with the advent of tacrolimus [37]. Cyclosporine use in non-heart

(i.e., renal/liver) transplant recipients does not produce Quilty lesions (in native hearts examined postmortem) [38].

Quilty lesions are composed of predominantly T lymphocytes which comprise more than 50% of the infiltrate with B lymphocytes and macrophages being present in lesser amounts. They also have a follicular dendritic cell framework which becomes increasingly more extensive with larger lesions [39]. There is an organization to Quilty lesions (Fig. 10.11) which have a central B lymphocyte component with supporting follicular dendritic cells surrounded by T lymphocytes. Small capillary-sized blood vessels, with high endothelial venule (HEV) features, are present within a Quilty lesion. The Quilty lesion has features of a tertiary lymphoid tissue suggesting an attempt to mount a local response to persistent alloantigen stimulation [40]. This is in contrast to rejection where the same cells are present, but without

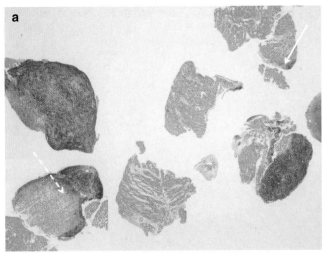
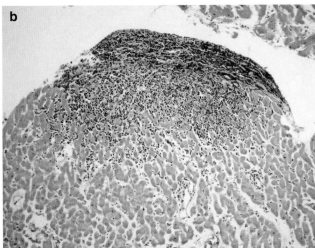

Fig. 10.10 (**a**) Low power of multiple biopsies showing prominent Quilty lesions (effect). Some can be seen to be confined to the endocardium (Quilty A) (*solid arrow*) and some extending into the myocardium (Quilty B) (*dashed arrow*) (Hematoxylin & eosin). (**b**) High power of a Quilty B lesion showing the typical dense inflammatory infiltrate. Entrapment of muscle fibers with apparent damage is readily apparent (Hematoxylin & eosin)

organization of the cells into compartments. Macrophages make up more than 50% of the infiltrate, and follicular dendritic cells and a vascular component are not present [39].

Early studies found not adverse outcome related to either Quilty A or B lesions, so required no augmentation of immunosuppression. Thus, it is vital to differentiate the Quilty lesion from rejection. It is generally accepted that most grade 2 rejections are tangentially cut Quilty B lesions [6, 41], and further levels should be cut or spares stained to try to confirm an endocardial component. Immunohistochemistry for CD3, CD68, and CD21 may also be helpful in identification of Quilty lesions. The most recent ISHLT guidelines no longer require distinction between A and B lesions.

More recently, studies have questioned the lack of adverse outcome of Quilty lesions [42–44], with variable findings on an association with the development of coronary vasculopathy [45, 46].

Previous Biopsy Site

These are common occurring in around 65% of all biopsies [47]. They vary in appearance depending on the time since the biopsy. Very recent previous biopsy sites often contain fibrin, a mixed inflammatory cell infiltrate and quite conspicuous muscle damage (Fig. 10.12a, b), and an overlying mural thrombus may be identified. With increasing time, the thrombus undergoes organization. The inflammation subsides, and later, the damaged muscle is removed by phagocytosis (Fig. 10.12c). The presence of hemosiderin-laden macrophages (Fig. 10.12d) is often the best indication of an area of inflammation in a previous biopsy site. Necrotic muscle fibers can be highlighted with C9 immunohistochemistry [20, 21]. In early post-transplant cases,

the differentiation from peritransplant injury and previous biopsy site may not be possible. Healed previous biopsy sites form fibrous scars indistinguishable from scars related to peritransplant injury or ischemia.

Peritransplant Injury

There are numerous mechanisms of injury to the donor heart in the peritransplant period. Injury can occur to the donor heart prior to transplantation as a result of the catecholamine surge ("storm") during donor brain death. This situation produces contraction band necrosis and microinfarcts similar to those seen with inotrope use for hemodynamic maintenance. The catecholamine surge is most pronounced in donor death from head injury, and it has long been recognized that patients with head injuries can die from a cardiac event [48–51]. Contrastingly periods of hypotension, prior to organ procurement and hypothermic ischemia during cold storage after procurement, can also result in varying degrees of reversible and irreversible myocyte injury. After transplantation, a reperfusion injury occurs as a result of the release of free radicals.

The patterns of the myocyte injury from these various entities are slightly different and poorly understood. The catecholamine surge produces contraction band necrosis. This cannot be assessed in early post-transplant biopsies as contraction bands may occur artifactually. Microinfarcts occur as a result of vasospasm related to the catecholamine storm or inotrope usage and are identified initially by coagulative necrosis. These manifest as hypereosinophilic, often wavy, myocytes with loss of nuclei. They are readily seen in early post-transplant biopsies for variable periods of time but usually most pronounced

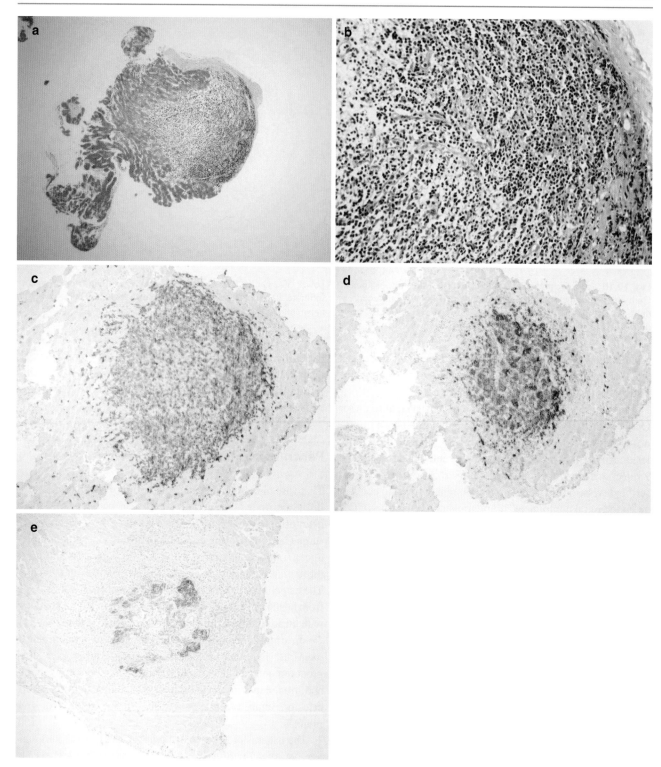

Fig. 10.11 (a) Low power of a Quilty lesion used for the immunohistochemistry stains (Hematoxylin & eosin). (b) Higher power of this Quilty lesion showing the extensive vascularity within the lesion (Hematoxylin & eosin). (c) CD3 T lymphocyte immunostain, when compared to (d); the T lymphocytes predominantly are forming a cuff around the central area where there are fewer T lymphocytes. (d) CD20 B lymphocyte immunostain showing the central part of the Quilty has a more dense B lymphocyte population. (e) CD21 immunostain to demonstrate the follicular dendritic cell framework within this well-developed Quilty lesion

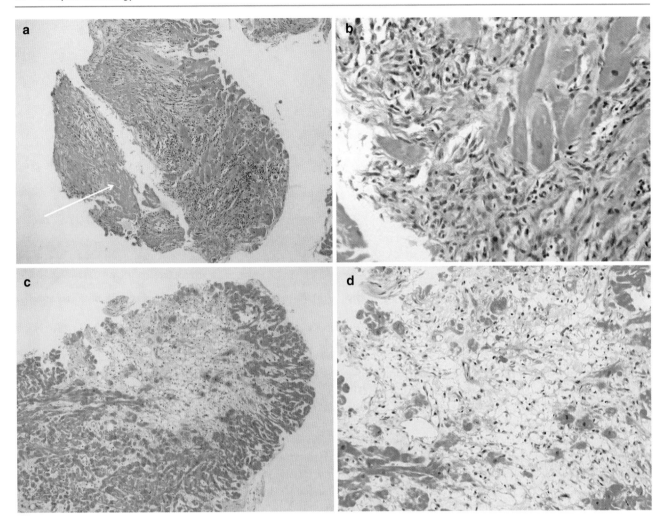

Fig. 10.12 (**a**) Low-power view of a recent previous biopsy site with marked inflammation and muscle damage and overlying thrombus (*arrow*) (Hematoxylin & eosin). (**b**) Higher-power view of the mixed infiltrate in a recent previous biopsy site (Hematoxylin & eosin). (**c**) An older previous biopsy site in the region of 2–4 weeks of age in which the inflammation has largely subsided and much of the damaged myocytes have been cleared (Hematoxylin & eosin). (**d**) A higher-power view of the biopsy site in (**c**) showing the brownish tinge of the hemosiderin-laden macrophages (Hematoxylin & eosin)

in the first few weeks (Fig. 10.13). Depending on the degree of immunosuppression, there is a variable inflammatory response. Unlike rejection, the muscle damage/necrosis is out of proportion to the inflammatory infiltrate (see Fig. 10.13), whereas in rejection, the muscle damage is very subtle. C9 highlights the necrotic muscle fibers [20, 21] which are often single cells or small groups of myocytes (see Fig. 10.13). This makes peritransplant injury readily identifiable, as pure cellular rejection does not result in C9-positive necrotic myocytes. Neutrophil infiltration is part of the reperfusion injury, though this is not usually conspicuous in cardiac transplant biopsies.

Problems Related to Specimen Orientation

As these tiny 2–3-mm biopsies are randomly orientated, there may be difficulties in distinguishing previous biopsy sites and Quilty lesions from rejection. A careful search for pigmented (hemosiderin laden) macrophages over the levels and serial sections helps confirm a previous biopsy site, while further levels or staining of spare sections may help confirm endocardial attachment for Quilty lesions. However, it should be recognized that a rejection infiltrate can also involve the endocardium.

Infection

Post-transplant infections are decreasing, reflecting better antimicrobial prophylaxis and refinements in immunosuppression allowing a lesser immunosuppressive burden, with 0.6 infective episodes per patient in the current era [52]. Infections involving the transplanted heart were rare, but are now very infrequent [3].

The most likely organisms to potentially cause histological changes in endomyocardial biopsies are viruses, with a viral

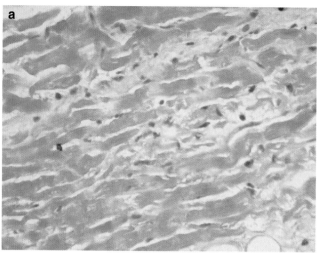
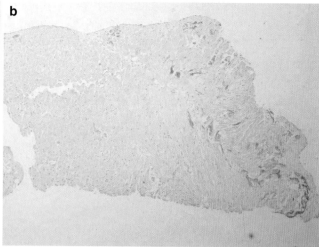

Fig. 10.13 (a) Hematoxylin & eosin section showing scattered necrotic myocytes which are hypereosinophilic with granular cytoplasm and a surrounding light inflammatory cell infiltrate – the muscle damage out of proportion to the inflammatory infiltrate. (b) C9-stained section staining scattered necrotic myocytes brown

myocarditis being indistinguishable from rejection in the majority of cases. With decreasing frequency, parvovirus B19, Epstein–Barr virus (EBV), cytomegalovirus (CMV), and adenovirus viral genome have been identified by nested polymerase chain reaction (PCR) in post-transplant endomyocardial biopsies [53, 54]. Parvovirus B19 is being increasingly reported, being often associated with an anemia and myocarditis in both the immunocompetent and immunosuppressed [55].

CMV viral titers are generally monitored serologically, and, if raised, a careful hunt for the characteristic inclusions within myocytes, endothelial, or stromal cells should be undertaken. CMV immunohistochemistry should also be performed, although it is unlikely that CMV myocarditis will be identified.

In both North and South America, Chagas' myocarditis should be considered. Chagas' disease can occur by transmission from the donor or reactivation in the recipient [56]. Amastigote nests can be seen on Hematoxylin & eosin and giemsa stains [56].

Toxoplasmosis is endemic in Europe and some tropical areas. Previous exposure of both the donor and recipient to toxoplasmosis is tested prior to transplantation, and routine prophylaxis is instituted using trimethoprim and sulfamethoxazole [57, 58]. Latent infection in the myocardium, in which there are cysts containing bradyzoites, is the most common method of donor transmission. However, reactivation and a primary infection can also occur in those not previously exposed [57, 58]. While the prophylaxis usually has largely prevented toxoplasmosis, case reports do occur in patients not given prophylaxis because of allergy to either of the drugs [59]. A chronic donor toxoplasma cyst is the most likely way of finding toxoplasmosis in an endomyocardial biopsy.

Post-transplant Lymphoproliferative Disorder

Post-transplant lymphoproliferative disorder (PTLD) is the most common malignancy following solid organ transplantation in children and second to skin cancers in adults [60]. Heart transplant recipients have one of the highest incidences of PTLD, in the vicinity of 2–5% [61, 62], with a higher incidence in children around 13% [63]. They occur most commonly within the first year post-transplant [60, 61, 64], but have been reported to develop as long as 20 years post-transplantation [62]. There is a 30–60% associated mortality rate [64]. Increased immunosuppression and EBV infection are two of the most important risk factors for the development of a PTLD [60, 61, 63, 64].

The lesions range from lymphocyte hyperplasia through to frank lymphomas, which have been divided into four basic histological types in the 2008 WHO classification of tumors of hematopoietic and lymphoid tissues [60, 61, 64, 65].

1. *Early lesions*: There is preservation of underlying tissue architecture with mixed B and T lymphocytes and plasma cells. There are two histological patterns seen – plasmacytic hyperplasia and infectious mononucleosis like. They are usually polyclonal and usually positive for EBV proteins by immunohistochemistry (LMP1) or EBV-encoded RNA (EBERs) by in situ hybridization.

2. *Polymorphic PTLD*: Destruction of underlying tissue architecture, full spectrum of B lymphocytes. Most express EBER or LMP1.

3. *Monomorphic PTLD*: There is architectural and cytological atypia of a degree readily classified as lymphoma on morphological features. It is usually B cell lineage, but some T cell and NK cell lymphomas occur. Most of the B

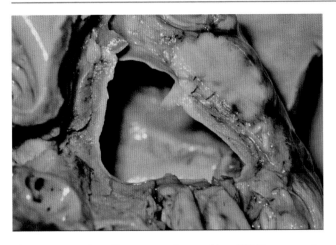

Fig. 10.14 Explanted/postmortem heart with a PTLD seen as the whitish nodule in the wall of the atrium involving the suture line

cell lymphomas are diffuse large B cell lymphomas, but Burkitt lymphoma, plasma cell myeloma, and plasmacytoma-like lesions also occur. The B cell and NK cell lymphomas are usually positive for EBV.

4. *Classical Hodgkin lymphoma – type PTLD:*. In this, the majority of Reed–Sternberg cells are positive for EBERs. The presentation is usually extranodal with involvement of the transplanted heart rare (Fig. 10.14) [66]. Cardiac involvement usually presents with heart dysfunction with the clinical suspicion of rejection. Endomyocardial biopsy will permit diagnosis usually.

Recurrent Disease

Recurrent disease is recurrence of the original disease process, which necessitated transplantation, in the transplanted heart. Histopathological assessment of the explanted heart is necessary to accurately diagnose as many histologically characterized causes of heart failure as possible. Pretransplant clinical diagnosis is incorrect in 30% of patients transplanted for conditions other than ischemic heart disease [67].

Amyloidosis of all types can recur in the transplanted heart, giving an overall lower survival rate of cardiac transplantation for other causes [68]. Patients currently transplanted for AL amyloid (light chain amyloid) should also be worked up for a bone marrow/stem cell transplant. Together with chemotherapy, this may provide complete remission in more than 60% of patients [68–74]. Combined kidney and cardiac transplantation is undertaken for non-AL variant Apo-A1 variants with recurrence occurring at 5 years, but the progression is slow with normal cardiac and renal function after 10 years [68, 70]. Combined liver and heart transplantation is performed for non-AL variant and wild-types of transthyretin amyloid. Recurrence does not occur as the liver was the source of the amyloid [68, 70].

Approximately 25% of patients transplanted for giant cell myocarditis recur at a mean of 3 years post-transplant with no impact on survival rates at 3 years post-transplant. Detection is by identification of giant cells in the routine endomyocardial biopsy. The earliest reported recurrence was at 3 weeks post-transplantation. Treatment is by initial steroid bolus and tapering course over several months [68, 75].

Sarcoidosis has been reported to recur in four patients, generally being identified on routine endomyocardial biopsy by the identification of non-caseating granulomas and exclusion of infective causes. They have been treated successfully with increased steroid dose [68, 76–79].

Graft Vasculopathy

Graft failure/patient survival after the first year has remained relatively unchanged [80] despite improvements in immunosuppressants with a steady 5–6% annual loss. The major cause for this is the development of graft vasculopathy (GV) – also known as graft vascular disease, coronary artery vasculopathy, chronic vascular rejection, and accelerated graft atherosclerosis. GV produces painless ischemia of the denervated graft, presenting as sudden death, silent myocardial infarcts, or heart failure [2]. There is diffuse involvement of all arteries, and veins may also be involved, with the second- and third-order intramyocardial branch arteries being the most affected [81–83]. The process is predominantly an intimal proliferative process and is considered to be a response to injury to the endothelium, although injury to the media may also contribute. The cause of the endothelial injury is multifactorial [80, 84], starting with systematic effects in the donor with brain death [85–87], endothelial and smooth muscle injury during the preservation period [88–91], and subsequent reperfusion injury [89, 92]. After that, there is continuing post-transplant related to antibody-mediated rejection and cell-mediated vascular rejection (endothelialitis), viral infections [54], hyperlipidemia, and more. The balance between the various injurious agents will vary from patient to patient.

The arteries involved are too large to be sampled in an endomyocardial biopsy, and the diffuse nature of the disease makes it difficult to identify on angiography [93]. Identification by angiography requires comparison of annual angiograms looking for a subtle decrease in caliber of the vessels. Intravascular ultrasound allows identification of intimal thickness and, if used in conjunction with other software, can produce a picture of the area of the intima (called virtual histology) [93]. Allowing GV lesions to be detected in early stages means potentially more patients might be amenable to treatment [80]. Examination of the explanted heart either at the time of retransplantation or postmortem allows identification of the arterial changes.

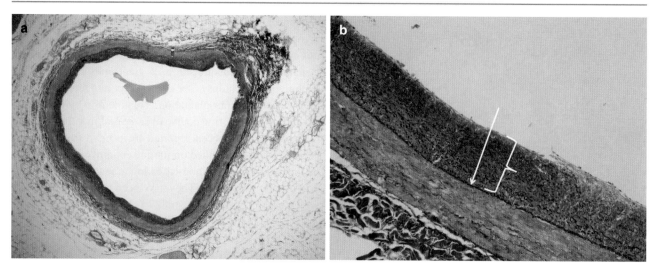

Fig. 10.15 (**a**) Low-power elastic van Gieson (Elastic van Gieson)-stained section showing the normal adaptive layer of concentric fibrointimal thickening in coronary arteries. (**b**) Higher-power view showing the internal elastic lamina (*arrow*) with adaptive fibroelastic intimal thickening (Elastic van Gieson)

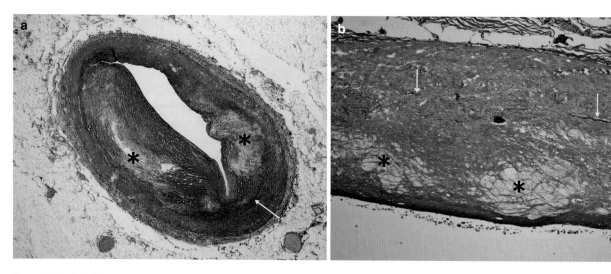

Fig. 10.16 (**a**) Low-power section showing naturally occurring atherosclerosis with eccentric plaques, lipid cores (*), and destruction of the underlying internal elastic lamina. An intact area of internal elastic

lamina (*arrow*) is seen (Elastic van Gieson). (**b**) Higher power showing lipid core (*) and destruction of the internal elastic lamina with fragments of the internal elastic lamina (*arrow*) still visible (Elastic van Gieson)

Differentiation from preexisting "normal" intimal thickening (Fig. 10.15) and preexisting atherosclerosis (Fig. 10.16), sometimes severe and requiring coronary bypass grafting at the time of transplantation, is important. Coronary arteries in adults have an adaptive layer of fibroelastic thickening between the endothelium and internal elastic lamina [94]. Atherosclerosis is focal and eccentric with destruction of the internal elastic lamina and involves the epicardial coronary arteries often with a lipid core and calcification (see Fig. 10.16). Graft vascular disease is diffuse and concentric, often most prominent in the intramyocardial arteries, with only focal disruption to the internal elastic lamina and rarely contains lipid or calcification (Fig. 10.17) [81–83, 95]. However, there is some evidence that progression of preexisting atherosclerotic plaques may also be accelerated.

Graft vasculopathy initially is loose and had a thin rim (Fig. 10.17a) and with time becomes thicker and more fibromuscular (Fig. 10.17b). There may be associated acute vascular rejection component (Fig. 10.17c, d) in which there is an intimal inflammatory cell infiltrate, sometimes with transmural inflammation. In this situation, a rejection component can be implied in the pathogenesis and the term "acute or chronic vascular rejection" used. However, other non-"rejection" causes are still possible.

Primary Graft Failure

Primary graft failure is a term used when the transplanted heart never functioned without medical support and results in patient death or the need for an urgent retransplant. The

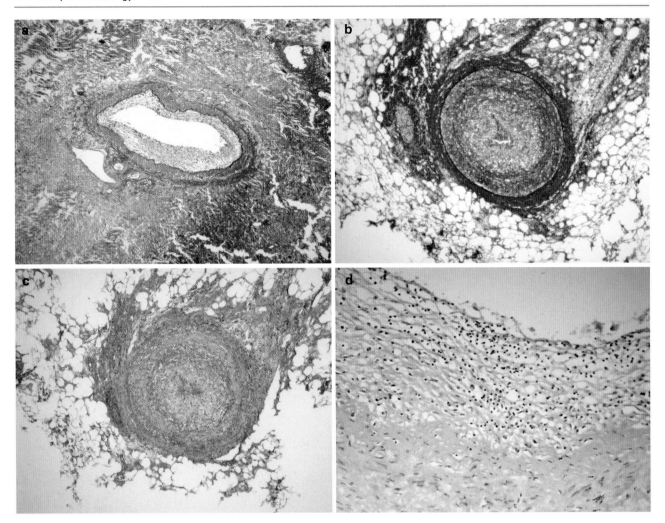

Fig. 10.17 (**a**) Low power of a relatively early graft vasculopathy with loose intimal thickening and intact internal elastic lamina (Elastic van Gieson). (**b**) More advanced graft vasculopathy with marked concentric narrowing of the lumen by fibromuscular intimal thickening (Elastic van Gieson). (**c**) Hematoxylin & eosin section of the same vessel as in Fig. 10.15b showing that there is transmural inflammation "acute or chronic vascular rejection." (**d**) Acute vascular rejection with intimal inflammation (Hematoxylin & eosin)

underlying problem is peritransplant injury which encompasses injury related to hypotension in the donor, brain death [85], preservation injury (hypothermic ischemia in preservation solutions), and reperfusion injury related to free radicals [92, 96, 97]. This can be exacerbated by a size mismatch between donor and recipient, particularly if there is an element of pulmonary hypertension in the recipient and if the right heart is unable to pump against these pressures.

The findings at autopsy can be a constellation of these different injuries, but often a mixture of contraction band necrosis and coagulative/ischemic necrosis is often seen (Fig. 10.18). Contraction band necrosis is related to hypercontraction and occurs during brain death, particularly when there is a rapid marked increase in intracranial pressure such as in closed head injuries [85, 98, 99], and as part of the reperfusion injury [100, 101]. Coagulative necrosis occurs during the various periods of ischemia in the donor and during storage [85, 98, 99] and mainly stain with C9 [19–21]. Cells with contraction band necrosis can secondarily progress to C9-positive necrosis [102], and so if the patient survives several days, there might be some C9-positive cells with contraction bands still apparent (Fig. 10.19).

Sampling of the Explanted or Postmortem Cardiac Transplant

Cardiac transplants either obtained at postmortem or explanted at the time of retransplantation should be examined diligently, similarly to a native heart in cases of sudden death [103–106] with the addition of an assessment of the anastomoses for evidence of dehiscence or stenosis. The

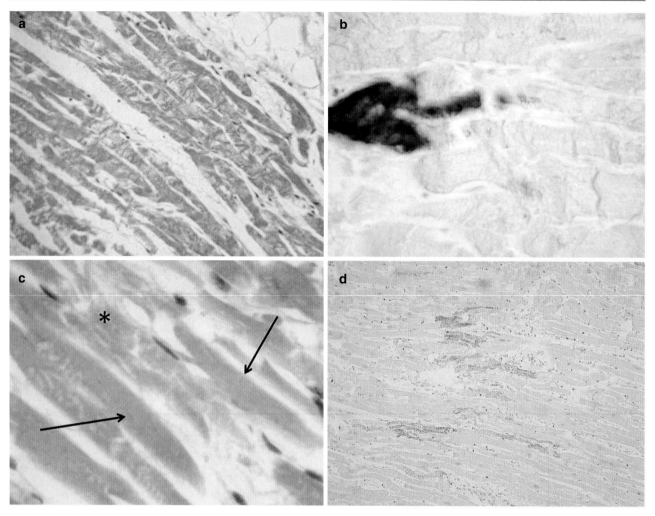

Fig. 10.18 (**a**) Contraction band necrosis with transverse contraction bands seen across many myocytes (Hematoxylin & eosin). (**b**) An ischemic necrotic fiber stains with C9 while adjacent fibers with contraction band necrosis do not stain. (**c**) Coagulative necrosis of myocytes with granular cytoplasm and a moth-eaten appearance (*). Cross striations can be seen in normal myocytes (*arrows*) (Hematoxylin & eosin). (**d**) C9 stains multiple necrotic fibers undergoing coagulative necrosis

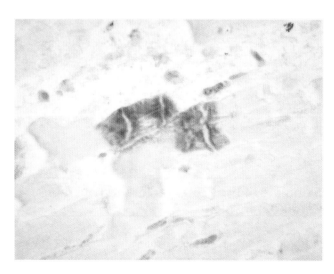

Fig. 10.19 A myocyte with contraction bands may become C9 positive with time

usual anastomoses are the aorta, pulmonary artery, superior and inferior vena cava, and left atrium (patch/cuff containing all four pulmonary veins). If the transplant is more than approximately 1 month old, there is usually fibrous obliteration of the pericardial space, making it difficult to remove which complicates identification and examination of the coronary arteries. A suture in the apex is usual from venting air at the end of the procedure, and there is often also one in the right auricular appendage from cardiopulmonary bypass. Coronary artery walls should be assessed macroscopically for discrete lesions of atherosclerosis. Inspection for diffuse thickening related to graft vascular disease should follow, with samples being taken throughout the length looking for both types of lesions. Areas of thrombosis should also be noted and sampled. Complete transverse sections through the ventricles from the apex to the midventricular level are made and focal lesions identified. Any discrete lesions should be sampled, together with a minimum of five samples from the transverse section at midventricular level.

Macroscopic photographs of the whole heart, from the stages during dissection of any focal lesion/s and those taken at the midventricular section, may be of particular use for case review with clinicians. Ideally, all cases should be managed by, or referred to, a specialist cardiac pathologist with transplant experience. The histological assessment will follow the above standards for cardiac graft histology review.

References

1. Hamour IM, Khaghani A, Kanagala PK, Mitchell AG, Banner NR. Current outcome of heart transplantation: a 10-year single centre perspective and review. QJM. 2010;104:335–43.
2. Crespo-Leiro MG, Barge-Caballero E, Marzoa-Rivas R, Paniagua-Martin MJ. Heart transplantation. Curr Opin Organ Transplant. 2010;15:633–8.
3. Tan CD, Baldwin III WM, Rodriguez ER. Update on cardiac transplantation pathology. Arch Pathol Lab Med. 2007;131:1169–91.
4. Billingham ME. Some recent advances in cardiac pathology. Hum Pathol. 1979;10:367–86.
5. Billingham ME, Cary NR, Hammond ME. A working formulation for the standardization of nomenclature in the diagnosis of heart and lung rejection: Heart Rejection Study Group. The International Society for Heart Transplantation. J Heart Transplant. 1990;9: 587–93.
6. Stewart S, Winters GL, Fishbein MC, et al. Revision of the 1990 working formulation for the standardization of nomenclature in the diagnosis of heart rejection. J Heart Lung Transplant. 2005;24: 1710–20.
7. Spiegelhalter DJ, Stovin PG. An analysis of repeated biopsies following cardiac transplantation. Stat Med. 1983;2:33–40.
8. Sharples LD, Cary NR, Large SR, Wallwork J. Error rates with which endomyocardial biopsy specimens are graded for rejection after cardiac transplantation. Am J Cardiol. 1992;70:527–30.
9. Kobashigawa J, Crespo-Leiro MG, Ensminger SM, et al. Report from a consensus conference on antibody-mediated rejection in heart transplantation. J Heart Lung Transplant. 2011;30:252–69.
10. Berry G, Angelini A, Burke M, et al. The ISHLT working formulation for pathological diagnosis of antibody-mediated rejection in heart transplantation: evolution and current status (2005–2011). J Heart Lung Transplant. 2011;30(6):601–11.
11. Behr TM, Feucht HE, Richter K, et al. Detection of humoral rejection in human cardiac allografts by assessing the capillary deposition of complement fragment C4d in endomyocardial biopsies. J Heart Lung Transplant. 1999;18:904–12.
12. Feucht HE, Schneeberger H, Hillebrand G, et al. Capillary deposition of C4d complement fragment and early renal graft loss. Kidney Int. 1993;43:1333–8.
13. Rodriguez ER, Skojec DV, Tan CD, et al. Antibody-mediated rejection in human cardiac allografts: evaluation of immunoglobulins and complement activation products C4d and C3d as markers. Am J Transplant. 2005;5:2778–85.
14. Reed EF, Demetris AJ, Hammond E, et al. Acute antibody-mediated rejection of cardiac transplants. J Heart Lung Transplant. 2006;25:153–9.
15. Stewart S, Cary NRB. The pathology of heart and lung transplantation. Curr Diagn Pathol. 1996;3:69–79.
16. Suvarna SK, Kennedy A, Ciulli F, Locke TJ. Revision of the 1990 working formulation for cardiac allograft rejection: the Sheffield experience. Heart. 1998;79:432–6.
17. Maleszewski JJ, Kucirka LM, Segev DL, Halushka MK. Survey of current practice related to grading of rejection in cardiac transplant recipients in North America. Cardiovasc Pathol. 2011;20:261–5.
18. Hook S, Caple JF, McMahon JT, Myles JL, Ratliff NB. Comparison of myocardial cell injury in acute cellular rejection versus acute vascular rejection in cyclosporine-treated heart transplants. J Heart Lung Transplant. 1995;14:351–8.
19. Howie AJ. C9 immunohistology in detection of myocardial infarction. J Pathol. 2001;193:421.
20. Robert-Offerman SR, Leers MP, van Suylen RJ, Nap M, Daemen MJ, Theunissen PH. Evaluation of the membrane attack complex of complement for the detection of a recent myocardial infarction in man. J Pathol. 2000;191:48–53.
21. Yasojima K, Schwab C, McGeer EG, McGeer PL. Human heart generates complement proteins that are upregulated and activated after myocardial infarction. Circ Res. 1998;83:860–9.
22. Fishbein MC, Kobashigawa J. Biopsy-negative cardiac transplant rejection: etiology, diagnosis, and therapy. Curr Opin Cardiol. 2004;19:166–9.
23. Hammond EH, Hansen JK, Spencer LS, Jensen A, Yowell RL. Immunofluorescence of endomyocardial biopsy specimens: methods and interpretation. J Heart Lung Transplant. 1993;12:S113–24.
24. Hammond EH, Yowell RL, Nunoda S, et al. Vascular (humoral) rejection in heart transplantation: pathologic observations and clinical implications. J Heart Transplant. 1989;8:430–43.
25. Olsen SL, Wagoner LE, Hammond EH, et al. Vascular rejection in heart transplantation: clinical correlation, treatment options, and future considerations. J Heart Lung Transplant. 1993;12:S135–42.
26. Bonnaud EN, Lewis NP, Masek MA, Billingham ME. Reliability and usefulness of immunofluorescence in heart transplantation. J Heart Lung Transplant. 1995;14:163–71.
27. Crespo M, Pascual M, Tolkoff-Rubin N. Acute humoral rejection in renal allograft recipients: I. Incidence, serology and clinical characteristics. Transplantation. 2001;71:652–8.
28. Chantranuwat C, Qiao JH, Kobashigawa J, Hong L, Shintaku P, Fishbein MC. Immunoperoxidase staining for C4d on paraffin-embedded tissue in cardiac allograft endomyocardial biopsies: comparison to frozen tissue immunofluorescence. Appl Immunohistochem Mol Morphol. 2004;12:166–71.
29. Miller DV, Roden AC, Gamez JD, Tazelaar HD. Detection of C4d deposition in cardiac allografts: a comparative study of immunofluorescence and immunoperoxidase methods. Arch Pathol Lab Med. 2010;134:1679–84.
30. Lones MA, Czer LS, Trento A, Harasty D, Miller JM, Fishbein MC. Clinical-pathologic features of humoral rejection in cardiac allografts: a study in 81 consecutive patients. J Heart Lung Transplant. 1995;14:151–62.
31. Ratliff NB, McMahon JT. Activation of intravascular macrophages within myocardial small vessels is a feature of acute vascular rejection in human heart transplants. J Heart Lung Transplant. 1995;14:338–45.
32. Takemoto SK, Zeevi A, Feng S, et al. National conference to assess antibody-mediated rejection in solid organ transplantation. Am J Transplant. 2004;4:1033–41.
33. Wu GW, Kobashigawa JA, Fishbein MC, et al. Asymptomatic antibody-mediated rejection after heart transplantation predicts poor outcomes. J Heart Lung Transplant. 2009;28:417–22.
34. Tan CD, Sokos GG, Pidwell DJ, et al. Correlation of donor-specific antibodies, complement and its regulators with graft dysfunction in cardiac antibody-mediated rejection. Am J Transplant. 2009;9:2075–84.
35. Kfoury AG, Hammond ME, Snow GL, et al. Cardiovascular mortality among heart transplant recipients with asymptomatic antibody-mediated or stable mixed cellular and antibody-mediated rejection. J Heart Lung Transplant. 2009;28:781–4.
36. Forbes RD, Rowan RA, Billingham ME. Endocardial infiltrates in human heart transplants: a serial biopsy analysis comparing four immunosuppression protocols. Hum Pathol. 1990;21:850–5.

37. Gajjar NA, Kobashigawa JA, Laks H, Espejo-Vassilakis M, Fishbein MC. FK506 vs. cyclosporin. Pathologic findings in 1067 endomyocardial biopsies. Cardiovasc Pathol. 2003;12:73–6.

38. Barone JH, Fishbein MC, Czer LS, Blanche C, Trento A, Luthringer DJ. Absence of endocardial lymphoid infiltrates (Quilty lesions) in nonheart transplant recipients treated with cyclosporine. J Heart Lung Transplant. 1997;16:600–3.

39. Sattar HA, Husain AN, Kim AY, Krausz T. The presence of a CD21+ follicular dendritic cell network distinguishes invasive Quilty lesions from cardiac acute cellular rejection. Am J Surg Pathol. 2006;30:1008–13.

40. Di Carlo E, D'Antuono T, Contento S, Di NM, Ballone E, Sorrentino C. Quilty effect has the features of lymphoid neogenesis and shares CXCL13-CXCR5 pathway with recurrent acute cardiac rejections. Am J Transplant. 2007;7:201–10.

41. Marboe CC, Billingham M, Eisen H, et al. Nodular endocardial infiltrates (Quilty lesions) cause significant variability in diagnosis of ISHLT Grade 2 and 3A rejection in cardiac allograft recipients. J Heart Lung Transplant. 2005;24:S219–26.

42. Hiemann NE, Knosalla C, Wellnhofer E, Lehmkuhl HB, Hetzer R, Meyer R. Quilty in biopsy is associated with poor prognosis after heart transplantation. Transpl Immunol. 2008;19:209–14.

43. Hiemann NE, Knosalla C, Wellnhofer E, Lehmkuhl HB, Hetzer R, Meyer R. Quilty indicates increased risk for microvasculopathy and poor survival after heart transplantation. J Heart Lung Transplant. 2008;27:289–96.

44. Chantranuwat C, Blakey JD, Kobashigawa JA, et al. Sudden, unexpected death in cardiac transplant recipients: an autopsy study. J Heart Lung Transplant. 2004;23:683–9.

45. Yamani MH, Ratliff NB, Starling RC, et al. Quilty lesions are associated with increased expression of vitronectin receptor (alphavbeta3) and subsequent development of coronary vasculopathy. J Heart Lung Transplant. 2003;22:687–90.

46. Zakliczynski M, Nozynski J, Konecka-Mrowka D, et al. Quilty effect correlates with biopsy-proven acute cellular rejection but does not predict transplanted heart coronary artery vasculopathy. J Heart Lung Transplant. 2009;28:255–9.

47. Sibley RK, Olivari MT, Ring WS, Bolman RM. Endomyocardial biopsy in the cardiac allograft recipient. A review of 570 biopsies. Ann Surg. 1986;203:177–87.

48. Connor RC. Heart damage associated with intracranial lesions. Br Med J. 1968;3:29–31.

49. Connor RC. Focal myocytolysis and fuchsinophilic degeneration of the myocardium of patients dying with various brain lesions. Ann N Y Acad Sci. 1969;156:261–70.

50. Connor RC. Myocardial damage secondary to brain lesions. Am Heart J. 1969;78:145–8.

51. Connor RC. Fuchsinophilic degeneration of myocardium in patients with intracranial lesions. Br Heart J. 1970;32:81–4.

52. Haddad F, Deuse T, Pham M, et al. Changing trends in infectious disease in heart transplantation. J Heart Lung Transplant. 2010;29:306–15.

53. Breinholt JP, Moulik M, Dreyer WJ, et al. Viral epidemiologic shift in inflammatory heart disease: the increasing involvement of parvovirus B19 in the myocardium of pediatric cardiac transplant patients. J Heart Lung Transplant. 2010;29:739–46.

54. Moulik M, Breinholt JP, Dreyer WJ, et al. Viral endomyocardial infection is an independent predictor and potentially treatable risk factor for graft loss and coronary vasculopathy in pediatric cardiac transplant recipients. J Am Coll Cardiol. 2010;56:582–92.

55. Kotton CN. Update on infectious diseases in pediatric solid organ transplantation. Curr Opin Organ Transplant. 2008;13:500–5.

56. Casadei D. Chagas' disease and solid organ transplantation. Transplant Proc. 2010;42:3354–9.

57. Kotton CN, Lattes R. Parasitic infections in solid organ transplant recipients. Am J Transplant. 2009;9 Suppl 4:S234–51.

58. Derouin F, Pelloux H. Prevention of toxoplasmosis in transplant patients. Clin Microbiol Infect. 2008;14:1089–101.

59. Sanchez MA, Debrunner M, Cox E, Caldwell R. Acquired toxoplasmosis after orthotopic heart transplantation in a sulfonamide-allergic patient. Pediatr Cardiol. 2011;32:91–3.

60. Parker A, Bowles K, Bradley JA, et al. Diagnosis of post-transplant lymphoproliferative disorder in solid organ transplant recipients – BCSH and BTS guidelines. Br J Haematol. 2010;149:675–92.

61. Tsao L, Hsi ED. The clinicopathologic spectrum of posttransplantation lymphoproliferative disorders. Arch Pathol Lab Med. 2007;131:1209–18.

62. Grivas PD. Post-transplantation lymphoproliferative disorder (PTLD) twenty years after heart transplantation: a case report and review of the literature. Med Oncol. 2011;28:829–34.

63. Manlhiot C, Pollock-Barziv SM, Holmes C, et al. Post-transplant lymphoproliferative disorder in pediatric heart transplant recipients. J Heart Lung Transplant. 2010;29:648–57.

64. Mucha K, Foroncewicz B, Ziarkiewicz-Wroblewska B, Krawczyk M, Lerut J, Paczek L. Post-transplant lymphoproliferative disorder in view of the new WHO classification: a more rational approach to a protean disease? Nephrol Dial Transplant. 2010;25:2089–98.

65. Swerdlow SH, Campo E, Harris NL, et al. WHO classification of tumours of haematopoietic and lymphoid tissues. Geneva: World Health Organization; 2008.

66. Turillazzi E, Pennella A, Di GG, Neri M, Fineschi V. Post-transplant lymphoproliferative disorder in the heart late after heterotopic transplantation: autopsy findings. J Heart Lung Transplant. 2010;29:904–6.

67. Luk A, Metawee M, Ahn E, Gustafsson F, Ross H, Butany J. Do clinical diagnoses correlate with pathological diagnoses in cardiac transplant patients? The importance of endomyocardial biopsy. Can J Cardiol. 2009;25:e48–54.

68. Neil D. Recurrent and de novo disease in kidney, heart, lung, pancreas and intestinal transplants. Curr Opin Organ Transpl. 2006;11:289–95.

69. Alloni A, Pellegrini C, Ragni T, et al. Heart transplantation in patients with amyloidosis: single-center experience. Transplant Proc. 2004;36:643–4.

70. Dubrey SW, Burke MM, Hawkins PN, Banner NR. Cardiac transplantation for amyloid heart disease: the United Kingdom experience. J Heart Lung Transplant. 2004;23:1142–53.

71. Kristen AV, Meyer FJ, Perz JB, et al. Risk stratification in cardiac amyloidosis: novel approaches. Transplantation. 2005;80:S151–5.

72. Kristen AV, Sack FU, Schonland SO, et al. Staged heart transplantation and chemotherapy as a treatment option in patients with severe cardiac light-chain amyloidosis. Eur J Heart Fail. 2009;11:1014–20.

73. Mignot A, Varnous S, Redonnet M, et al. Heart transplantation in systemic (AL) amyloidosis: A retrospective study of eight French patients. Arch Cardiovasc Dis. 2008;101:523–32.

74. Sattianayagam PT, Gibbs SD, Pinney JH, et al. Solid organ transplantation in AL amyloidosis. Am J Transplant. 2010;10:2124–31.

75. Moloney ED, Egan JJ, Kelly P, Wood AE, Cooper Jr LT. Transplantation for myocarditis: a controversy revisited. J Heart Lung Transplant. 2005;24:1103–10.

76. Luk A, Lee A, Ahn E, Soor GS, Ross HJ, Butany J. Cardiac sarcoidosis: recurrent disease in a heart transplant patient following pulmonary tuberculosis infection. Can J Cardiol. 2010;26:e273–5.

77. Oni AA, Hershberger RE, Norman DJ, et al. Recurrence of sarcoidosis in a cardiac allograft: control with augmented corticosteroids. J Heart Lung Transplant. 1992;11:367–9.

78. Strecker T, Zimmermann I, Wiest GH. Pulmonary and cardiac recurrence of sarcoidosis in a heart transplant recipient. Dtsch Med Wochenschr. 2007;132:1159–62.

79. Yager JE, Hernandez AF, Steenbergen C, et al. Recurrence of cardiac sarcoidosis in a heart transplant recipient. J Heart Lung Transplant. 2005;24:1988–90.

80. Vassalli G, Gallino A, Weis M, et al. Alloimmunity and nonimmunologic risk factors in cardiac allograft vasculopathy. Eur Heart J. 2003;24:1180–8.

81. Demetris AJ, Zerbe T, Banner B. Morphology of solid organ allograft arteriopathy: identification of proliferating intimal cell populations. Transplant Proc. 1989;21:3667–9.

82. Billingham ME. Cardiac transplant atherosclerosis. Transplant Proc. 1987;19:19–25.

83. Billingham ME. Graft coronary disease: the lesions and the patients. Transplant Proc. 1989;21:3665–6.

84. Eisen HJ. Pathogenesis and management of cardiac allograft vasculopathy. Curr Opin Organ Transpl. 2004;9:448–52.

85. Pratschke J, Volk HD. Brain death-associated ischemia and reperfusion injury. Curr Opin Organ Transpl. 2004;9:153–8.

86. Mehra MR, Uber PA, Ventura HO, Scott RL, Park MH. The impact of mode of donor brain death on cardiac allograft vasculopathy: an intravascular ultrasound study. J Am Coll Cardiol. 2004;43:806–10.

87. Cohen O, De La Zerda DJ, Beygui R, Hekmat D, Laks H. Donor brain death mechanisms and outcomes after heart transplantation. Transplant Proc. 2007;39:2964–9.

88. Neil DA, Lynch SV, Hardie IR, Effeney DJ. Cold storage preservation and warm ischaemic injury to isolated arterial segments: endothelial cell injury. Am J Transplant. 2002;2:400–9.

89. Neil DA, Maguire SH, Walsh M, Lynch SV, Hardie IR, Effeney DJ. Progression of changes in arteries following cold storage preservation in UW and Collins solution in a syngeneic aortic transplant model. Transplant Proc. 1997;29:2561–2.

90. Hiemann NE, Musci M, Wellnhofer E, Meyer R, Hetzer R. Light microscopic biopsy findings after heart transplantation and possible links to development of graft vessel disease. Transplant Proc. 1999;31:149–51.

91. Koch A, Bingold TM, Oberlander J, et al. Capillary endothelia and cardiomyocytes differ in vulnerability to ischemia/reperfusion during clinical heart transplantation. Eur J Cardiothorac Surg. 2001; 20:996–1001.

92. Kupiec-Weglinski JW. Ischemia and reperfusion injury. Curr Opin Organ Transpl. 2004;9:130–1.

93. Logani S, Saltzman HE, Kurnik P, Eisen HJ, Ledley GS. Clinical utility of intravascular ultrasound in the assessment of coronary allograft vasculopathy: a review. J Interv Cardiol. 2011;24:9–14.

94. Stary HC, Blankenhorn DH, Chandler AB. A definition of the intima of human arteries and of its atherosclerosis-prone regions. A report from the Committee on Vascular Lesions of the Council on Arteriosclerosis, American Heart Association. Circulation. 1992;85:391–405.

95. Gao SZ, Schroeder JS, Alderman EL, et al. Clinical and laboratory correlates of accelerated coronary artery disease in the cardiac transplant patient. Circulation. 1987;76:V56–61.

96. Becker LB. New concepts in reactive oxygen species and cardiovascular reperfusion physiology. Cardiovasc Res. 2004;61: 461–70.

97. Turer AT, Hill JA. Pathogenesis of myocardial ischemia-reperfusion injury and rationale for therapy. Am J Cardiol. 2010;106: 360–8.

98. Nijboer WN, Schuurs TA, Van der Hoeven JAB, Ploeg RJ. Effect of brain death and donor treatment on organ inflammatory response and donor organ viability. Curr Opin Organ Transpl. 2004;9:110–5.

99. Van der Hoeven JAB, Ploeg RJ. Effects of brain death on donor organ viability. Curr Opin Organ Transpl. 2001;6:75–82.

100. Rodriguez-Sinovas A, Abdallah Y, Piper HM, Garcia-Dorado D. Reperfusion injury as a therapeutic challenge in patients with acute myocardial infarction. Heart Fail Rev. 2007;12:207–16.

101. Inserte J, Garcia-Dorado D, Ruiz-Meana M, et al. Effect of inhibition of Na(+)/Ca(2+) exchanger at the time of myocardial reperfusion on hypercontracture and cell death. Cardiovasc Res. 2002;55: 739–48.

102. Miller DL, Li P, Dou C, Armstrong WF, Gordon D. Evans blue staining of cardiomyocytes induced by myocardial contrast echocardiography in rats: evidence for necrosis instead of apoptosis. Ultrasound Med Biol. 2007;33:1988–96.

103. Boyle JJ, Rassl DM, Neil D, Suvarna K, Doran H. Heart dissection – explants post cardiac transplantation. In: Boyle JJ, editor. Tissue pathways for cardiovascular pathology. Royal College of Pathologists, London; 2008. http://www.rcpath.org/Resources/RCPath/Migrated%20Resources/Documents/G/g074tpcvsfinal.pdf p. 20–1.

104. Boyle JJ, Rassl DM, Neil D, Suvarna K, Doran H. Autopsy cardiac dissection. In: Boyle JJ, editor. Tissue pathways for cardiovascular pathology. Royal College of Pathologists, London; 2008. http://www.rcpath.org/Resources/RCPath/Migrated%20Resources/Documents/G/g074tpcvsfinal.pdf p. 22–7.

105. Basso C, Burke M, Fornes P, et al. Guidelines for autopsy investigation of sudden cardiac death. Virchows Arch. 2008;452:11–8.

106. Suvarna SK. National guidelines for adult autopsy cardiac dissection and diagnosis–are they achievable? A personal view. Histopathology. 2008;53:97–112.

Cardiomyopathies

11

Siân Hughes

Abstract

This chapter focuses on the primary cardiomyopathies. These heterogeneous group of diseases occur intrinsically to the myocardium and most have an underlying genetic basis. This chapter describes in detail dilated cardiomyopathy, hypertrophic cardiomyopathy, arrhythmogenic right ventricular cardiomyopathy, restrictive cardiomyopathy, as well as isolated left ventricular noncompaction, a more recently recognized entity. This chapter provides macroscopic and microscopic images of the various cardiomyopathies and describes in detail current concepts surrounding their pathogenesis and genetic basis.

Keywords

Cardiomyopathy • Hypertrophy • Myocyte disarray • Autosomal dominant • Arrhythmogenic right ventricular cardiomyopathy • Isolated left ventricular noncompaction • Endomyocardial fibrosis • Sarcoidosis • Fabry's disease • Amyloidosis

Introduction

The cardiomyopathies are a heterogeneous group of heart diseases, which are currently classified as either primary or secondary according to the World Health Organization's 1995 Task Force classification [1]. The primary cardiomyopathies are defined as diseases intrinsic to the myocardium, whereas the secondary cardiomyopathies are due to diseases such as coronary vascular disease or rheumatic valve pathology, which impair cardiac function. The primary cardiomyopathies are commonly subclassified by their echocardiographic and morphological characteristics and in contrast to secondary cardiomyopathies are often familial in nature, arising as a consequence of single gene mutations. This primary cardiomyopathy group includes dilated cardiomyopathy (DCM), hypertrophic cardiomyopathy (HCM), restrictive cardiomyopathy (RCM), arrhythmogenic right ventricular cardiomyopathy (ARVC), and other unclassified

cardiomyopathy [1, 2]. The last subgroup encompasses more recently described entities such as isolated left ventricular noncompaction (LVNC) cardiomyopathy, which could be regarded as a primary genetic cardiomyopathy [3]. This chapter will focus on the primary cardiomyopathies and how the pathologist can accurately diagnose each by performing a detailed macroscopic and microscopic examination of the heart, as described in Chapter 1.

Dilated Cardiomyopathy (DCM)

DCM is the most common cause of congestive heart failure in the adult population worldwide and is usually classified as either idiopathic (i.e., primary) or acquired (i.e., following other disorders). Clinically, it is associated with progressive congestive heart failure during life and in contrast to other primary cardiomyopathies does not usually present with sudden cardiac death (SCD) without antemortem symptoms. DCM is often classified as familial when it is observed in two or more family members [4]. It is now known that over 20% cases of idiopathic DCM are familial in origin pointing to a variety of underlying familial pathologies [5, 6].

S. Hughes, MBBS, M.Sc., Ph.D., FRCPath
Department of Histopathology, University College Hospital London, 21 University St., Rockefeller Building London, WC1E 6JJ, UK
e-mail: sian.hughes@ucl.ac.uk, rmkdshu@ucl.ac.uk

However, the majority of familial and nonfamilial cases are of unknown etiology [7]. Several single gene defects in a wide variety of different genes encoding structural proteins of the myocyte cytoskeleton, sarcolemma, nuclear membrane, or ion channels have been identified as linked to DCM, but these account for only a small number of cases [8–11]. Mutations in cardiac actin, cardiac β-myosin heavy chain, metavinculin, troponin T, and α(alpha)-tropomyosin cause a pure DCM phenotype without multisystem disease [11]. In contrast, mutations in lamin A/C cause DCM with predominant conduction system disease [12] and mutations in δ-sarcoglycan, dystrophin, and the mitochondrial respiratory chain cause DCM with associated skeletal myopathy [7].

The mode of inheritance of familial DCM appears complex and includes autosomal dominant, X-linked and autosomal recessive forms, as well as inheritance through maternal mitochondrial DNA [2, 8, 9, 13, 14]. Familial DCM tends to exhibit incomplete or age-related penetrance, and many cases of DCM do not present until the fifth or sixth decade of life [15]. Although single mutations responsible for familial DCM have been identified, diagnostic molecular genetic tests are available for the identification of only a limited number of genes, (i.e., dystrophin) in routine clinical practice [11]. Furthermore, the majority of causative mutations are private mutations, which are not observed between unrelated families increasing the genetic complexity of familial DCM [11]. In a series of 101 patients with familial or nonfamilial DCM, the prognosis and 5-year survival were found to be similar between the two groups, being 55% in the nonfamilial group and 51% for familial patients [7].

Acquired causes of DCM are more common, and ventricular dilatation may occur in the setting of coronary artery

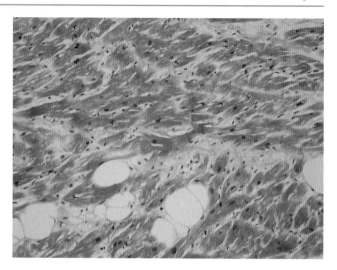

Fig. 11.2 A case of sudden death in myotonic dystrophy. The macroscopy was minimally dilated, but there was histological diffuse fibrous and fatty tissue replacement seen across the ventricular tissues, more easily discerned in the left ventricle (hematoxylin and eosin stain)

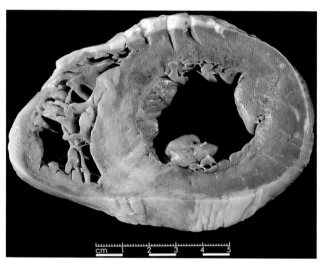

Fig. 11.3 Macroscopic view in a case of sarcoidosis. The chambers are mildly dilated and there is also some wall thickening. Focal scarring is seen mainly in the septum and left ventricle wall towards the base of the image (Courtesy of Dr. PJ Gallagher)

disease/valvular disease, hypertension, postviral myocarditis, chronic alcoholic intake, following chemotherapy (in particular, doxorubicin), in relation to pregnancy and with Duchenne's/Becker's muscular dystrophies (Fig. 11.1), myotonic dystrophy (Fig. 11.2), and infiltrative diseases of the heart (e.g., sarcoidosis, amyloidosis, and hemochromatosis) (Fig. 11.3). In the pediatric population, metabolic cardiomyopathy accounts for a significant proportion of cases [11].

The macroscopic (Fig. 11.4) and microscopic phenotypes of DCM are similar in the vast majority of cases, irrespective of the underlying cause. DCM is manifest by an increase in heart weight and thinning of the left ventricular wall with enlargement of both ventricular cavities. The normal trabecular

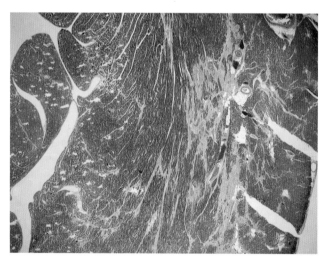

Fig. 11.1 Left ventricle tissues in a case of Duchenne-type muscular dystrophy. The masson trichrome highlights the scarred/fibrous element (*green*) as compared with the viable muscular tissue (*red*). Clearly electrical depolarization and cardiac contractility will be degraded by this amount of fibrous tissue replacement

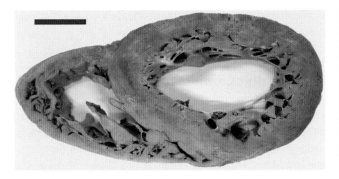

Fig. 11.4 Dilated cardiomyopathy in a case of prior myocarditis. There is generalized ventricular dilatation (bar marker 3 cm). This pattern of chamber enlargement is the standard format seen in many toxic, inflammatory, and degenerative disorders as an end point

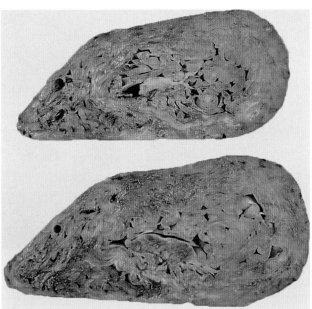

Fig. 11.5 Photograph of left ventricular myocardium from the autopsy of a patient with LVNC. The noncompacted endocardial layer is composed of a complex meshwork of elongated and thinned trabeculations with deep intertrabecular recesses imparting a spongelike appearance to the left ventricular wall

pattern is effaced, and there may often be diffuse endocardial thickening. Mural thrombus due to nonlaminar blood flow is also frequently present. It is evident surrounding the ventricular trabeculations and within the atrial appendages.

The microscopic features of DCM are often nonspecific, and some, but not all, histological changes may be seen. Classically, the myocytes are thinned with nuclear hypertrophy and pleomorphism. There is often loss of myofibrils leading to myocyte vacuolation imparting an empty appearance. There are varying degrees of either coarse or diffuse interstitial fibrosis within the ventricular myocardium depending on the duration of the disease. A patchy lymphocytic infiltrate accompanied by histiocytes associated with myocyte dropout can exist. It is noteworthy that there are no histological features specific to distinguish between the acquired or familial forms of DCM, and a detailed examination and clinical/family/occupational history is mandatory in pinpointing the underlying cause. Provided that acquired causes of DCM have been excluded, then it is important to refer first-degree relatives of potential index cases of familial DCM for cardiac screening, given the increasingly apparent inherited nature of this type of cardiomyopathy.

Isolated Left Ventricular Noncompaction (LVNC)

Isolated LVNC is a congenital myocardial disorder first described in 1984 by Engberding and Bender [16] that can present in either childhood or adulthood with congestive heart failure, arrhythmia, or the complications of thromboembolism [17]. Isolated LVNC is becoming increasingly recognized as an important cause of cardiomyopathy and has an underlying genetic basis although the molecular pathology has yet to be fully defined. In the pediatric population, isolated LVNC was detected in 9.2% of children with cardiomyopathy and was the third most common type [18]. Its incidence in the general population is estimated between 0.05%

and 0.25% [19, 20]. It occurs due to persistence of the noncompacted endocardial layer characteristic of the early fetal period before myocardial compaction is complete [21]. The left ventricle is usually affected, and it may be either dilated or hypertrophied. Echocardiography or MRI is the diagnostic method of choice for detecting LVNC cardiomyopathy, which is characterized by at least four prominent trabeculations associated with deep intertrabecular recesses with a characteristic bilaminar structure.

The pathologist may encounter LVNC cardiomyopathy as an incidental finding at autopsy [19] but more commonly in the setting of heart failure [22]. However, it can also present as SCD. At autopsy, the complex pattern of prominent trabeculation in association with deep intertrabecular recesses imparts a spongelike appearance to the wall of the left ventricle (Fig. 11.5). It is also frequently associated with overlying mural thrombus due to stasis. It is important to confine the diagnosis of LVNC to the assessment of trabeculae in the left ventricle where the compaction during development is greatest, rather than those in the right ventricle, which are less compacted and may simulate pathological noncompaction. Histologically, LVNC is characterized by prominent and thinned trabecula manifest as fingerlike processes (Fig. 11.6). Subendocardial fibrosis is usually evident due to the impaired coronary microcirculation associated with this disease (Fig. 11.7) [23].

LVNC cardiomyopathy may occur sporadically, but some studies indicate a familial origin, and cardiac screening of

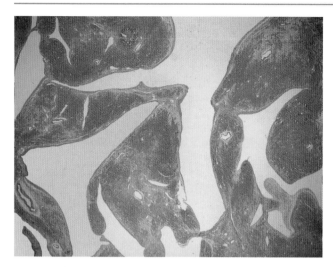

Fig. 11.6 Low-power hematoxylin- and eosin-stained photograph of LVNC showing that the noncompacted layer is composed of "fingerlike" projections

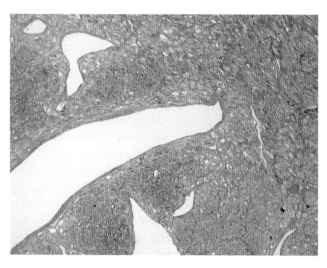

Fig. 11.7 A Masson's trichrome stain confirms the prominent endocardial and subendocardial fibrosis, which is a feature of this disease due to abnormal myocardial microperfusion

first-degree relatives is advised. In one family, LVNC was associated with mutations in the G4.5 gene, which encodes tafazzin, an enzyme involved in the metabolism of cardiolipin [24]. Other disease-causing mutations include those identified in sarcomeric protein genes including the cardiac β(beta)-myosin heavy chain gene, α(alpha)-dystrobrevin, the α(alpha)-cardiac actin gene, and FKBP-12 [25–31]. However, another study of 48 patients with this disease indicated that isolated LVNC is rarely caused by mutations in G4.5, α(alpha)-dystrobrevin, or FKBP-12 [31].

The prognosis of LVNC is generally poor with one study following up 34 patients with isolated LVNC over a 44-month period. Of these patients, six suffered SCD and four died of heart failure [32]. The registry of the Italian Society of

Echocardiography indicates that patients with symptomatic disease have a worse outcome [33].

Hypertrophic Cardiomyopathy (HCM)

HCM is a common autosomal dominant genetic disorder affecting 1:500 of the population and is more prevalent in males [34, 35]. It is an important cause of SCD in the young and in athletes. HCM is predominantly a disease affecting the cardiac contractile apparatus [36] and is caused by mutations in the genes encoding sarcomeric proteins as well as genes involved in myocyte energy homeostasis [2, 9, 37]. Mutations in the PRKAG2 gene, which encodes the β(beta)-2 subunit of AMP-activated-protein kinase (AMPK), have been found to cause HCM with Wolff-Parkinson-White syndrome [38]. Similarly, in certain types of mitochondrial cardiomyopathy, it has been shown that mutations in the mitochondrial tRNA(Lys) gene (G8363A) involved in energy production lead to HCM associated with sensorineural hearing loss and encephalomyopathy [39]. However, in clinical practice, most cases of HCM are due to mutations in the sarcomeric genes encoding cardiac β(beta)-myosin heavy chain, cardiac troponin T, myosin binding protein-C, cardiac troponin I, regulatory and essential light chains, α(alpha)-tropomyosin, and actin [2, 40, 41].

The clinical spectrum of HCM as shown by genotype-phenotype correlation analyses is highly variable. For each gene, many different mutations have been identified, and different mutations in the same gene may be associated with different disease severity and prognosis. For example, "malignant" mutations (Arg403Gln, Arg453Gln, Arg719Trp), which cause a severe form of HCM with early onset, complete penetrance, and high risk of SCD, have been identified in the cardiac β(beta)-myosin heavy chain gene. Conversely, other mutations (Leu908Val and Val606Met) are considered low risk and associated with near-normal life expectancy [41–45]. Similarly, mutations in different contractile protein genes often carry very different prognoses. For example, mutations in the troponin T gene cause minimal ventricular hypertrophy and have a poor prognosis in that they are associated with a high risk of SCD. Furthermore, HCM may exhibit significant phenotypic variation within the same family, and it has been observed that individuals with identical mutations can exhibit different clinical and morphological phenotypes [46]. The latter is likely to be due to the complex interplay between lifestyle factors (e.g., exercise) and polymorphisms in modifier genes such as TNF-α(alpha) and the renin-angiotensin-aldosterone system [47, 48] modulating the hypertrophic response and thereby the subsequent risk of SCD.

At autopsy in cases of SCD, it is important to be aware that, despite its name, HCM does not invariably present with hypertrophy. This is certainly the case with troponin T mutations where hypertrophy may be minimal or absent.

Conversely, "big hearts" are not exclusive to HCM. Hypertrophy may occur as a consequence of essential hypertension, valvular heart disease, and athletic training. Thus, from the practical point of view, it is unwise to reach a diagnosis of HCM on macroscopic assessment of the heart alone. It is also important that the pathologist is aware of the effects of agonal contraction. When death coincides with systolic contraction, the resulting increase in left ventricular wall thickness can be very exaggerated, leading to a misdiagnosis of HCM. It is thus essential to correlate heart mass with body weight to provide an accurate indicator of genuine left ventricular hypertrophy rather than relying on measurements of left ventricular wall thickness alone.

Classical HCM is characterized macroscopically by left ventricular hypertrophy, which may be asymmetrical (Fig. 11.8) or symmetrical [49, 50]. First described in 1958, this type of HCM is characterized by hypertrophy of the basal anterior septum, which protrudes beneath the subaortic valvular apparatus causing outflow obstruction and mitral regurgitation [51, 52]. This is accompanied by systolic anterior motion (SAM) of the mitral valve and endocardial fibrosis over the septum, leading to a subaortic mitral impact lesion, which resembles a mirror image of the anterior cusp of the mitral valve (Fig. 11.9). Previously, this lesion was regarded as pathognomonic of HCM [49]. However, it may occur in hypertrophied hearts due to hypertension and prominence of the basal septum in the hearts of the elderly [50]. This is why it is important to interpret macroscopic features in conjunction with histology and other data.

The symmetrical type of HCM is characterized by concentric thickening of the left ventricle [49]. At autopsy, it is indistinguishable from hypertrophy due to essential hypertension and aortic stenosis or even athletic training. Adequate

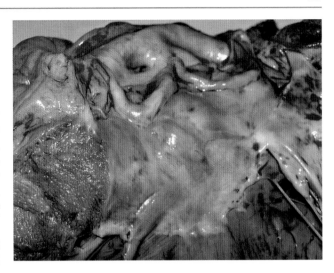

Fig. 11.9 Photograph of a subaortic mitral impact lesion, which resembles a mirror image of the anterior cusp of the mitral valve in a patient with familial HCM

histological sampling is essential in this situation [50]. In true HCM, often the right ventricle may also be involved by the hypertrophic process [53]. Other morphological variants have been described including apical HCM and a variant of HCM with midventricular cavity obstruction and segmental hypertrophy confined to the posterobasal left ventricular free wall [54]. Though rare, these subtypes are of relevance since patients with midventricular HCM are severely symptomatic, whereas those with the apical type tend to exhibit mild disease [55–58]. A further subgroup of HCM patients with left ventricular apical aneurysms and adverse clinical outcomes has recently been described [59]. End-stage HCM often manifest as ventricular dilatation due to myocyte loss with extensive replacement-type fibrosis may also simulate DCM. This occurs in approximately 10–15% of affected individuals. Furthermore, some patients with familial HCM due to mutations in the troponin I gene can also present clinically with RCM [60–62]. In this subset of patients, disarray with, or without, hypertrophy was evident. In general, HCM has a good prognosis and near-normal life expectancy provided SCD does not occur. Unfortunately, patients with the restrictive phenotype of HCM carry a poor prognosis [63].

Classically, HCM is characterized by microscopy by myocyte hypertrophy and myocyte disarray (Fig. 11.10) [50]. The latter occurs due to the loss of the normal parallel arrangement of myocytes within the myocardium, and the myocytes are distributed at odd angles to one another assuming either a cartwheel or herringbone pattern due to abnormal cell-to-cell contacts. Within individual myocytes, there is disruption of the myofibrillary architecture, with crisscrossing of the myofibrils (Fig. 11.11). This can be demonstrated by phosphotungstic acid-hematoxylin (PTAH) staining or electron microscopy. Depending on the longevity of the disease process, there may be either coarse or fine interstitial

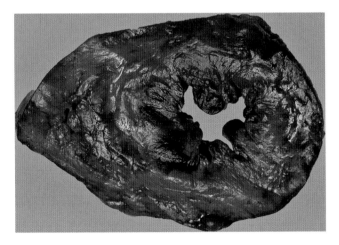

Fig. 11.8 Photograph of a transverse slice of the heart at midseptal level from a patient with familial HCM. This is the asymmetrical variant with disproportionate left ventricular hypertrophy affecting the interventricular septum. The right ventricle is also involved by the hypertrophic process

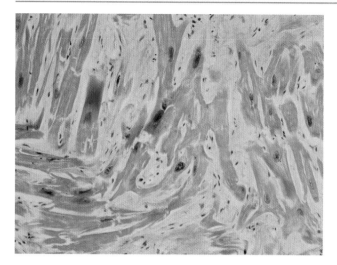

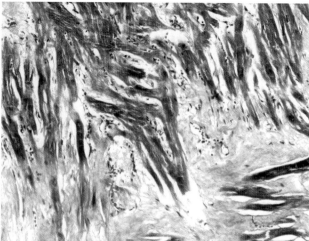

Fig. 11.10 Hematoxylin and eosin-stained section showing florid myocyte disarray and fibrosis in familial HCM. Disarray is characterized by hypertrophic myocytes with enlarged and pleomorphic nuclei aligned at odd angles to one another

Fig. 11.12 Masson's trichrome stain confirming the marked increase in interstitial collagen, which is an integral part of the disease process and a hallmark of familial HCM

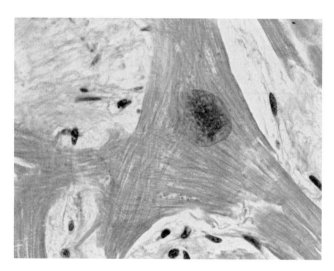

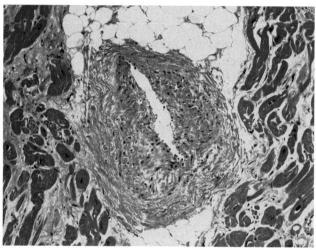

Fig. 11.11 Within individual myocytes, there is disruption of the myofibrillary architecture with crisscrossing of the myofibrils (hematoxylin & eosin)

Fig. 11.13 The small intramural branches of coronary arteries exhibit luminal narrowing and medial hypertrophy (dysplasia) in HCM, contributing to myocardial ischemia and myocyte loss leading to increased fibrosis (hematoxylin & eosin)

fibrosis or a combination of these patterns due to increased amounts of collagen (Fig. 11.12). Fibrosis is a hallmark of HCM and is associated with poor clinical outcomes including an increased risk of arrhythmic events and progression to heart failure [64–66], which occurs in approximately 10% of patients. In vivo, fibrosis can be measured by late gadolinium enhancement cardiac MRI. Similarly, at autopsy, fibrosis can be assessed by histochemical stains for collagen including picrosirius red and Masson's trichrome staining [65].

In cases of HCM, provided an entire circumferential left ventricular slice of myocardium at midseptal level is sampled (generating between six and eight blocks of tissue or large geographic blocks), disarray will usually be evident in more

than 20% of the myocardium in at least two blocks. HCM is not a histologically subtle or focal disease, and myocyte disarray is usually obvious. If the pathologist has to search carefully for aberrant myocardial architecture, it is probably not genuine HCM. A common error is to sample the area where the left and right ventricles interdigitate. The myocytes are not usually parallel here in healthy hearts, and misinterpretation of this as disarray can lead to an erroneous diagnosis of HCM. Similarly, mild degrees of nonparallelism in normal hearts can be seen around trabeculations, adjacent to blood vessels, and where large muscle bundles converge.

HCM is also characterized by abnormal myocardial vasculature. The small intramural branches of coronary arteries often

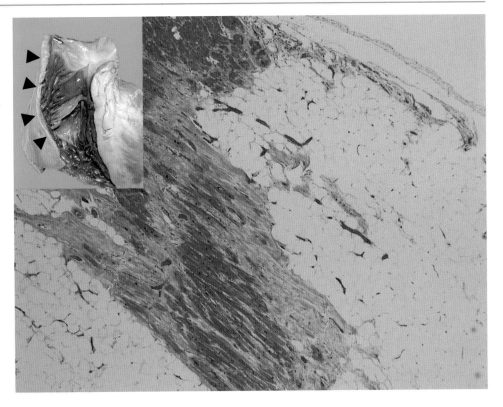

Fig. 11.14 Classical ARVC is characterized by fibroadipose infiltration of the right ventricle, seen in the inset macroscopically *top right, arrowed*. Histology shows the adipose and fibrous tissue replacement of the myocyte architecture (hematoxylin & eosin)

exhibit so-called dysplasia characterized by luminal narrowing and medial hypertrophy (Fig. 11.13). It is likely that this contributes to ischemia and myocyte loss with replacement fibrosis. Furthermore, it may contribute to electrical instability leading to arrhythmia and SCD [67–69] or a DCM-like picture culminating in congestive heart failure [67, 68, 70].

HCM is a common genetic disorder. Accurate diagnosis will help to identify those families who will need cardiac screening, mutation analysis, and genetic counseling. SCD may be the initial presentation of HCM in a family, and it is inevitable that the pathologist will encounter index cases as part of their coronial autopsy practice.

Arrhythmogenic Right Ventricular Cardiomyopathy (ARVC)

Arrhythmogenic right ventricular cardiomyopathy (ARVC) is an inherited cardiomyopathy characterized by progressive myocardial loss and fibroadipose replacement, primarily affecting the right ventricle (Figs. 11.14 and 11.15) and causing ventricular tachycardia, syncope, cardiac failure, and SCD [71]. ARVC is a rare disease with an estimated prevalence of 1:5,000, but it is one of the most common causes of unheralded SCD in young people, and athletes and may account for up to 20% of cases [72–76].

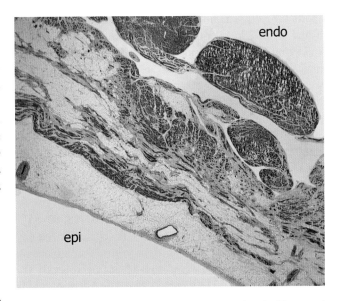

Fig. 11.15 Masson trichrome histology demonstrating the fibrous and fatty tissue replacement that has swept inwards from the epicardial (*epi*) aspect to the endocardial (*endo*) aspect of the ventricle chamber

A broad spectrum of structural and functional abnormalities has been described in ARVC depending upon the stage of the disease, ranging from an initial subclinical phase to an overt electrical disorder culminating in right and/or left

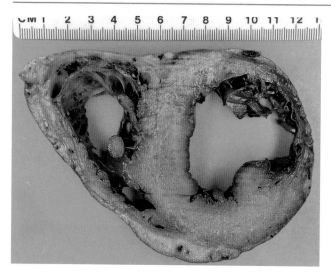

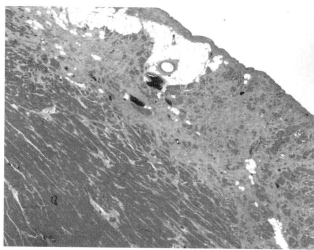

Fig. 11.16 Photograph of a transverse slice of the heart at midseptal level from a patient with the left ventricular predominant type of ARVC. There is thinning of the lateral wall of the left ventricle and fibroadipose replacement involving the outer third of the posterior wall of the left ventricle. This phenotype is associated with mutations in the desmoplakin gene

Fig. 11.17 Low-power hematoxylin-stained photomicrograph showing myocardial substitution and replacement by fibroadipose tissue involving the outer third of the posterior wall of the left ventricle in a patient with ARVC with predominant left ventricular involvement. The fibroadipose replacement is advancing from the epicardium towards the endocardium

ventricular failure [77]. The early phase of ARVC is often clinically silent and difficult to diagnose. There may be minimal symptoms, but later, there is a disproportionate risk of arrhythmic events, especially during strenuous activities and sports [78, 79]. The first clinical profile of ARVC was published in 1982 in a series of patients with advanced disease and symptomatic ventricular tachycardias [80]. The pathological changes of early ARVC are localized, with a predilection for the apical, subtricuspid, and pulmonary outflow regions of the right ventricle: the so-called triangle of dysplasia manifest as segmental aneurysms or wall thinning [72, 80–82]. With disease progression, right ventricular dilation and involvement of the left ventricular myocardium may follow. Left ventricular wall involvement typically begins as subepicardial posterior wall fibrosis, which subsequently becomes diffuse, leading to end-stage ARVC, which can be difficult to distinguish from DCM (Fig. 11.16) [78, 82–85].

Histologically, classical ARVC is characterized by fibroadipose infiltration of the right ventricle commencing in the outer epicardial layer and advancing towards the endocardium (Figs. 11.14 and 11.15). The left ventricle is also involved in up to 50% of cases [71]. The presence of fibrosis is the diagnostic hallmark [86, 87], and it is likely that earlier reports in the literature describing pure adipose replacement represented the extreme end of the spectrum observed in normal right ventricular myocardium [72, 81, 86]. Adipose replacement of the right ventricular wall occurs with advancing age and may be especially prominent in the hearts of middle-aged and elderly women and/or obese individuals [88]. Moreover, significant fatty infiltration of the heart may be observed in the anteroapical and subtricuspid

regions of the right ventricle of normal hearts [87]. It is therefore essential at autopsy to sample the right ventricle adequately and record the site from where blocks are taken from to avoid misinterpretation of the significance of fatty tissue within the heart.

Although predominant right ventricular disease is one of the defining features of ARVC, an increasingly recognized variant characterized by subepicardial and mediomural fibroadipose replacement confined to the left ventricle has been identified at autopsy as a cause of SCD in the young (Fig. 11.17) [83, 84, 89, 90]. Despite extensive disease involvement of the left ventricle, most of these young people were asymptomatic during life, with SCD being the initial presenting symptom. This variant of ARVC may be caused by mutations in the desmoplakin gene, further supporting the notion that this phenotypic variant is part of the ARVC spectrum, rather than a separate disease entity. Furthermore, evaluation of affected relatives shows both left- and classic right-sided disease [74].

At autopsy, a subepicardial distribution pattern of fibroadipose replacement should alert the pathologist to the possibility of ARVC with predominant or exclusive left ventricular involvement since left ventricular subepicardial myocardial lesions are rare in other cardiac diseases [91] but frequent in ARVC. Fibrosis secondary to myocardial ischemia or hypertensive heart disease typically favors the subendocardial zone with sparing of the epicardial region of the heart. Furthermore, fibrosis as a consequence of postviral myocarditis is patchy rather than zonal and randomly distributed throughout the entire ventricular wall of both ventricles.

The pathogenesis of ARVC has been the subject of much investigation. It has become increasingly apparent that most cases of ARVC are familial with an autosomal dominant mode of inheritance and incomplete penetrance [92, 93]. Gene linkage analysis of large families affected by ARVC has revealed multiple chromosomal loci, indicating genetic heterogeneity. The more common autosomal dominant form of ARVC has been linked with mutations in desmosomal proteins including desmoplakin, plakophilin-2 and desmoglein-2, desmocollin-2, and plakoglobin [74, 94–102]. These are all key structural components of desmosomes, which are located at the intercalated disc and provide mechanical coupling between the intermediate filaments and cytoplasmic membranes of neighboring cardiac myocytes. It is likely that a complex interplay between intercellular signaling pathways and desmosomal proteins under conditions of mechanical stress leads to myocyte detachment/damage and death by apoptosis [103, 104]. There may be accompanying inflammation and hence induction of adipogenic and fibrogenic genes [102, 105]. Repair by fibroadipose replacement occurs as a response to myocyte loss, thereby providing the pathological substrate for electrical instability and arrhythmias, which are a manifestation of this disease [102].

Mutations in plakophilin-2 were found to be present in 22% of individuals in one series of 108 patients with ARVC [79]. Interestingly, in this study, 34% of the probands presenting with symptomatic disease were athletes, supporting the hypothesis that exercise-induced repetitive stretching of a diseased right ventricle may promote the phenotypic expression of ARVC [79, 106–108]. Genotype-phenotype correlation analyses have also revealed that mutations in desmoplakin are associated with a high risk of SCD and left ventricular involvement [74, 109], whereas mutations in plakoglobin and plakophilin-2 predominantly affect the right ventricle [110].

Mutations in cell adhesion proteins also cause several autosomal recessive cardiocutaneous forms of ARVC [97, 111, 112]. These include Naxos disease and Carvajal syndrome. The former was initially described in cases from the Hellenic island of Naxos, but cases have also been reported in Israel, Turkey, and Saudi Arabia [113]. Carvajal syndrome is similar to Naxos disease but occurs at a younger age with more prominent left ventricular involvement, mainly in Ecuador and India. These autosomal recessive forms of ARVC are characterized by the triad of ARVC, palmoplantar keratoderma, and woolly hair and are due to mutations in the plakoglobin and desmoplakin genes [111, 114, 115]. Other genes have been implicated in causing ARVC including mutations in cardiac ryanodine receptor 2 [116], transforming growth factor-β(beta)3 [117] and the TMEM43 gene [118]. However, compared with the desmosomal protein genes, there is controversy as to whether mutations in these genes cause classical ARVC, and less is known about the underlying pathogenetic mechanism by which they may induce the ARVC phenotype.

Restrictive Cardiomyopathy (RCM)

RCM is essentially caused by a variety of myocardial or endomyocardial diseases, which stiffen the heart by infiltration or fibrosis leading to restrictive filling [119, 120]. The primary restrictive cardiomyopathies include tropical endomyocardial fibrosis (EMF), Loeffler's endomyocarditis, and idiopathic or primary RCM. These are less common than the secondary types of RCM due to diseases where the heart is affected as part of a multisystem disorder. Primary RCM is rare and may occur sporadically or can occur in families where it is inherited as an autosomal dominant trait with/without skeletal myopathy and heart block [121, 122]. It is an important disease requiring orthotopic cardiac transplantation in children. However, primary RCM is characterized by a lack of specific myocardial pathology in either endomyocardial biopsy or autopsy specimens [123].

Tropical EMF is a restrictive obliterative cardiomyopathy of unknown cause and occurs in tropical and subtropical Africa affecting children and adolescents [124, 125]. EMF is an indolent disease but is a common cause of heart failure and death in endemic regions, where it is often associated with hypereosinophilia [126, 127]. It is characterized by endocardial thickening of one or both ventricles with mural thrombi in the apices causing partial cavity obliteration and disease involvement of the atrioventricular valves, leading to mitral and tricuspid regurgitation. Microscopically there is a thick layer of endocardial acellular/hyalinized collagen and granulation tissue extending into the myocardium [128]. Despite immunosuppressive therapy and surgical treatment for EMF, this disease carries a poor prognosis and is a significant cause of mortality [129, 130]. It has recently been proposed that in a subset of EMF patients, autoimmunity may be involved, as shown by the identification of IgG and IgM class antimyosin antibodies [131].

Loeffler's endomyocarditis is an uncommon debilitating disease, which tends to affect males (Fig. 11.18). It occurs in temperate climates, usually resulting in death within months. It is related to hypereosinophilic states including idiopathic hypereosinophilic syndrome, eosinophilic leukemia, and Churg-Strauss syndrome. The initial stages of the disease are characterized by an acute inflammatory myocarditis involving the endocardium and myocardium with a prominent eosinophilic component and endocardial thrombus formation associated with underlying granulation tissue (Fig. 11.19). In patients that survive, there may be extensive fibrosis of the endocardium similar to tropical EMF. It is therefore likely that both diseases represent a continuum,

Fig. 11.18 Photograph of a transverse slice of the heart at midseptal level from a patient with hypereosinophilic syndrome and Loeffler's endomyocarditis. A shaggy coat of thrombus is seen coating the right ventricle, and there is fibrosis and white endocardial thickening of the left ventricle

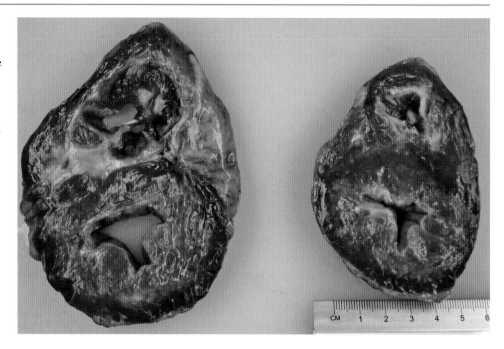

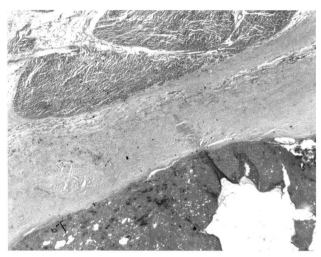

Fig. 11.19 Hematoxylin- and eosin-stained photomicrograph showing that in the acute phase, the endocardial thickening is due to granulation tissue covered by more recently formed thrombus imparting a layered appearance

whereby eosinophils play an essential role in the evolution of tissue damage [132–134] due to degranulation and the release of "toxic" proteins [126, 133, 134, 135, 136, 137]. The more indolent course of tropical EMF may be related to the less pronounced hypereosinophilia, compared with that observed in patients with Loeffler's endomyocarditis [132, 134].

The secondary forms of RCM can be subclassified as either infiltrative or noninfiltrative. In RCM due to infiltrative disease, the infiltrates are extracellular and localize in the myocyte interstitium, whereas in other forms, such as stor-

age disorders, the deposits are intracellular and found within myocytes [119]. Amyloidosis and sarcoidosis are the prototypical cardiac infiltrative disorders. Common storage disorders with myocardial involvement include hemochromatosis, glycogen storage disease(s), and Fabry's disease. The noninfiltrative secondary causes of RCM include carcinoid heart disease and iatrogenic disorders, in particular, following radiotherapy and anthracycline chemotherapy [119]. In the latter conditions, restrictive dynamics ensue as a consequence of diffuse fibrosis.

Cardiac amyloidosis is the most common infiltrative type of secondary RCM [119] and is caused by the deposition of insoluble amyloid protein fibrils in the interstitium of the myocardium and/or walls of blood vessels. It may be acquired or inherited. Cardiac amyloidosis may be classified according to the type of amyloid fibril protein deposited. The major fibrillar protein is designated protein A followed by an abbreviation of the amyloidogenic protein name. Over 18 different types of protein causing amyloid have been identified [135], but this chapter will focus only on those that primarily involve the heart. It is noteworthy that amyloidosis due to chronic infections and inflammatory disease leading to serum amyloid A formation rarely involves the heart.

The most common type of amyloidosis to affect the heart is AL amyloidosis. This is due to the deposition of amyloid fibrils complexed with monoclonal kappa and lambda immunoglobulin light chains. It is principally associated with plasma cell dyscrasias, (B cell lymphoma, Waldenstrom's macroglobulinemia, multiple myeloma, etc.). Extracardiac manifestations such as nephrotic syndrome,

Fig. 11.20 The myocardium is heavily infiltrated by eosinophil matrix around cells and throughout the interstitium. The *inset* macroscopic view of cardiac amyloidosis shows a semirigid structure that is self-supporting, even in the fresh postmortem state. This macroscopic quality often provides a clue to the ultimate histology

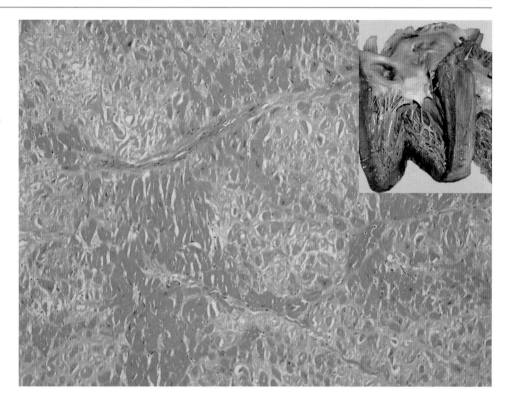

hepatosplenomegaly, and macroglossia are common. Cardiac involvement and death due to congestive heart failure or arrhythmias occur in more than 50% of patients with AL amyloidosis. It has a poor prognosis despite treatment with melphalan [137].

Systemic senile amyloidosis affects more than 25% of the population over the age of 80 and is a common incidental finding at autopsy [137, 138, 139, 140]. It is caused by the deposition of normal transthyretin (TTR) in the heart [139]. This form of cardiac amyloidosis tends to run a relatively benign clinical course, and only a minority of patients develop heart failure or conduction disturbances [137, 139, 141]. Another form of age-related amyloidosis is isolated atrial amyloidosis (IAA). In IAA, the amyloid fibril is composed predominantly of atrial natriuretic factor (ANF). This is an extremely common finding in the atria of individuals over 90 years of age, and these patients often have atrial fibrillation [142, 143].

Hereditary or familial amyloidosis is less common, and the heart is less frequently involved than with AL amyloidosis. It is due to the deposition of mutant TTR in the majority of cases, but mutations in other proteins including apoprotein AI (ApoAI) [144, 145] and apoprotein AII (ApoAII) [146] have been described. TTR-related amyloidosis may occur sporadically but is usually inherited as an autosomal dominant trait. More than 70 mutations in the TTR gene have been described [147], but the clinical phenotype and presence or absence of cardiac disease depend on the type of TTR mutation. For example, cardiac disease predominates with TTRThr45, TTRMet111, and TTRLys92 mutations [148–150], and individuals with TTRMet30 often have isolated conduction system disease [151].

Macroscopically cardiac amyloidosis may present with biatrial dilatation, and the ventricular cavity may be of normal size or hypertrophied and mimic HCM [152].

The cut surface of the myocardium has a waxy appearance, and the heart has a noncompliant "rubbery" consistency due to the matrix deposited around cells and through the local connective tissues (Fig. 11.20). IAA is characterized by the presence of translucent tiny pearl-like nodules coating the atrial surface [153]. Microscopically, in H&E-stained sections, there are interstitial infiltrates of homogeneous eosinophilic material surrounding individual myocytes forming a honeycomb pattern as well as nodular myocardial deposits. The material can be highlighted by Sirius or Congo red histochemistry (Fig. 11.21). Within the media and adventitia of the intramural coronary vessels, nodular amyloid deposits may be observed, which may cause luminal narrowing [152, 154]. Amyloid deposition may occur in all layers of the heart, and the pattern of deposition can be classified as nodular, pericellular, or mixed type with or without vascular involvement [153].

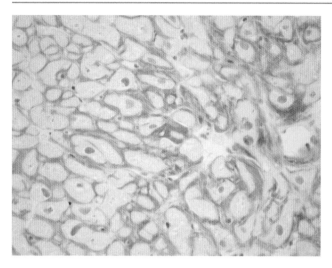

Fig. 11.21 Sirius red histochemistry highlights the case of amyloid deposition around individual myocytes

Fig. 11.22 Electron micrograph of amyloid fibrils which typically have a diameter of 7.5–10 nm

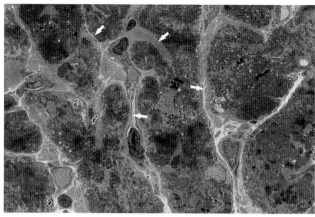

Fig. 11.23 Ultrastructural view of cardiac myocytes, externally coated by amyloid fibrils (marked by *arrows*)

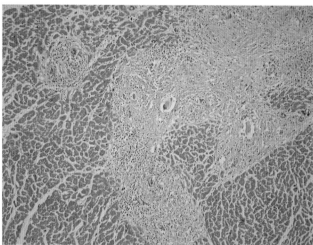

Fig. 11.24 Histological view of left ventricle tissues affected focally by noncaseating granulomatous inflammation, in a known case of sarcoidosis (Courtesy of Dr. PJ Gallagher) (hematoxylin & eosin)

The amyloid deposits classically display apple-green birefringence when stained with Sirius or Congo red and viewed under polarized light and appear red/orange when viewed by light microscopy (see Chap. 5). Further diagnostic confirmation and analysis of the amyloid fibril subtype can be obtained using electron microscopy and immunocytochemistry, respectively. The former reveals the presence of linear nonbranching fibrils with a diameter of 7.5 to 10 nm (Fig. 11.22) externally coating myocytes (Fig. 11.23). Immunocytochemistry can be used to identify the major protein component of the amyloid fibril, and this is an important technique for amyloid diagnosis, permits assessment of prognosis, and guides treatment.

Cardiac sarcoidosis is a granulomatous disorder of unknown etiology, which often affects the heart and has a prevalence of cardiac involvement in 5–10% of patients with known sarcoid [155]. A study of 41 sarcoidosis patients showed that the most common presenting symptom was heart failure [156]. Ventricular arrhythmias and conduction disturbances are also common (e.g., atrioventricular block, type1/2 heart block, and complete heart block) [156]. However, in up to 25% of patients, the sarcoid granulomas are clinically silent and may be found incidentally at autopsy [157, 158].

The macroscopic phenotype may range from massive tumorlike infiltrates with replacement of the myocardium to small granulomas that can only be detected by microscopy [157, 159]. The left ventricular free wall is the most commonly affected site. The granulomas are typically noncaseating and comprised of epithelioid histiocytes with multinucleated giant cells accompanied by a lymphocytic infiltrate (Fig. 11.24). The multinucleated giant cells are

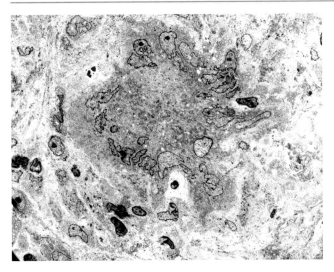

Fig. 11.25 Electron microscopy in a case of a dilated mixed pattern cardiomyopathy clinically identified a sarcoid granuloma, in a case of unexpected sarcoidosis. The Langhans giant cell has a peripheral rim of nuclei

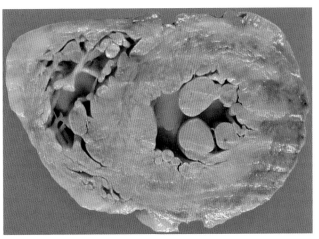

Fig. 11.26 Macroscopic photograph of the cardiac variant of Fabry's disease with asymmetrical ventricular hypertrophy. This can mimic HCM and needs histology and other tests to distinguish this diagnosis

initially foreign body type with haphazardly arranged central nuclei, but over time, Langhans type giant cells with peripherally arranged nuclei (Fig. 11.25) become evident [160]. Schaumann and asteroid bodies may also be observed. These are suggestive, but not specific, for sarcoidosis. Over time, the granulomas undergo fibrosis leading to patchy scar formation with a distortion of normal myocardial architecture.

Infiltrative cardiomyopathies causing secondary RCM include storage disorders, such as hemochromatosis, glycogen storage disease, and Fabry's disease, where the deposits occur within myocytes. Hemochromatosis is an iron-storage disorder and may be hereditary or secondary [161]. Hereditary hemochromatosis is usually inherited as an autosomal recessive disease and corresponds to a diverse spectrum of genetic abnormalities affecting iron metabolism [162]. Secondary hemochromatosis occurs due to excessive iron intake, following multiple blood transfusions or in abnormalities of hemoglobin synthesis leading to aberrant erythropoiesis. With both types of disease, there is iron deposition in multiple organs including the heart [163, 164].

Glycogen storage disease and Fabry's disease are autosomal recessive disorders of carbohydrate and glycolipid metabolism, respectively, and may cause RCM. In glycogen storage disease, there is deposition of glycogen in the cardiac myocytes and skeletal muscle. Fabry's disease is characterized by the deposition of neutral glycosphingolipids within myocytes. It is an X-linked autosomal recessive metabolic storage disorder due to deficiency of the enzyme lysosomal α(alpha)-galactosidase A [165]. This leads to the clinically widespread accumulation of neutral glycosphingolipid in

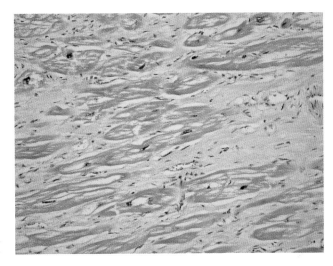

Fig. 11.27 Hematoxylin- and eosin-stained photomicrograph showing sarcoplasmic vacuolization which is characteristic of Fabry's disease

multiple organs and leads to angiokeratomas, corneal opacities, and peripheral and central CNS disorders. A variant of Fabry's disease has been described with late onset, which predominantly affects the heart without multiorgan involvement. Morphologically, cardiac Fabry's disease presents with concentric ventricular hypertrophy disease, but asymmetrical hypertrophy may also occur (Fig. 11.26) [165]. Histologically, stained sections feature prominent myocyte sarcoplasmic vacuolation (Fig. 11.27). However, this is not invariably present, and evaluation of the myocardium by electron microscopy is required [166–170]. This shows numerous concentric lamellar bodies or "myelinoid" figures within the myocyte sarcoplasm (Fig. 11.28). The diagnosis can also be made by measurement of α(alpha)-galactosidase A activity in plasma or leukocytes [166, 168].

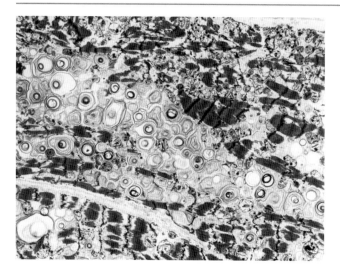

Fig. 11.28 Electron micrograph of "myelinoid" figures within the myocyte sarcoplasm in a case of Fabry's disease

Conclusion

The pathologist plays a pivotal role in the diagnosis of primary cardiomyopathy and may be the first to encounter index cases as part of coronial autopsy practice. Due to increased knowledge, coupled with the identification of single gene mutations, it is now known that many of the primary cardiomyopathies have an underlying genetic basis with implications for screening, risk stratification, and counseling of affected families. Furthermore, overlap between the different subsets of cardiomyopathy may occur as exemplified by the discovery of mutations in the troponin I gene that can cause HCM with features of a pure RCM. The pathology of ARVC is more complex than previously anticipated with the emergence of a phenotype with predominant left ventricular involvement. LVNC is a relatively recently described cardiomyopathy but is gradually gaining increased recognition as a significant cause of cardiac morbidity. It is therefore essential that the pathologist is able to provide a detailed analysis and diagnosis, being familiar with the pathoanatomical presentation of this heterogeneous group of cardiac diseases.

References

1. Richardson P, McKenna WJ, Bristow M, et al. Report of the 1995 WHO/ISFC Task Force on the definition and classification of cardiomyopathies. Circulation. 1996;93:841–2.
2. Franz W-M, Muller OJ, Katus HA. Cardiomyopathies: from genetics to the prospect of treatment. Lancet. 2001;358:1627–37.
3. Maron BJ, Towbin JA, Thiene G, et al. Contemporary definitions and classifications of the cardiomyopathies: an American Heart Association Scientific Statement from the Council on Clinical Cardiology, Heart Failure and transplantation Committee: Quality of Care and Outcomes Research and functional genomics and trans-

lational biology interdisciplinary working groups; and the Council on Epidemiology and Prevention. Circulation. 2006;113:1807–16.
4. Mestroni L, Maisch B, McKenna WJ, et al. Guidelines for the study of familial dilated cardiomyopathies. Eur Heart J. 1999;20: 93–102.
5. Michels VV, Moll PP, Miller FA, et al. The frequency of familial dilated cardiomyopathy in a series of patients with idiopathic dilated cardiomyopathy. N Engl J Med. 1992;326:77–82.
6. Keeling PJ, Gang Y, Smith G, et al. Familial dilated cardiomyopathy in the United Kingdom. BMJ. 1995;73:417–21.
7. Michels VV, Driscoll DJ, Miller FA, Olson TM, Atkinson EJ, Olswold CL, Schaid DJ. Progression of familial and non-familial dilated cardiomyopathy: long term follow up. Heart. 2003;89: 757–61.
8. Grunig E, Tasman JA, Kucherer H, et al. Frequency and phenotypes of familial dilated cardiomyopathy. J Am Coll Cardiol. 1998;31: 186–94.
9. Towbin JA, Bowles NE. The failing heart. Nature. 2002;415: 227–33.
10. Bowles NE, Bowles KR, Towbin JA. The "final common pathway" hypothesis and inherited cardiovascular disease. The role of cytoskeletal proteins in dilated cardiomyopathy. Herz. 2000;25: 168–75.
11. Taylor MRG, Carniel E, Mestroni L. Cardiomyopathy, familial dilated. Orphanet J Rare Dis. 2006;1:27.
12. Taylor MRG, Fain P, Sinagra G, et al. Natural history of dilated cardiomyopathy due to lamin A/C gene mutations. J Am Coll Cardiol. 2003;41:771–80.
13. Sinagra G, Di Lenarda A, Brodsky GL. Current perspective new insights into the molecular basis of familial dilated cardiomyopathy. Ital Heart J. 2001;2:280–6.
14. Arbustini E, Diegoli M, Fasani R, et al. Mitochondrial DNA mutations and mitochondrial abnormalities in dilated cardiomyopathy. Am J Pathol. 1998;153:1501–10.
15. Mestroni L, Krajinovic M, Severini GM, et al. Familial dilated cardiomyopathy. Br Heart J. 1994;72:35–41.
16. Engberding R, Bender F. Identification of a rare congenital anomaly of the myocardium by two-dimensional echocardiography: persistence of isolated myocardial sinusoids. Am J Cardiol. 1984;53: 1733–4.
17. Chin TK, Perloff JK, Williams R, et al. Isolated noncompaction of left ventricular myocardium. A study of eight cases. Circulation. 1990;82:507–13.
18. Andrews RE, Fenton MJ, Ridout DA, Burch M. British Congenital Cardiac Association. New-onset heart failure due to heart muscle disease in childhood: a prospective study in the United Kingdom and Ireland. Circulation. 2008;117:79–84.
19. Boyd MT, Seward JB, Tajik AJ, et al. Frequency and location of prominent left ventricular trabeculations at autopsy in 474 normal human hearts: implications for evaluation of mural thrombi by two-dimensional echocardiography. J Am Coll Cardiol. 1987;9:323–6.
20. Stollberger C, Finsterer J. Trabeculation and left ventricular hypertrabeculation/non-compaction. J Soc Echocardiogr. 2004;17:1120–1.
21. Sedmera D, Pexieder T, Vuillemin M, et al. Developmental patterning of the myocardium. Anat Rec. 2000;258:319–37.
22. Engberding R, Yelbuz MT. Breithardt G. Isolated noncompaction of the left ventricular myocardium. A review of the literature two decades after the initial case description. Clin Res Cardiol. 2007;96:481–8.
23. Jenni R, Wyss CA, Oechslin EN, Kaufman PA. Isolated ventricular noncompaction is associated with coronary microcirculatory dysfunction. JACC. 2002;39:450–4.
24. Bleyl SB, Mumford BR, Brown-Harrison MC, et al. Xq28-linked noncompaction of the left ventricular myocardium: prenatal diagnosis and pathologic analysis of affected individuals. Am J Med Genet. 1997;72:257–65.

25. Budde BS, Binner P, Waldmuller S, et al. Noncompaction of the ventricular myocardium is associated with a de novo mutation in the β(beta)-myosin heavy chain gene. PloS One. 2007;2(12): e1362.

26. Hoedemaekers YM, Caliskan K, Majoor-Krakauer D, et al. Cardiac β-myosin heavy chain defects in two families with non-compaction cardiomyopathy: linking non-compaction to hypertrophic, -restrictive, and dilated cardiomyopathies. Eur Heart J. 2007;28:2732–7.

27. Monserrat L, Hermida-Prieto M, Fernandez X, et al. Mutation in the alpha-cardiac actin gene associated with apical hypertrophic cardiomyopathy, left ventricular non-compaction, and septal defects. Eur Heart J. 2007;28:1953–61.

28. Klaassen S, Probst S, Oechslin E, et al. Mutations in sarcomere protein genes in left ventricular noncompaction. Circulation. 2008;117:2893–901.

29. Chrissoheris MP, Ronan A, Vivas Y, et al. Isolated noncompaction of the ventricular myocardium: contemporary diagnosis and management. Clin Cardiol. 2007;30:156–60.

30. Xing Y, Ichida F, Matsuoka T, et al. Genetic analysis in patients with left ventricular noncompaction and evidence for genetic heterogeneity. Mol Genet Metab. 2006;88:71–7.

31. Kenton AB, Sanchez X, Coveler KJ. Isolated left ventricular noncompaction is rarely caused by mutations in G4.5, α(alpha)-dystrobrevin and FK Binding Protein-12. Mol Genet Metab. 2004;82: 162–6.

32. Oechslin EN, Attenhofer Jost CH, Rojas JR. Long-term follow-up of 34 adults with isolated left ventricular noncompaction: a distinct cardiomyopathy with poor prognosis. J Am Coll Cardiol. 2000;36:493–500.

33. Corrado G, Fazio G, Zachara E, et al. Natural history of isolated noncompaction of the ventricular myocardium in adults. Data from the Societa Italiana di Ecografia Cardiovascolare (SIEC) Registry. Circulation 2008;118:S_948

34. Maron BJ. Hypertrophic cardiomyopathy. A systematic review. JAMA. 2002;287:1308–20.

35. Maron BJ, Gardin JM, Flack JM. Prevalence of hypertrophic cardiomyopathy in a general population of young adults. Echocardiographic analysis of 4111 subjects in the CARDIA study. Circulation. 1995;92:785–9.

36. Thierfelder L, Watkins H, MacRae C, et al. Alpha-tropomyosin and cardiac troponin T mutations cause familial hypertrophic cardiomyopathy: a disease of the sarcomere. Cell. 1994;77:701–12.

37. Bonne G, Carrier L, Richard P, et al. Familial hypertrophic cardiomyopathy: from mutations to functional defects. Circ Res. 1998;83: 580–93.

38. Blair E, Redwood C, Ashrafian H, et al. Mutations in the γ2 subunit of AMP-activated protein kinase cause familial hypertrophic cardiomyopathy: evidence for the central role of energy compromise in disease pathogenesis. Hum Mol Genet. 2001;10:1215–20.

39. Santorelli FM, Mak SC, El-Schahawi M, et al. Maternally inherited cardiomyopathy and hearing loss associated with a novel mutation in the mitochondrial tRNA (Lys) gene (G8363A). Am J Hum Genet. 1996;58:933–9.

40. Marian AJ, Salek L, Lutucuta S. Molecular genetics and pathogenesis of hypertrophic cardiomyopathy. Minerva Med. 2001;92: 435–51.

41. Watkins H, McKenna WJ, Thierfelder L, et al. Mutations in the genes for cardiac troponin T and α-tropomyosin in hypertrophic cardiomyopathy. New Engl J Med. 1995;332:1058–64.

42. Anan R, Greve G, Thierfelder L, et al. Prognostic implication of novel β cardiac myosin heavy chain gene mutations that cause familial hypertrophic cardiomyopathy. J Clin Invest. 1994;93: 280–5.

43. Watkins H, Rosenzweig T, Hwang DS, et al. Characteristics and prognostic implications of myosin missense mutations in familial hypertrophic cardiomyopathy. N Engl J Med. 1992;326:1106–14.

44. Vikstrom KL, Leinwand LA. Contractile protein mutations and heart disease. Curr Op Cell Biol. 1996;8:97–105.

45. Marian AJ, Roberts R. The molecular genetic basis for hypertrophic cardiomyopathy. J Mol Cell Cardiol. 2001;33:655–70.

46. Solomon SD, Wolff S, Watkins H, et al. Left ventricular hypertrophy and morphology in familial hypertrophic cardiomyopathy associated with mutations of the beta-myosin heavy chain gene. J Am Coll Cardiol. 1993;22:498–505.

47. Patel R, Lim DS, Reddy D, et al. Variants of trophic factors and expression of hypertrophic cardiomyopathy in patients with hypertrophic cardiomyopathy. J Mol Cell Cardiol. 2000;32:2369–77.

48. Perkins MJ, Van Driest SL, Ellsworth ML, et al. Gene-specific modifying effects of pro-LVH polymorphisms involving the renin-angiotensin-aldosterone system among 389 unrelated patients with hypertrophic cardiomyopathy. Eur Heart J. 2005;26:2457–62.

49. Davies MJ, McKenna WJ. Hypertrophic cardiomyopathy – pathology and pathogenesis. Histopathology. 1995;26:493–500.

50. Hughes SE. The pathology of hypertrophic cardiomyopathy. Histopathology. 2004;44:412–27.

51. Teare D. Asymmetrical hypertrophy of the heart in young adults. Br Heart J. 1958;20:1–8.

52. Yu EHC, Omran AS, Wigle ED, et al. Mitral regurgitation in hypertrophic obstructive cardiomyopathy; Relationship to obstruction and relief with myectomy. J Am Coll Cardiol. 2000;36:2219–25.

53. Mozaffarian D, Caldwell JH. Right ventricular involvement in hypertrophic cardiomyopathy: a case report and literature review. Clin Cardiol. 2001;24:2–8.

54. Maron BJ, Sherrid MV, Haas TS, et al. Novel hypertrophic cardiomyopathy phenotype: segmental hypertrophy isolated to the posterobasal left ventricular free wall. Am J Cardiol. 2010;106:750–2.

55. Falicov RE, Resnekov L, Bharati S, Lev M. Mid-ventricular obstruction: a variant of obstructive cardiomyopathy. Am J Cardiol. 1976;37:432–7.

56. Fighali S, Krajcer Z, Edelman S, Leachman RD. Progression of hypertrophic cardiomyopathy into a hypokinetic left ventricle: higher incidence in patients with midventricular obstruction. J Am Coll Cardiol. 1987;9:288–94.

57. Ando H, Imaizumi T, Urabe Y, et al. Apical segmental dysfunction in hypertrophic cardiomyopathy: subgroup with unique clinical features. J Am Coll Cardiol. 1990;16:1579–88.

58. Barbosa MM, Coutinho AH, Motta MS, et al. Apical hypertrophic cardiomyopathy: a study of 14 patients and their first degree relatives. Int J Cardiol. 1996;56:41–51.

59. Maron MS, Finley JJ, Bos M, et al. Prevalence, clinical significance, and natural history of left ventricular apical aneurysms in hypertrophic cardiomyopathy. Circulation. 2008;118:1541–9.

60. Mogensen J, Kubo T, Duque M, et al. Idiopathic restrictive cardiomyopathy is part of the clinical expression of cardiac troponin I mutations. J Clin Invest. 2003;111:209–16.

61. Kaski JP, Syrris P, Burch M, et al. Idiopathic restrictive cardiomyopathy in children is caused by mutations in cardiac sarcomere protein genes. Heart. 2008;94:1478–84.

62. Gambarin FI, Tagliasni M, Arbustini E. Pure restrictive cardiomyopathy associated with cardiac troponin I gene mutation: mismatch between the lack of hypertrophy and the presence of disarray. Heart. 2008;94:1257.

63. Kubo T, Gimeno JR, Bahl A, et al. Prevalence, clinical significance, and genetic basis of hypertrophic cardiomyopathy with restrictive phenotype. J Am Coll Cardiol. 2007;49:2419–26.

64. Kwon DH, Smedira NG, Rodriguez ER, et al. Cardiac magnetic resonance detection of myocardial scarring in hypertrophic cardiomyopathy: correlation with histopathology and prevalence of ventricular tachycardia. J Am Coll Cardiol. 2009;54:242–9.

65. O'Hanlon R, Grasso A, Roughton M, et al. Prognostic significance of myocardial fibrosis in hypertrophic cardiomyopathy. J Am Coll Cardiol. 2010;56:867–74.

66. Moon JC, McKenna WJ, McCrohon JA, et al. Toward clinical risk assessment in hypertrophic cardiomyopathy with gadolinium cardiovascular magnetic resonance. J Am Coll Cardiol. 2003;41:1561–7.

67. Basso C, Thiene G, Corrado D, Buja G, et al. Hypertrophic cardiomyopathy and sudden death in the young: pathologic evidence of myocardial ischemia. Hum Pathol. 2000;31:988–98.

68. Takemura G, Takatsu Y, Fujiwara H. Luminal narrowing of coronary capillaries in human hypertrophic hearts: an ultrastructural morphometrical study using endomyocardial biopsy specimens. Heart. 1998;79:78–85.

69. Cannon 3rd RO, Rosing DR, Maron BJ, et al. Myocardial ischaemia in patients with hypertrophic cardiomyopathy: contribution of inadequate vasodilator reserve and elevated left ventricular filling pressures. Circulation. 1985;71:234–43.

70. Iida K, Yutani C, Imakita M, et al. Comparison of percentage area of myocardial fibrosis and disarray in patients with classical form and dilated phase of hypertrophic cardiomyopathy. J Cardiol. 1998;32:173–80.

71. Sen-Chowdhry S, Lowe MD, Sporton SC, et al. Arrhythmogenic right ventricular cardiomyopathy: clinical presentation, diagnosis and management. Am J Med. 2004;117:685–95.

72. Thiene G, Nava A, Corrado D, et al. Right ventricular cardiomyopathy and sudden death in young people. N Engl J Med. 1988;318:129–33.

73. Maron BJ. Cardiovascular risks to young persons on the athletic field. Ann Int Med. 1998;129:379–86.

74. Norman N, Simpson M, Mogensen J, et al. Novel mutation in desmoplakin causes arrhythmogenic left ventricular cardiomyopathy. Circulation. 2005;112:636–42.

75. Corrado D, Basso C, Rizzoli G, et al. Does sports activity enhance the risk of sudden death in adolescents and young adults? J Am Coll Cardiol. 2003;42:1959–63.

76. Blomstrom-Lundquist C, Sabel K, Olsson S. A long term follow-up with arrhythmogenic right ventricular dysplasia. Br Heart J. 1987;58:477–88.

77. Thiene G, Basso C. Arrhythmogenic right ventricular cardiomyopathy. An update. Cardiovasc Pathol. 2001;10:109–11.

78. Corrado D, Basso C, Thiene G. Arrhythmogenic right ventricular cardiomyopathy: diagnosis, prognosis and treatment. Heart. 2000;83:588–95.

79. Marcus FI, Wojciech Z, Calkins H, et al. Arrhythmogenic right ventricular cardiomyopathy/dysplasia, clinical presentation and diagnostic evaluation: results from the North American multidisciplinary study. Heart Rhythm. 2009;6:984–92.

80. Marcus FI, Fontaine G, Guiraudon G. Right ventricular dysplasia. A report of 24 adult cases. Circulation. 1982;65:384–99.

81. Basso C, Thiene G, Corrado D. Arrhythmogenic right ventricular cardiomyopathy. Dysplasia, dystrophy or myocarditis? Circulation. 1996;94:983–91.

82. Corrado D, Basso C, Thiene G, et al. Spectrum of clinicopathologic manifestations of arrhythmogenic right ventricular cardiomyopathy/dysplasia: a multicenter study. J Am Coll Cardiol. 1997;30:1512–20.

83. Gallo P, D'Amati G, Pellicia F. Pathologic evidence of extensive left ventricular involvement in arrhythmogenic right ventricular cardiomyopathy. Hum Pathol. 1992;23:948–52.

84. Pinamonti B, Sinagra GF, Salvi A, et al. Left ventricular involvement in right ventricular dysplasia. Am Heart J. 1992;123:711–24.

85. Miani D, Pimamonti B, Bussani R, et al. Right ventricular dysplasia: a clinical and pathological study of two families with left ventricular involvement. Br Heart J. 1993;69:151–7.

86. D'Amati G, Leone O, di Gioa CR, et al. Arrhythmogenic right ventricular cardiomyopathy: clinicopathologic correlation based on a revised definition of pathologic patterns. Hum Pathol. 2001;32:1078–86.

87. Burke AP, Farb A, Tashko G, et al. Arrhythmogenic right ventricular cardiomyopathy and fatty replacement of the right ventricular myocardium: are they different diseases? Circulation. 1998;97:1571–80.

88. Shirani J, Berezowski K, Roberts WC. Quantitative measurement of normal adipose and excessive (cor adiposum) subepicardial adipose tissue, its clinical significance and its effect on electrocardiographic QRS voltage. Am J Cardiol. 1995;76:414–8.

89. De Pasquale CG, Heddle WF. Left sided arrhythmogenic ventricular dysplasia in siblings. Heart. 2001;86:128–30.

90. Michalodimitrakis M, Papadomanolakis A, Stiakakis J, et al. Left side right ventricular cardiomyopathy. Med Sci Law. 2002;42:313–7.

91. Shirani J, Roberts WC. Subepicardial myocardial lesions. Am Heart J. 1993;125:1346–52.

92. Nava A, Bauce B, Basso C, et al. Clinical profile and long-term follow-up of 37 families with arrhythmogenic right ventricular cardiomyopathy. J Am Coll Cardiol. 2000;36:2226–33.

93. Nava A, Thiene G, Canciani B, et al. Familial occurrence of right ventricular dysplasia: a study involving nine families. J Am Coll Cardiol. 1988;12:1222–8.

94. Syrris P, Ward D, Asimaki A, et al. Clinical expression of plakophilin-2 mutations in familial arrhythmogenic right ventricular cardiomyopathy. Circulation. 2006;113:356–64.

95. Syrris P, Ward D, Asimaki A, et al. Desmoglein-2 mutations in arrhythmogenic right ventricular cardiomyopathy: a genotype-phenotype characterization of familial disease. Eur Heart J. 2007;28:581–8.

96. Rampazzo A, Nava A, Malacrida S, et al. Mutation in human desmoplakin binding domain binding to plakoglobin causes a dominant form of arrhythmogenic right ventricular cardiomyopathy. Am J Hum Genet. 2002;71:1200–6.

97. Kaplan SR, Gard JJ, Carvajal-Huerta L, et al. Structural and molecular pathology of the heart in Carvajal syndrome. Cardiovasc Pathol. 2004;13:26–32.

98. Heuser A, Plovie ER, Ellinor PT, et al. Mutant desmocollin-2 causes arrhythmogenic right ventricular cardiomyopathy. Am J Hum Genet. 2006;79:1081–8.

99. Pilichou K, Nava A, Basso C, et al. Mutations in desmoglein-2 gene are associated with arrhythmogenic right ventricular cardiomyopathy. Circulation. 2006;113:1171–9.

100. Sen-Chowdhry S, Syrris P, McKenna W. Genetics of right ventricular cardiomyopathy. J Cardiovasc Electrophysiol. 2005;16:927–35.

101. Dokuparti MV, Pamuru PR, Thakkar B, et al. Etiopathogenesis of arrhythmogenic right ventricular cardiomyopathy. J Hum Genet. 2005;50:375–81.

102. MacRae CA, Birchmeier W, Thierfelder L. Arrhythmogenic right ventricular cardiomyopathy; moving towards mechanism. J Clin Invest. 2006;116:1825–8.

103. Mallat Z, Tedgui A, Fontaliran F, et al. Evidence of apoptosis in arrhythmogenic right ventricular dysplasia. N Engl J Med. 1996;335:1190–6.

104. Valente M, Calabrese F, Thiene G, et al. In vivo evidence of apoptosis in arrhythmogenic right ventricular cardiomyopathy. Am J Pathol. 1998;152:479–84.

105. Garcia-Gras E, Lombardi R, Giocondo MJ, et al. Suppression of canonical Wnt/beta-catenin signaling by nuclear plakoglobin recapitulates phenotype of arrhythmogenic right ventricular cardiomyopathy. J Clin Invest. 2006;116:2012–21.

106. Heidbuchel H, Hoogsteen J, Fagard R, et al. High prevalence of right ventricular involvement in endurance athletes with ventricular arrhythmias. Role of an electrophysiologic study in risk stratification. Eur Heart J. 2003;24:1473–80.

107. Marcus F, Towbin JA. The mystery of arrhythmogenic right ventricular dysplasia/cardiomyopathy: from observation to mechanistic explanation. Circulation. 2006;114:1794–5.

108. Kirchhof P, Fabritz L, Zwiener M, et al. Age and training dependent development of arrhythmogenic right ventricular cardiomyopathy in heterozygous plakoglobin deficient mice. Circulation. 2006;113:1799–806.

109. Bauce B, Basso C, Rampazzo A, et al. Clinical profile of four families with arrhythmogenic right ventricular cardiomyopathy caused by dominant desmoplakin mutations. Eur Heart J. 2005;26:1666–75.

110. Antoniades L, Tsatsopoulou A, Anastasakis A. Arrhythmogenic right ventricular cardiomyopathy caused by deletions in plakophilin-2 and plakoglobin (Naxos disease) in families from Greece and Cyprus: genotype-phenotype relations, diagnostic features and prognosis. Eur Heart J. 2006;27:2208–16.

111. McKoy G, Protonotarios N, Crosby A, et al. Identification of a deletion in plakoglobin in arrhythmogenic right ventricular cardiomyopathy with palmoplantar keratoderma and woolly hair (Naxos disease). Lancet. 2000;355:2119–24.

112. Alcalai R, Metzger S, Rosenheck S, et al. A recessive mutation in desmoplakin causes arrhythmogenic right ventricular dysplasia, skin disorder and woolly hair. J Am Coll Cardiol. 2003;42:319–27.

113. Protonotarios P, Tsatsopoulou A. Naxos disease and Carvajal syndrome: cardiocutaneous disorders that highlight the pathogenesis and broaden the spectrum of arrhythmogenic right ventricular cardiomyopathy. Cardiovasc Pathol. 2004;13:418–21.

114. Coonar AS, Protonoarius N, Tsatsopoulou A, et al. Gene for arrhythmogenic right ventricular cardiomyopathy with diffuse nonepidermolytic palmoplantar keratoderma and woolly hair (Naxos disease) maps to 17q21. Circulation. 1998;97:2049–58.

115. Norgett EE, Hatsell SJ, Carvajal-Huerta L, et al. Recessive mutation in desmoplakin disrupts desmoplakin-intermediate filament interactions and causes dilated cardiomyopathy, woolly hair and keratoderma. Hum Mol Genet. 2000;9:2761–6.

116. Tiso N, Stephan DA, Nava A, et al. Identification of mutations in the cardiac ryanodine receptor gene in families affected with arrhythmogenic right ventricular cardiomyopathy type 2 (ARVD2). Hum Mol Genet. 2001;10:189–94.

117. Beffagna G, Occhi G, Nava A, et al. Regulatory mutations in transforming growth factor-[beta]3 gene cause arrhythmogenic right ventricular cardiomyopathy type 1. Cardiovasc Res. 2005;65:366–73.

118. Merner ND, Hodgkinson KA, Haywood AFM, et al. Arrhythmogenic right ventricular cardiomyopathy type 5 is a fully penetrant, lethal arrhythmic disorder caused by a missense mutation in the TMEM43 gene. Am J Hum Genet. 2008;82:809–21.

119. Klein AL, Asher CR. Diseases of the Pericardium, Restrictive Cardiomyopathy and Diastolic Dysfunction. In: Topol EJ, editor. Textbook of cardiovas-cular medicine. Philadelphia: Lippincott-Raven Publishers; 1998, p595–646.

120. Child JS, Perloff JK. The restrictive cardiomyopathies. Cardiol Clin. 1988;6:289–316.

121. Fitzpatrick AP, Shapiro LM, Rickards AF, et al. Familial restrictive cardiomyopathy with atrioventricular block and skeletal myopathy. Br Heart J. 1990;63:114–8.

122. Cubero GI, Larraya GL, Reguero JR. Familial restrictive cardiomyopathy with atrioventricular block without skeletal myopathy. Exp Clin Cardiol. 2006;12:54–5.

123. Benotti JR, Grossman W, Cohn PF. Clinical profile of restrictive cardiomyopathy. Circulation. 1980;61:1206–12.

124. Spry CJ, Take M, Tai PC. Eosinophilic disorders affecting the myocardium and endocardium: a review. Heart Vessels Suppl. 1985;1:240–2.

125. Davies JNP. Endomyocardial fibrosis. A heart disease of obscure aetiology in Africans. MD thesis. Bristol: Bristol University; 1948

126. Parrillo JE. Heart disease and the eosinophil. N Engl J Med. 1990;323:1560–1.

127. Gupta PN, Valiathan MS, Balakrishnan KG, et al. Clinical course of endomyocardial fibrosis. Br Heart J. 1989;62:450–4.

128. Chopra P, Narula J, Talwar KK, et al. Histomorphologic characteristics of endomyocardial fibrosis: an endomyocardial biopsy study. Hum Pathol. 1990;21:613–6.

129. Mady C, Pereira Barretto AC, de Oliveira SA, et al. Effectiveness of operative and nonoperative therapy of endomyocardial fibrosis. Am J Cardiol. 1989;63:1281–2.

130. de Oliveira SA, Pereira Barretto AC, Mady C. Surgical treatment of endomyocardial fibrosis: a new approach. J Am Coll Cardiol. 1990;16:1246–51.

131. Mocumbi AO, Latif N, Yacoub MH. Presence of circulating anti-myosin antibodies in endomyocardial fibrosis. PloS Negl Trop Dis. 2010;20:e661.

132. Andy JJ. Aetiology of endomyocardial fibrosis (EMF). West Afr J Med. 2001;20:199–207.

133. Roberts WC, Buja LM, Ferrans VJ. Loeffler's fibroplastic parietal endocarditis, eosinophilic leukaemia, and Davies' endomyocardial fibrosis: the same disease at different stages? Pathol Microbiol (Basel). 1970;35:90–5.

134. Davies J, Spry CJ, Vijayaraghavan G, De Souza JA. A comparison of the clinical and cardiological features of endomyocardial disease in temperate and tropical regions. Postgrad Med J. 1983;59:179–85.

135. De Mello DE, Liapis H, Jureidini S, et al. Cardiac localization of eosinophil-granule major basic protein in acute necrotizing myocarditis. N Engl J Med. 1990;323:1542–5.

136. Kholova I, Niessen HWM. Amyloid in the cardiovascular system: a review. J Clin Pathol. 2005;58:125–33.

137. Bigoni R, Cuneo A, Roberti MG, et al. Cytogenetic and molecular cytogenetic characterization of 6 new cases of idiopathic hypereosinophilic syndrome. Haematologica. 2000;85: 486–91.

138. Kyle RA. Amyloidosis. Circulation. 1995;91:1269–71.

139. Westermark P, Bergstrom J, Solomon A. Transthyretin-derived senile systemic amyloidosis: clinicopathologic and structural considerations. Amyloid. 2003;10(Suppl I):48–54.

140. Cornwell III GG, Murdoch W, Kyle RA, et al. Frequency and distribution of senile cardiovascular amyloid. A clinicopathologic correlation. Am J Med. 1983;75:618–23.

141. Pitkanen P, Westermark P, Cornwell III GG. Senile systemic amyloidosis. Am J Path. 1984;117:391–9.

142. Steiner I. The prevalence of isolated atrial amyloid. J Pathol. 1987;153:395–8.

143. Rocken C, Peters B, Juenemann G, et al. Atrial amyloidosis. An arrhythmogenic substrate for persistent atrial fibrillation. Circulation. 2002;106:2091–7.

144. Hamidi Asl, Liepniks JJ, Hamidi Asl K. Hereditary amyloid cardiomyopathy caused by a variant apolipoprotein A1. Am J Pathol. 1999;154:221–7.

145. Arbustini E, Gavazzi A, Merlini G. Fibril-forming proteins: the amyloidosis. New hopes for a disease that cardiologists must know. Ital Heart J. 2002;3:590–7.

146. Yazaki M, Liepniks JJ, Barats MS, et al. Hereditary systemic amyloidosis associated with a new apolipoprotein AII stop codon mutation Stop78Arg. Kidney Int. 2003;64:11–6.

147. Saraiva MJ. Transythretin mutations in health and disease. Hum Mutat. 1995;5:191–6.

148. Saito F, Nakazato M, Akiyama H, et al. A case of late onset cardiac amyloidosis with a new transthyretin variant (Lysine 92). Hum Pathol. 2001;32:237–9.

149. Saraiva MJ, Almeida MdoR, Sherman W. A new transthyretin mutation associated with amyloid cardiomyopathy. Am J Hum Genet. 1992;50:1027–30.

150. Magnus JH, Stenstad K, Kolset SO. Glycosaminoglycans in extracts of cardiac amyloid fibrils from familial amyloid cardiomyopathy of Danish origin related to variant transthyretin Met 111. Scand J Immunol. 1991;34:63–9.

151. Falk RH, Comenzo RL, Skinner M. The systemic amyloidoses. N Engl J Med. 1997;337:898–909.
152. Roberts WC, Waller BF. Cardiac amyloidosis causing cardiac dysfunction: analysis of 54 necropsy patients. Am J Cardiol. 1983;52:137–46.
153. Smith TJ, Kyle RA, Lie JT. Clinical significance of histopathologic patterns of cardiac amyloidosis. Mayo Clin Proc. 1984;59:547–55.
154. Booth DR, Tan SY, Hawkins PN, et al. A novel variant of transthyretin, 59Thr-Lys, associated with autosomal dominant cardiac amyloidosis in an Italian family. Circulation. 1995;91:962–7.
155. Newman LS, Rose CS, Maier LA. Sarcoidosis. New Engl J Med. 1997;336:1224–34.
156. Chapelon-Abric C, de Zuttere D, Duhaut P, et al. Cardiac sarcoidosis: a retrospective study of 41 cases. Medicine (Baltimore). 2004;83:315–34.
157. Silverman KJ, Hutchins GM, Bulkley BH. Cardiac sarcoid: a clinicopathologic study of 84 unselected patients with systemic sarcoidosis. Circulation. 1978;58:1204–11.
158. Perry A, Vuitch F. Causes of death in patients with sarcoidosis: a morphologic study of 38 autopsies with clinicopathologic correlations. Arch Pathol Lab Med. 1995;119:1767–72.
159. Roberts WC, McAllister HA, Ferrans VJ. Sarcoidosis of the heart. Am J Med. 1977;63:86–108.
160. Lagana SM, Parwani A, Nichols LC. Cardiac sarcoidosis. A pathology-focused review. Arch Pathol Lab Med. 2010;134:1039–46.
161. Hauser SC. Hemochromatosis and the heart. Heart Dis Stroke. 1993;2:487–91.
162. Zaahl MG, Merryweather-Clarke AT, Kotze MJ, et al. Analysis of genes implicated in iron regulation in individuals presenting with primary iron overload. Hum Genet. 2004;115:409–17.
163. Olson LJ, Edwards WD, McCall JT, et al. Cardiac iron deposition in idiopathic hemochromatosis: histologic and analytic assessment of 14 hearts from autopsy. J Am Coll Cardiol. 1987;10:1239–43.
164. Cecchetti G, Binda A, Piperno A, et al. Cardiac alterations in 36 consecutive patients with idiopathic hemochromatosis: polygraphic and echocardiographic evaluation. Eur Heart J. 1991;12:224–30.
165. Linhart A, Palecek T, Bultas J, et al. New insights in cardiac structural changes in patients with Fabry's disease. Am Heart. 2000;139:1101–8.
166. Beer G, Reinecke P, Gabbert HE, Hort W, Kuhn H. Fabry disease in patients with hypertrophic cardiomyopathy (HCM). Z Kardiol. 2002;91:992–1002.
167. Ommen SR, Nishimura RA, Edwards WD. Fabry disease: a mimic for obstructive hypertrophic cardiomyopathy? Heart. 2003;89:929–30.
168. Nakao S, Takenaka T, Maeda M, et al. An atypical variant of Fabry's disease in men with left ventricular hypertrophy. N Engl J Med. 1995;333:288–93.
169. Nagueh SF. Fabry disease. Heart. 2003;89:819–20.
170. Frustaci A, Chimenti C, Ricci R, et al. Improvement in cardiac function in the cardiac variant of Fabry's disease with galactose-infusion therapy. N Engl J Med. 2001;345:25–32.

Cardiac Tumors

Doris M. Rassl and Susan J. Davies

Abstract

Primary cardiac tumors are rare, and metastases are in fact the commonest tumors within the heart. Malignancies associated with metastasis to the heart include melanoma, sarcoma, and carcinomas of the lung, breast, stomach, colon, liver, kidney, thyroid, as well as lymphomas.

The commonest primary cardiac tumor is the benign cardiac myxoma. Other benign lesions of the heart include papillary fibroelastoma, rhabdomyoma, cardiac fibroma, cystic tumor of the atrioventricular node, cardiac lipoma, and hemangioma.

Malignant cardiac tumors comprise rhabdomyosarcoma, angiosarcoma, and other types of sarcoma. The heart may rarely be involved by inflammatory myofibroblastic tumor, and other primary cardiac entities considered to be of hamartomatous etiology include histiocytoid cardiomyopathy and lipomatous hypertrophy.

Clinical presentation of cardiac tumors is varied and is usually dependent upon the site and size of the lesion and any associated complications such as pericardial effusion, systemic, or pulmonary emboli.

Keywords

Cardiac tumors • Metastases • Cardiac myxoma • Papillary fibroelastoma • Rhabdomyoma Rhabdomyosarcoma • Histiocytoid cardiomyopathy

Introduction

Cardiac tumors are rare and accounted for only 0.7% of cardiac surgical procedures at one specialist center [1]. By far the commonest cardiac tumor is actually metastatic malignancy, which has been found to be approximately 100 times more common than primary tumors [1] in autopsy studies. However, in surgical series, metastatic disease of the heart is still uncommon (3.3%) [1].

The vast majority of primary cardiac tumors are benign; however, one should always be alert to the possibility of malignancy, in particular sarcomas, which are the commonest primary malignant tumors of the heart and are often a histological mimic of the commonest benign cardiac tumor, the cardiac myxoma.

In cases of cardiac tumors, clinical presentation is myriad but is generally related to the presence of a mass lesion affecting the heart. Both benign and malignant cardiac tumors may present with sudden death, chest pain, cardiac failure, superior vena cava syndrome, valvular abnormalities, or arrhythmias. The presentation depends mainly upon the site and size of the lesion. However, many tumors are completely asymptomatic and are discovered incidentally.

Systemic or pulmonary emboli can be seen in both benign and malignant intracavity lesions, although only soft, friable tumor types generally present a risk of embolus. Pericardial

D.M. Rassl, MBBS, FRCPath (✉)
Department of Histopathology, Papworth Hospital,
Papworth Everard, Cambridge CB23 3RE, UK
e-mail: doris.rassl@papworth.nhs.uk

S.J. Davies, MBBS, FRCPath
Consultant Histopathologist Cumberland Infirmary, North Cumbria
University Hospitals NHS Trust, Newtown Road, Carlisle CA2 7HY, UK

S.K. Suvarna (ed.), *Cardiac Pathology*,
DOI 10.1007/978-1-4471-2407-8_12, © Springer-Verlag London 2013

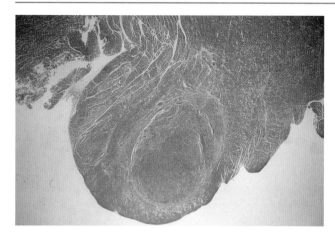

Fig. 12.1 Low-power view of a subendocardial deposit of metastatic malignant melanoma (Hematoxylin and eosin)

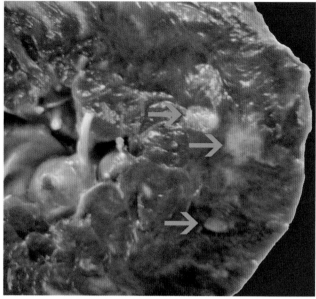

Fig. 12.2 Macroscopic view of the heart at autopsy showing areas of metastatic tumor (arrows), which in this case is metastatic mesothelioma. This patient suffered ventricular tachycardias and a final ventricular fibrillation arrest.

effusions tend to be associated with malignancy. Occasionally, protean systemic symptoms may arise. This is thought to be related to the release of cytokines, but a systemic response may occur secondary to embolus or infective vegetation related to the tumor.

Tumors Metastatic to the Heart

Metastases are by far the commonest tumor of the heart. The following malignancies are most strongly associated with metastasis to the heart: lymphoma, leukemia, melanoma (Fig. 12.1), sarcoma, and carcinomas of the lung, breast, stomach, colon, liver, kidney, and thyroid. Metastatic deposits may be diffuse or multifocal (Fig. 12.2) or may consist of a single mass lesion. The diagnostic criteria reflect those of the primary tumor. The presentation mostly reflects the site involved in the heart and the volume of the tumor. There is a predictable poor prognosis.

Cardiac Myxoma

Cardiac myxomas are generally accepted as being neoplastic, although some have previously suggested they are reactive lesions or hamartomas [2]. The cell of origin is postulated to be either from mesenchymal "embryonic rests," possibly entrapped foregut derivatives or subendothelial reserve cells present within the fossa ovalis and/or surrounding endocardium. It is believed that these cells are capable of divergent differentiation, hence the presence of "heterologous" elements in some myxomas and the eclectic immunohistochemical profile. Others have suggested cardiac myxomas are possibly of neural origin and arise from neural tissue within the endocardium [3].

Myxoma is the commonest primary heart tumor, accounting for 36–76% of cases in surgical series, with lesions most commonly found in the atria [4, 5]. The highest incidence is in women (F:M ratio 1.9:1) [6, 7], in the age range 30–60 years, but it occurs in all age groups. Cardiac myxoma can sometimes occur in the context of a familial syndrome, Carney's complex, which has an autosomal dominant mode of inheritance and is associated with the following: cardiac and cutaneous myxomas, cutaneous lentiginosis and blue nevi, myxoid fibroadenomas of the breast, pituitary adenomas, primary pigmented adrenocortical disease, thyroid tumors, psammomatous melanotic schwannomas, and Sertoli cell tumors of the testes, in particular, large-cell calcifying Sertoli cell tumor [8, 9]. Cardiac myxomas occurring in the context of Carney's syndrome tend to occur in a younger age group than sporadic cases and may be multifocal, metachronous [10, 11], and found at sites other than the left atrial septum. The possibility of Carney's syndrome should be considered if any of the above features are present.

Myxoma may be asymptomatic. Symptoms, when they occur, are usually related to the location of the lesion within the cardiac chambers. They can result in obstruction of the mitral or tricuspid valves, leading to cardiac failure or palpitations. The classical clinical signs on auscultation are of a murmur which changes with time and position [12] and/or an early diastolic "tumor plop" caused by prolapse of the lesion through the valve orifice [13]. Pulmonary or systemic emboli of tumor are seen in 30–40% of cases, with or without thrombus. Systemic emboli to the brain, coronary arteries, kidney,

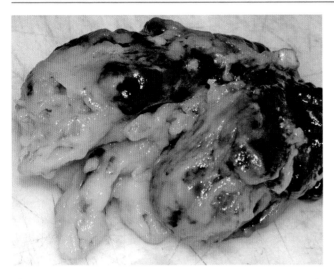

Fig. 12.3 Cardiac myxoma (37-mm maximal diameter) macroscopic view showing irregular surface with variable areas of hemorrhage and myxoid change (white zones). This type of myxoma can fragment and embolize

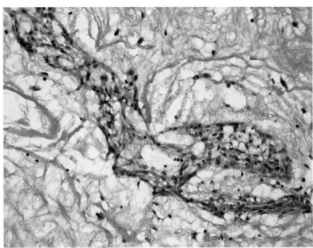

Fig. 12.4 Cardiac myxoma demonstrating perivascular cuffing by lepidic cells, set within a background myxoid matrix (Hematoxylin and eosin)

spleen, and extremities are documented [13]. Systemic symptoms may occur and are thought to be the result of interleukin 6 production by the tumor, which may cause fever and malaise [13]. Secondary infection of the tumor may also cause systemic symptoms.

Cardiac myxomas most commonly occur on the left side of the intra-atrial septum in the region of the foramen ovale, but may also occur at other sites within both atria and, rarely, in the ventricles. However, if the lesion arises from a heart valve, an alternate diagnosis should be considered [14]. Myxomas arise from the endocardium and project into the cardiac chamber as a sessile or pedunculated mass. Involvement of the underlying myocardium is not a feature. The tumors are usually rounded polypoid masses, but may have a villous architecture. They range in size from about 1–15 cm [15] and are usually variegated in appearance, with opaque gray and yellow areas, as well as red/brown areas, corresponding to zones of hemorrhage. They have a gelatinous consistency, and the cut surface may be solid or contain cystic spaces.

It is important for the pathologist to identify and sample the base of the lesion (Fig. 12.3), as the surgeon will generally take a cuff of myocardium along with the tumor to ensure complete excision. This should be inked and processed in its entirety in order to confirm excision and also to exclude the differential diagnosis of an infiltrating malignancy.

Microscopically, myxomas are usually covered by a single layer of flattened endothelial cells. The bulk of the lesion is composed of bland stellate or polygonal (lepidic) cells in a copious metachromatic myxoid stroma. The cells have small round, oval, or sometimes spindled nuclei and a moderate amount of eosinophilic cytoplasm. They are scattered singly,

but are also seen in cords and surrounding vascular spaces within the stroma (Fig. 12.4). This latter feature is pathognomonic and is helpful in excluding the differential diagnosis of organizing thrombus. Mitoses are not normally seen and, if present, should alert the pathologist to an alternative, malignant diagnosis.

There is usually prominent hemorrhage with hemosiderin deposition within the stroma. On occasion, calcium-encrusted elastic fibers, known as Gamna–Gandy bodies, may be observed. A stromal inflammatory infiltrate, which includes lymphocytes and plasma cells, as well as macrophages, is usually present. This inflammatory component often extends into the underlying myocardium. At the base of the lesion, there are often one or two thick-walled vessels. There is a glandular variant which contains cysts lined by a single layer of bland mucin-secreting or ciliated epithelial cells (Fig. 12.5) [8]. Some myxomas contain aggregates of cells with the morphological and immunostaining characteristics of fibroblasts, myofibroblasts, or smooth muscle [8]. Myxomas have an eclectic immunohistochemical profile, being variably positive for markers of neural differentiation [3], endothelial markers, and calretinin [13]. Epithelial cells within the glandular variant are positive for cytokeratin.

The differential diagnosis of myxoma includes primary or metastatic sarcoma. A myxomatous neoplasm that does not conform to the histological pattern described above or tumors showing mitotic activity, cytological atypia, or invasion should not be diagnosed as benign myxoma. The concept of "malignant myxoma" is rejected by many [16], although one report of a sarcoma arising within an otherwise typical myxoma is noted [17]. However, it is stressed that one must exclude low-grade myxoid areas in a cardiac sarcoma.

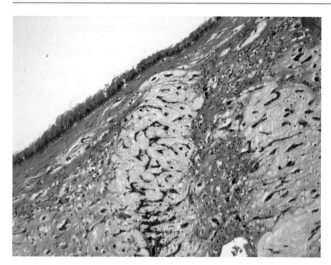

Fig. 12.5 Glandular variant of cardiac myxoma. Note the layer of columnar epithelium towards the *left-hand side* of the image (Hematoxylin and eosin)

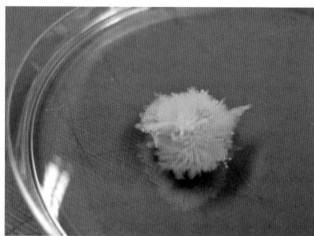

Fig. 12.6 Papillary fibroelastoma: macroscopic appearance resembling a sea anemone (11-mm diameter). The lesion is best appreciated when suspended in a Petri dish with formalin

Papillary Fibroelastoma

Papillary fibroelastomas are the second commonest primary cardiac tumor after myxoma, accounting for 10% of tumors [18]. They are rarely reported in children [19]. They do not recur following excision, which is usually performed as a shave excision of the lesion [19]. Although it is generally accepted that papillary fibroelastomas are nonneoplastic, there is lack of agreement about whether the lesions are hamartomatous, represent a peculiar kind of reactive phenomenon, or simply organized thrombi [18–21]. They are commonly asymptomatic and are often found incidentally at autopsy or cardiac surgery.

A hamartomatous derivation has been suggested on the basis of the similarity of the entity to normal chordae tendineae [20], although the rarity of this lesion in childhood argues against this concept. On the basis of the similarity of papillary fibroelastoma to Lambl's excrescences, which are composed of fibrin, others have suggested the lesion is caused by a reactive response in endothelial cells, which undergo hyperplasia, with excessive basement membrane formation, possibly secondary to trauma [20]. The increased incidence of these lesions in structurally abnormal hearts, where there is disruption to the normal flow of blood potentially leading to repetitive hemodynamic trauma, supports this theory [22]. Abnormal blood flow might also explain the presence of organized thrombus. Papillary fibroelastoma has been shown to contain fibrin, hyaluronic acid, and elastic fibers, in keeping with organized thrombus [18].

Although not neoplastic, papillary fibroelastomas can cause considerable morbidity as a result of systemic or pulmonary emboli, which is a more common complication than

with myxoma (emboli occur in 34% of papillary fibroelastomas compared to 24% of myxomas) [19]. This is probably due to the location of the lesion, commonly in the left ventricular outflow tract, which has a high blood flow rate [19]. It is believed that emboli originate from thrombus associated with the lesion, as much as from the lesion itself [19, 23], leading to the proposal that anticoagulation be considered as a therapeutic option in patients unfit for surgery [23, 24]. There is also the risk of obstruction of the coronary artery ostia, in those lesions situated on the aortic valve [20], and of valvular dysfunction [19]. However, many are asymptomatic and are discovered incidentally. Interestingly, mortality rates may be higher with fibroelastomas than with myxomas. This is postulated to be because of the overall older age at which they occur and the increased risk of embolism [19].

Papillary fibroelastomas tend to occur in structurally abnormal hearts, most commonly on valve leaflets, and are most frequently found on the aortic valve [19, 20, 22]. About 23% arise from the atrial or ventricular endocardial surface [19]. Rarely, they may be multiple [19, 22], and in whole heart specimens, it is important to consider this possibility, even if the patient has undergone echocardiography, since second smaller lesions may be missed using this technique [23, 25]. Papillary fibroelastomas generally are around 1.0 cm in diameter, but range in size from 0.2 to 7 cm [18, 19, 21]. They are cream in color and have a characteristic appearance when immersed in formalin, resembling a sea anemone (Fig. 12.6). This is due to the multiple fine strand-like fronds, of which the lesions are composed, emanating from a central core at the base. The lesions may act as a nidus for thrombus formation and are sometimes associated with infective vegetations [19, 21], which may alter the classical macroscopic appearance.

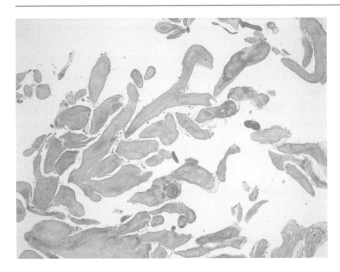

Fig. 12.7 Papillary fibroelastoma showing a villous architecture with bland fibrous stromal cores (Hematoxylin and eosin)

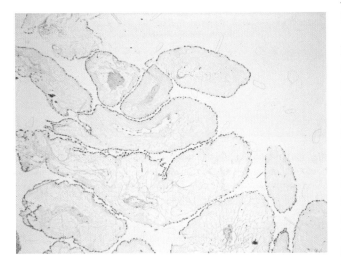

Fig. 12.8 Papillary fibroelastoma at high magnification showing a bland endothelial surface (Hematoxylin and eosin)

The fine strands seen macroscopically are composed of hypocellular or acellular hyalinized material and are covered by a monolayer of endothelial cells (Figs. 12.7 and 12.8). In some cases, the hyalinized core is surrounded by a myxomatous rim. Stains for elastin reveal the presence of elastic fibers, from which the lesion derives its name. There is no infiltration of the underlying valve leaflet.

The differential diagnosis includes cardiac myxoma, Lambl's excrescence, and thrombus. Although cardiac myxoma can sometimes have a fronded appearance, the fronds are much thicker than those of papillary fibroelastoma. Myxomas arise from the atrial or occasionally from the ventricular wall, and only a handful of case reports describe myxomas arising from a cardiac valve. Myxomas differ histologically from fibroelastomas, although there may be some

confusion between the two entities macroscopically, especially if there is associated thrombus [26].

Lambl's excrescences are 0.1–2.0 cm in size and occur exclusively at the line of closure of the semilunar valves, whereas fibroelastomas occur anywhere on the valve surface [18]. Although fibroelastomas are morphologically similar (hence the synonym "giant Lambl's excrescence"), Lambl's excrescences are composed of fibrin and lack the acid-mucopolysaccharide matrix of fibroelastomas [21]. However, many transitional forms exist, where the similarities between the two lesions are striking, making the distinction between the two somewhat arbitrary [20].

Papillary fibroelastomas may be associated with thrombus, and it is important to exclude an underlying fibroelastoma in any valvular/mural thrombi or in embolic material. This requires processing all the material submitted for histological examination.

Rhabdomyoma

Rhabdomyomas are benign striated muscle tumors, regarded as hamartomas without malignant potential [27]. They are usually classified as cardiac or extracardiac based on their location and unique histology [28]. Extracardiac rhabdomyomas are very rare (<2%) and are classified into the adult type, the fetal type, the genital type, and rhabdomyomatous mesenchymal hamartomas [29]. Cardiac rhabdomyoma is the most common cardiac tumor seen in infancy and childhood (60–86% of primary fetal cardiac tumors [30]). About 75% occur before the age of 1 year [28]. The UK incidence of symptomatic rhabdomyomas in infancy has been estimated to be 1 in 326,000 [27]. They are strongly associated with tuberous sclerosis (TS) with 51–85% patients having this genetic condition. It is estimated that 43–72% of patients with TS will have or develop cardiac rhabdomyomas [27, 31, 32].

The clinical presentation and hemodynamic findings depend on the number, size, and location of the lesions. They can be detected prenatally by ultrasound (as early as 20 weeks). Rhabdomyomas may cause fetal dysrhythmias or nonimmune hydrops fetalis [33]. Postnatally they may be asymptomatic. However, clinical examination may reveal a murmur, reduced peripheral pulses, cyanosis, or congestive cardiac failure. Arrhythmias occur in approximately 16–47% of cases, with frequent atrial or ventricular arrhythmias and a higher incidence of Wolff–Parkinson–White syndrome [31]. Life-threatening situations may arise if inflow or ventricular outflow tract obstruction occurs [34].

Echocardiographically rhabdomyomas appear as well-circumscribed, homogenous echogenic masses. The finding of multiple cardiac masses is highly suggestive of rhabdomyomas, especially in patients with TS. On MRI, rhabdomyomas have signal characteristics similar to normal myocardium, but they are hypointense on postgadolinium imaging. On CT they may appear hyper or hypoattenuated compared to the surrounding myocardium [33].

Cardiac rhabdomyomas have a tendency for spontaneous regression (54–100%), especially throughout the first year, and up to 5 years of age [34]. Once fetal somatic growth is complete, hamartomas lose their mitotic potential and undergo apoptosis. Therefore, most rhabdomyomas will regress, although rarely some may continue to grow in early childhood before doing so [31]. Surgical resection is only indicated if serious symptoms (e.g., significant obstruction, arrhythmia) occur. Antiarrhythmic drugs may be used to control symptoms until lesions regress.

Cardiac rhabdomyomas are single or multiple, well-circumscribed, nonencapsulated, white or gray nodules which can range from a few millimeters to several centimeters in size [33, 35]. The lesions have a uniform cut surface, being lighter than the surrounding myocardium (Fig. 12.9). They can occur anywhere in the heart, including the atria and atriocaval junction, but are most commonly found in the ventricles and interventricular septum. They can be intramural or pedunculated, encroaching on the intracavitary space [27]. Rare case reports of involvement of the mitral valve annulus and valve leaflets exist [34].

The lesions are composed of enlarged myocytes with clear cytoplasm (Figs. 12.9 and 12.10). The majority of the cells show vacuolization and sparse myofilaments, but in some cells, strands of eosinophilic cytoplasm radiate from the central nucleus to the cell membrane, so-called spider cells which are considered pathognomonic of cardiac

rhabdomyoma (Fig. 12.11) [33]. The cells contain abundant glycogen, staining positively for periodic acid-Schiff (PAS) reagent [33]. Rhabdomyomas show immunoreactivity with myoglobin, desmin, actin, vimentin, hamartin, and tuberin. The cells do not express proliferation markers, such as Ki67, but the "spider cells" stain for ubiquitin. This may provide insight into the mechanisms involved in the regression of rhabdomyomas, as the ubiquitin pathway is associated with degradation of myofilaments, vacuolization, enlargement of glycogen vacuoles, apoptosis, and myxoid degeneration [31]. By electron microscopy, the cells of rhabdomyomas

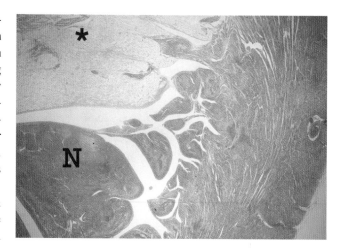

Fig. 12.10 Low-power view showing a subendocardial rhabdomyoma composed of enlarged myocytes with clear cytoplasm (*) with normal (*N*) endomyocardial tissue adjacent (Hematoxylin and eosin)

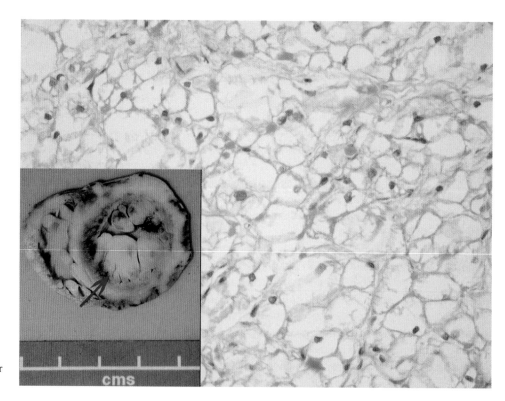

Fig. 12.9 Histology of the cardiac rhabdomyoma with characteristic clear cells. The macroscopic sample is seen in the *low left corner*, showing several nonencapsulated gray-white areas representing rhabdomyomas (*one arrowed*). These project into the ventricular lumen focally

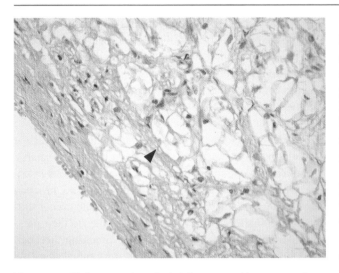

Fig. 12.11 High-power view of a rhabdomyoma with myocytes showing vacuolization and sparse myofilaments, often termed "spider cells" (*arrowhead*) (Hematoxylin and eosin)

resemble altered myocytes, possessing small and sparse mitochondria, abundant glycogen, and cell junctions all around the periphery, instead of exclusively at the poles of the cell as seen in differentiated myocytes [33].

Over half of cardiac rhabdomyomas are associated with TS and may be the earliest sign of TS in utero. The genetic basis of TS is heterogenous and may be caused by mutation of the tumor suppressor genes TSC1 at chromosome 9q34 (encoding hamartin) and TSC2 at chromosome 16p13 (encoding tuberin) [30, 33]. TS is autosomal dominant with variable expression, but studies indicate 50–80% of childhood cases result from spontaneous mutations [30]. TSC1 and TSC2 gene mutations have been associated with the combination of cardiac rhabdomyomas and TS. Therefore, in case of a family history of TS, a search for cardiac rhabdomyomas is required. Similarly, a fetus with cardiac lesions should prompt a search for TS in other family members [35].

The differential diagnosis includes histiocytoid cardiomyopathy and hamartoma of mature cardiac myocytes. Histiocytoid cardiomyopathy shows collections of oncocytic cells rich in mitochondria rather than vacuolated cells, and the cell nests are less discrete and smaller. Hamartomas of mature cardiac myocytes lack circumscription and "spider cells" [33].

Primary Cardiac Fibroma

Primary cardiac fibroma is a benign lesion containing fibroblasts or myofibroblasts [36, 37]. There is some debate as to whether the lesion is hamartomatous or neoplastic [37, 38]. Although rare, accounting for only 3.2% of all primary cardiac tumors [38], the cardiac fibroma is the second commonest primary cardiac tumor of childhood.

The peak incidence is in infants (under 1 year old) [39], but may occur at any age, including in the fetus and in the elderly [36, 40]. However, only 15% occur in adulthood [41]. Since many consider the lesion to be congenital [41], it is possible that those discovered in older patients may actually have been present since birth. There is no sex predilection, but there is an association with Gorlin syndrome, and cardiac fibroma occurs in 3% of patients with this autosomal dominant disease [37].

As stated, the tumor is benign and may be asymptomatic. However, sudden death can occur, secondary to arrhythmia. There may be serious morbidity if the tumor is large enough to form a significant space-occupying lesion.

Cardiac fibroma is not associated with tumor emboli. Cardiac fibroma does not spontaneously regress [37, 42], but it often ceases to grow [38], so that the enlarging, developing heart favorably alters the heart to tumor size ratio, possibly obviating the need for surgery. A "watch and wait" approach is therefore valid in symptomatic but stable pediatric patients. Partial excision of symptomatic lesions is possible to preserve the integrity of the heart [36].

The most common location for fibroma is within the myocardium of the left ventricular free wall or septum [38], although cases do occur in the right ventricle and, rarely, the atria. The lesions range in size from a few millimeters to over 12 cm [38].

Multiple fibromas have been reported, but these must be distinguished from outgrowths at the periphery of the main tumor mass [38]. Careful sectioning is required to demonstrate continuity of "satellite" lesions with the main tumor.

The tumor appears macroscopically well circumscribed and is usually solid, white, and fibrous, although cystic degeneration may be apparent at the center of larger lesions. When examined microscopically, cardiac fibromas are unencapsulated and usually show myocardial infiltration at the periphery, with entrapment of myocytes, which are sometimes seen quite deeply within the lesion [37].

The tumor histologically is composed of spindle cells in a collagenous background. The cellularity of the lesion varies with age (Figs. 12.12 and 12.13). Fibromas in neonates tend to be highly cellular, and there may even be rare mitoses, whereas those occurring in adulthood are predominantly composed of collagen, with only sparse bland spindle cells [37]. Foci of dystrophic calcification are common, especially in tumors from older individuals. The more cellular tumors sometimes contain foci of extramedullary hematopoiesis [36, 37]. Myxoid change and foci of chronic inflammation may also occur [37]. Stains for elastin reveal the presence of elastic fibers. Cardiac fibromas are positive for vimentin and actin and negative for desmin, CD34, and S100 [37].

The differential diagnosis includes sarcoma, inflammatory myofibroblastic tumor, and rhabdomyoma. Sarcoma may come into the differential, especially in more cellular, lesions. Mitoses are extremely rare in fibromas, and their presence

Fig. 12.12 Low-power view of a cardiac fibroma showing bland spindle cells in a collagenous background (Hematoxylin and eosin)

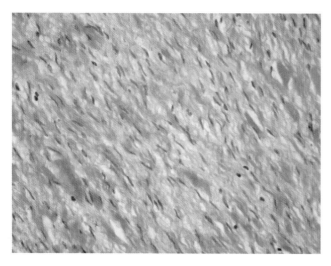

Fig. 12.13 Higher magnification of the cardiac fibroma demonstrating relatively uniform spindle cells, without mitotic activity (Hematoxylin and eosin)

warrants consideration of malignancy. Inflammatory fibroblastic tumors are very rare in the heart, and their diagnosis is often suggested by significant numbers of inflammatory cells [39]. Entrapped myocytes within a fibroma may show degenerative vacuolation, and the lesion could be mistaken for a rhabdomyoma [39].

Cystic Tumor of the Atrioventricular (AV) Node

Cystic tumor of the atrioventricular node is a benign cystic mass at the base of the atrial septum, in the region of the atrioventricular node [43]. It is considered a form of endodermal heterotopia with differentiation towards an upper foregut phenotype [44]. It is believed to reflect alterations in the development of the cardiac neural crest which could

explain the presence of ultimobranchial rests in the AV node region [43]. In 10% of cases, the lesions occur in association with other midline defects, and there is evidence that limited cell proliferation occurs in some cases [45]. Possible familial occurrence, as well as the association with other congenital and midline defects, may suggest a genetic defect involving the migration of embryologic tissues [43].

Cystic tumors of the AV node are rare, with a mean age at presentation of 38 years (age range from birth to 86 years). They are more commonly found in women (F:M = 3:1) [45]. The precise incidence is difficult to determine as in some cases the lesions are asymptomatic until presentation or sudden death. There are rarely macroscopic clues to their presence at autopsy if the lesions are small, requiring thorough blocking of this tissue if one is not to miss this lesion (see Chap. 5).

Due to their location, the lesions can cause variable degrees of heart block, including complete heart block in up to 66% of patients, with 10% of cases being associated with sudden death [45]. Ventricular tachycardia or fibrillation is experienced by some patients, but there appears to be no relationship between size and the occurrence of lethal arrhythmia [46]. In a small number of cases, which presented with atrial fibrillation and atrioventricular block, the lesions have been successfully resected, usually requiring subsequent pacemaker support [46, 47].

Cystic tumors of the AV node may be visualized by transesophageal echocardiography, computed tomography, or cardiac magnetic resonance imaging (CMR). With the latter modality, the lesions have been reported to be of high intensity on T1-weighted images and isointense with myocardium on T2-weighted images [46].

The lesions, which are located in the inferior interatrial septum in the region of the AV node, vary in size, ranging from 0.05 to 3 cm [46]. They are multicystic, although some cysts may be barely visible macroscopically, and not infrequently contain a small volume of yellow/brown, semisolid material [46, 48].

Microscopically, tumor cell nests and variably sized cystic spaces lined by tumor cells are set within a fibrous stroma, which may show foci of chronic inflammation (Figs. 12.14 and 12.15). The tumor cells may have a cuboidal, transitional, or squamoid morphology and rarely show features of sebaceous differentiation [45]. A minor population of neuroendocrine cells may also be apparent [43]. The cysts may contain amorphous material and keratinous debris [48]. Generally there is no involvement of the central fibrous body or significant extension into the ventricular myocardium by the lesion.

The main tumor cells express many cytokeratins (CAM5.2, 34βE12, AE1/AE3, CK7), as well as EMA, B72.3, CEA, CA19.9, p63, bcl-2, and galectin 3 [43, 45]. A second, minor population, as described in some reports, may be present which stains for calcitonin, chromogranin, and

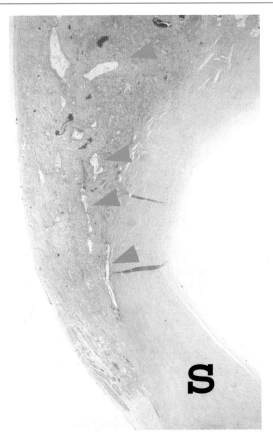

Fig. 12.14 Low-power view of a cystic tumor of the atrioventricular node (*arrowed*) above the membranous septum (*S*) (Hematoxylin and eosin)

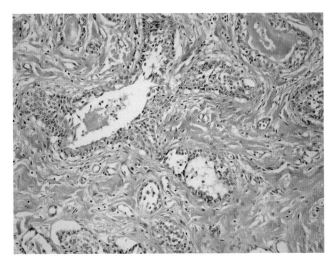

Fig. 12.15 Cystic tumor of the atrioventricular node with variably sized cystic spaces lined by tumor cells set within fibrous stroma (Hematoxylin and eosin)

synaptophysin, as well as cytokeratins, EMA, and CEA. The tumor cells are reported to be negative for CK20, thyroglobulin, vimentin, CD31, calretinin, estrogen, and progesterone receptor [43], although one case report found focal positivity

for progesterone and strong staining for estrogen receptor [48], suggesting that the lesions may be hormone sensitive.

On electron microscopic examination, the solid cell nests demonstrate a well-formed basement membrane, desmosomes, and cytoplasmic tonofilaments. Cells lining the spaces also have short microvilli and some may contain electron-dense material [45], consistent with the finding that neuroendocrine markers stain some of the cells.

The differential diagnosis includes metastatic carcinoma and teratoma. In comparison to metastatic carcinoma, cystic tumor of the atrioventricular node is a benign lesion with histologically bland epithelial cells, lacking significant mitotic activity or pleomorphism. Teratomas by contrast should show elements derived from the different embryonic cell layers (ecto-, endo-, and mesoderm) and so should be easily excluded.

Cardiac Lipoma and Lipomatous Hypertrophy

Together lipomatous hypertrophy and lipoma represent 6–10% of benign cardiac lesions. CT and MRI scans are helpful in establishing the fatty nature of these lesions and the exact anatomical location.

Lipomatous hypertrophy is found almost exclusively in older (>50 years), obese patients [49]. It is defined as fatty infiltration (>2cm in thickness), is usually brown and firm in consistency, and generally affects the interatrial septum, although it may involve the entire atrial wall [50, 51]. It typically spares the foramen ovale, giving the lesion a characteristic dumbbell shape [50]. It is often located anterior to the foramen ovale, but may extend into the region of the atrioventricular node. The histogenesis of lipomatous hypertrophy is uncertain. It may result from a metabolic disturbance associated with obesity, increasing age, starvation, or anemia or simply represent a hamartoma of adipocytes [52].

Lipomatous hypertrophy is usually asymptomatic and most often an incidental finding at autopsy. It may uncommonly be the cause of atrial arrhythmias (atrial fibrillation and atrioventricular block) [49], congestive cardiac failure, and if large, superior vena cava obstruction [53].

Lipomatous hypertrophy does not represent a neoplastic process and is a nonencapsulated lesion composed of varying proportions of mature adipocytes and brown fat cells, which contain multiple small vacuoles with a central nucleus. Myocytes are usually entrapped within the mass, especially at the periphery, and these may show bizarre hypertrophic and degenerative changes, but mitoses are absent [52–56]. Often areas of fibrosis and focal collections of chronic inflammatory cells are present (Fig. 12.16) [52].

Cardiac lipomas, by contrast, are well-defined, benign masses composed of mature, white adipocytes. Cardiac lipomas are rare and account for only 0.5–3% of excised heart

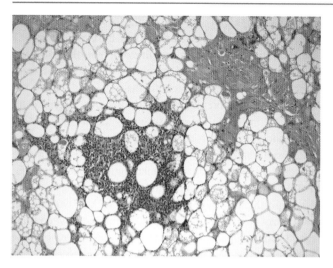

Fig. 12.16 Lipomatous hypertrophy including fetal (brown) fat cells, entrapped myocytes, and a collection of chronic inflammatory cells (Hematoxylin and eosin)

It should be noted that the intramuscular variant of hemangioma may contain variable numbers of adipocytes [53] and could be confused with a true lipomatous lesion.

Hibernoma is a rare, benign tumor of brown adipose tissue composed of multivacuolated adipocytes. Hibernomas are encapsulated and slow growing. They possibly arise from vestiges of brown fat that can persist around the great vessels or at unusual sites. Aberrant differentiation of mesenchymal cells, ectopic growth, or migration of adipose tissue may account for their occurrence. Four variants have been identified: the typical hibernoma, a mixture of hibernoma cells and white fat cells; the lipoma-like variant, with only scattered hibernoma cells amongst mature adipocytes; the myxoid variant; and the spindle cell variant [58]. A diagnosis of hibernoma should only be considered where the macroscopic appearances do not fit lipomatous hypertrophy and where microscopically the lesion is predominantly composed of multivacuolated cells [54].

tumors [53]. They can occur at any age with equal frequency in both sexes [50].

The presentation of cardiac lipomas is varied and depends on their location. Many are incidental findings, but they can cause arrhythmias, syncope, embolization, and even compression of the coronary arteries or blood flow within the heart [57]. Echocardiographic abnormalities may also be encountered [53]. Excision of cardiac lipomas is indicated if clinical symptoms develop or it is not possible to confidently exclude liposarcoma. Surgical excision generally provides complete cure and a good long-term prognosis [50].

Lipomas are encapsulated and can occur throughout the heart, including the visceral and parietal pericardium [49]. Most are subendocardial (50%), and the remaining tumors have a pericardial (25%) or intramyocardial (25%) position [50].

The size of cardiac lipomas varies, and those that are left in situ when they are asymptomatic may grow to large dimensions [55]. Although typically solitary, multiple cardiac lipomas may be found in association with TS [54].

Similar to extracardiac lipomas, those in the heart are circumscribed and composed of bland, mature adipocytes. A few myocytes may be entrapped at the margin, but a capsule is usually present [56]. Unusual histologic variants of lipoma are generally not encountered within the heart [53]. The presence of fat droplets may be demonstrated with an oil-red O stain, which requires frozen section.

The differential diagnosis includes liposarcoma, intramuscular variant of hemangioma [53], and hibernoma. The brown fat cells of lipomatous hypertrophy should not be mistaken for the lipoblasts of liposarcoma, which have indented, hyperchromatic, atypical nuclei [56]. Liposarcomas usually grow quickly and infiltrate into surrounding cardiac and thoracic structures.

Cardiac Hemangioma

It is uncertain whether hemangiomas are true neoplasms or developmental vascular anomalies [59]. They represent a benign proliferation of endothelial cells, which form vascular channels, often separated by varying amounts of supporting connective tissue, in a nonencapsulated but relatively well demarcated structure without necrosis [60]. Primary cardiac hemangiomas are infrequent and only account for about 2–3% of all primary cardiac tumors and up to 5% of all benign cardiac tumors [61]. They can occur at any age, but are more common in children and adolescents [62]. Some studies suggest a female predominance [60], whilst others report an equal sex incidence [61].

The clinical presentation of cardiac hemangiomas depends primarily on the tumor location, size, and extension. The lesions may involve any part of the heart, including the endocardium and heart valves [63], myocardium, epicardium, and pericardium.

Cardiac hemangiomas are usually asymptomatic and discovered incidentally, either radiologically, during cardiac surgery, or at autopsy. In symptomatic cases, the most common symptoms include shortness of breath, atypical chest pain, palpitations, and arrhythmias [61], but pericardial effusion or hemopericardium, cardiac tamponade, congestive heart failure, right ventricular outflow tract obstruction, coronary insufficiency, systemic embolization, valvular stenosis, and sudden death have also been reported [59, 62, 64]. Intracavitary tumors may produce a triad of obstruction, embolization, and constitutional symptoms [60]. Genetic susceptibility to cardiac hemangiomas has not been described [65]. Most cardiac hemangiomas are sporadic, and without associated extracardiac lesions. However, giant cardiac hemangiomas can show associated thrombosis and coagulopathies (Kasabach–Merritt syndrome) [65].

Diagnosis can be made using transthoracic or transesophageal echocardiography, CT, or cardiac MR imaging. Coronary angiography may reveal the feeding vessel to the tumor and a characteristic tumor blush [66]. In many cases, a definitive diagnosis is only made after surgical excision and histological examination.

The natural history of these hemangiomas is unpredictable. They can regress, remain static, or enlarge over time. Surgical resection is the treatment of choice for symptomatic lesions, and the outcome and prognosis are usually good. Follow-up is recommended to allow for the detection of tumor recurrence, although the rate of recurrence is unknown [61].

Most hemangiomas have been reported to represent small, endocardial nodules ranging from 0.2 to 3.5 cm in diameter, either polypoid or sessile, and without evidence of infiltration [60]. Intramural hemangiomas tend to be poorly circumscribed masses with a hemorrhagic or congested appearance [63]. Pericardial hemangiomas typically are solitary and well defined. They arise from the visceral pericardium and range in size from 1 to 14 cm [59].

The most frequent locations are the anterior wall of the right ventricle, the lateral wall of the left ventricle, and the interventricular septum, and sometimes the right ventricular outflow tract is involved [65].

Histologically hemangiomas have been subdivided into three types. Firstly, cavernous hemangioma – composed of multiple dilated, thin-walled vascular channels. Secondly, capillary hemangioma – composed of small vessels resembling capillaries in a lobular or grouped arrangement, with an associated feeder vessel; mast cells and factor XIII-positive interstitial cells are present [65]. Finally, arteriovenous hemangioma or cirsoid aneurysm – composed of malformed arteries and veins [62, 66].

Most of the lesions have overlapping features, and many contain variable amounts of interspersed adipose and fibrous tissue [63, 65], especially the intramuscular lesions. They parallel similar hemangiomas elsewhere in the body. Intramural lesions are also often surrounded by hypertrophied myocytes. The tumor cells stain positively for standard endothelial markers such as CD31, CD34, and factor VIII. The pericytic framework of cells surrounding the endothelial-lined vascular channels stains for smooth muscle actin.

The differential diagnosis includes cardiac myxoma and angiosarcoma. In hemangiomas, the classic myxoma cells are absent; more importantly, there is a well-developed pericytic framework of cells surrounding the endothelial structures, and cellular areas with numerous capillaries are usually present. Some low-grade angiosarcomas may be difficult to differentiate from hemangiomas, but lack of cellular pleomorphism, mitotic activity, necrosis, and cellularity may aid in distinguishing hemangioma from angiosarcoma [62].

Inflammatory Myofibroblastic Tumor

The etiology of inflammatory myofibroblastic tumor (IMT), also known as "plasma cell granuloma" or "inflammatory pseudotumor," is uncertain. The lesions are composed of differentiated myofibroblastic cells accompanied by inflammatory cells [67]. Historically it has been suggested that IMTs arise secondary to immune or inflammatory dysregulation or represent an exaggerated response to tissue injury [68]. Postviral cell cycle dysregulation has also been suggested as a possible etiology. Polymerase chain reaction (PCR) assays and in situ hybridization (ISH) studies for evidence of Epstein–Barr virus (EBV) and human herpes virus 8 (HHV8) have not shown a clear association [68, 69]. Although cardiac and extracardiac IMTs share many features, there are differences in that cardiac IMTs usually behave in a benign fashion, lacking metastatic potential, whereas atypical and aggressive cases of extracardiac IMTs have been reported [67].

Cardiac IMT is an extremely uncommon tumor, and the exact incidence is unknown due to very different terms used to designate the lesion and the lack of uniform diagnostic criteria [67, 70]. The majority of these lesions have been described in children and young adults, although there have been infrequent reports in older adolescents [70]. There is no apparent sex predilection.

The presentation of the tumor is related to its size and location, and depending on the intracardiac location, it may be associated with syncope, myocardial infarction, or even sudden death [68]. Peripheral embolization of IMT has also been described [70]. There may be an associated inflammatory syndrome of fever, malaise, anemia, weight loss, vasculitis, thrombocytosis, and polyclonal hypergammaglobulinemia, thought to stem from IMT-mediated cytokine expression (IL-6) [71, 72]. These symptoms often resolve once the lesion is excised. IMTs may be identified by echocardiography and appear bright on ultrasound.

Treatment options depend on the location of the tumor and associated symptoms, but complete surgical resection is the favored option, with a good prognosis. Tumor recurrence is rare (8% overall) but may be more likely if resection is incomplete [68]. Steroids, chemotherapy, and radiotherapy have been used, mainly in patients with unresectable or incompletely resected tumors [68].

Up to 60% of extracardiac IMTs show a clonal cytogenetic aberration that activates the ALK receptor kinase gene (chromosome 2p23), leading to ALK protein overexpression, which is detectable immunohistochemically with cytoplasmic staining [67]. Several ALK fusion products involving tropomyosin genes and the clathrin heavy-chain gene have been reported [69]. In extracardiac IMTs, ALK reactivity has been associated with a more favorable prognosis. However, ALK expression appears different in

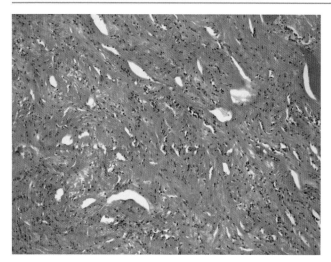

Fig. 12.17 Inflammatory myofibroblastic tumor with relatively bland spindle cells set within a fibrous stroma, alongside other areas with more dense cellularity (Hematoxylin and eosin)

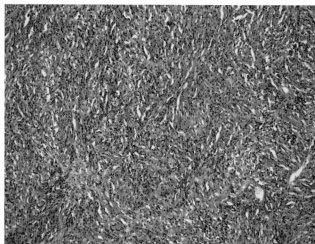

Fig. 12.18 Inflammatory myofibroblastic tumor showing a more cellular background with a prominent inflammatory cell infiltrate (Hematoxylin and eosin)

cardiac and extracardiac IMTs, with little or no ALK expression and no evidence of a prognostic role in cardiac cases. No other specific cytogenetic abnormality, to correlate with biological behavior or clinical presentation, has been described.

There appears to be no predilection for either side of the heart [67, 70, 72], and although some reports have suggested a right-sided predominance, these may have included a heterogenous group of tumors [70]. IMTs tend to arise from endocardial surfaces, including the valves [72], to form polypoid, broad-based lesions, generally with a smooth surface, which may show overlying fibrin [70]. Nonluminal masses are very rare [67]. The lesions range from approximately 1.5 to 6 cm in size [70].

Grossly, IMTs exhibit textural variation, including fleshy and fibrous portions [72]. The cut surface usually has a tan-white, sometimes whorled appearance and may show myxoid areas, focal punctuate hemorrhage, and softer, yellow foci, the latter being sometimes related to areas of coagulative necrosis or infarction possibly due to torsion [67].

The histological appearance of cardiac IMT is heterogenous with a variable degree of cellularity and collagen deposition, including myxoid areas, areas with densely collagenized stroma and focal areas of compact cellularity (Fig. 12.17) [70, 72]. The tumors contain a mixture of spindle cells showing fibroblastic and myofibroblastic differentiation, arranged in fascicles, or exhibiting a storiform architecture [73]. The spindle cells possess oval nuclei, fine chromatin, and mostly inconspicuous nucleoli, although occasional prominent nucleoli may be seen. Cytological atypia is low grade and mitotic activity infrequent (<2/10 hpf) [72], with no abnormal mitotic figures. Admixed with the

spindle cell proliferation is a variable inflammatory cell infiltrate, comprising plasma cells and lymphocytes with a smaller number of granulocytes, including eosinophils (Fig. 12.18).

The spindle cells are positive for smooth muscle actin and vimentin and show focal immunoreactivity for calponin, whilst staining for myogenin, caldesmon, S100, synaptophysin, CD56, cytokeratin AE1/AE3, CD34, CD117, and bcl-2 is generally negative. Desmin is rarely weakly positive [6], and only scanty (<1%) p53-positive nuclei are present [67]. The lack of staining for anaplastic lymphoma kinase (ALK-1) in most cases and lack of apparent locally aggressive behavior suggest that cardiac IMT may be biologically different from other IMTs at other sites [70]. ALK-1-reactivity does not have a diagnostic or prognostic role in cardiac IMT [67]. CD68-positive macrophages and CD138-positive plasma cells are variably distributed within the lesion.

The differential diagnosis is naturally wide and includes myxoma, myxofibrosarcoma, low-grade fibromyxosarcoma, inflammatory leiomyosarcoma, inflammatory sarcomatoid carcinoma, and inflammatory fibrous histiocytoma. IMT lacks the cords and perivascular rings of "myxoma" cells in a loose matrix. In comparison to myxofibrosarcoma and low-grade fibromyxosarcoma, IMT shows diffuse inflammation, and there is an absence of the "curvilinear" vessels seen in these sarcomas [72]. In general, inflammatory leiomyosarcoma, inflammatory sarcomatoid carcinoma, and inflammatory malignant fibrous histiocytoma show a greater degree of cytological atypia than is seen in IMTs and occur in adults. The immunoprofiles also differ from those of myofibroblastic proliferations [71].

Histiocytoid Cardiomyopathy

The name of this entity reflects the original belief that the lesion was composed of histiocytes due to the morphological appearance of lesional cells microscopically [74]. However, it has since become apparent that the cells are possibly derived either from myocytes or Purkinje cells [75, 76], hence the alternative name "Purkinje cell tumor." Although classified as a "tumor" in most textbooks, with consideration given to a neoplastic or hamartomatous etiology, some dispute this designation and suggest instead that the entity is a cardiomyopathy [76], probably resulting from a mitochondrial disorder [77–79]. A possible viral etiology has also been mooted, but evidence for this is lacking [76, 77].

This process is a very rare entity which occurs only in the very young. It is uncommon to see a case in a child over the age of 2 years [75]. There is a strong predilection for females [76, 79], and there appears to be an overlap between histiocytoid cardiomyopathy and microphthalmia with linear skin defect (MLS) – a genetic disease which shows monosomy for Xp22, with many patients sharing similar features. This has led to speculation that histiocytoid cardiomyopathy has an X-linked pattern of inheritance. The predominance of females would be explained by prenatal lethality in affected males [77]. Five percent of cases are familial [75].

Histiocytoid cardiomyopathy usually presents with arrhythmias, including supraventricular tachycardia and atrial or ventricular fibrillation [75, 79]. It may present with sudden death and is an important entity to consider at autopsy before classifying a case as "sudden infant death syndrome." Occasional patients present with a flu-like prodrome [77]. Several congenital cardiac anomalies are associated with histiocytoid cardiomyopathy, including ventricular and atrial septal defects and hypoplastic left heart syndrome. Extracardiac malformations occur in 17% of cases, including cataract, corneal opacities, microcephaly, hydrocephalus, cleft palate, laryngeal web, linear skin defect, aphakia, and agenesis of the corpus callosum [75]. In 7% of cases, "histiocytoid" cells are seen in other organs [75]. Untreated, histiocytoid cardiomyopathy is usually fatal by the age of 2 years. However, since the introduction of surgical excision and cryoablation therapies, the survival rate has now risen to approximately 80% [75, 77].

On examination of the heart, there is usually cardiomegaly [77]. A congenital structural abnormality may also be present. Single or multiple yellow nodules 0.1–1.5 cm in size are seen, most commonly beneath the endocardium, and tend to be distributed along the course of the cardiac conduction system [75]. However, nodules may occur within the myocardium, subepicardium, or on cardiac valves. Occasionally, no discrete lesion is identifiable macroscopically, although in some cases the myocardium may have a mottled appearance in

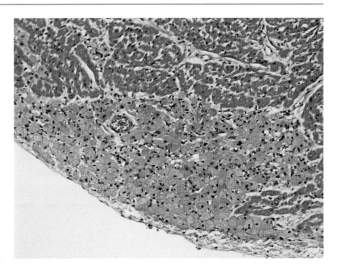

Fig. 12.19 Histiocytoid cardiomyopathy showing aggregates of large polygonal cells with copious granular or vacuolated cytoplasm and small bland nuclei (Hematoxylin and eosin) (Courtesy of Dr M Ashworth)

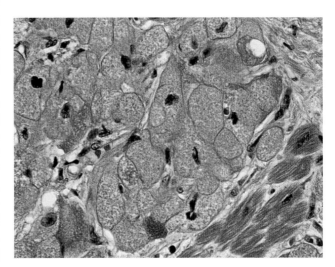

Fig. 12.20 High magnification of histiocytoid cardiomyopathy (Hematoxylin and eosin) (Courtesy of Dr. M Ashworth)

places [75]. The lesions are composed of aggregates of large polygonal cells, with copious granular or bubbly cytoplasm and small bland nuclei (Figs. 12.19 and 12.20). No mitoses are seen. The PAS stain for glycogen and stains for lipid show only faint positivity [77]. Immunohistochemistry for histiocytic markers such as CD68 are negative, and staining for S100 is variable [75]. Studies have shown positive staining with cholinesterase antibody, which lends support to the hypothesis that the lesions are of Purkinje cell origin [77]. Ultrastructural studies have shown markedly increased and sometimes morphologically abnormal mitochondria [75, 77].

The differential diagnosis includes storage disorders, mitochondrial cardiomyopathy, and rhabdomyoma. Glycogen and lipid storage disorders show strong staining with PAS and Sudan black respectively. Only weak staining is seen with these markers in histiocytoid cardiomyopathy [77, 79]. Although it has been suggested that histiocytoid cardiomyopathy may be a mitochondrial cardiomyopathy of some description, this term should be reserved for cases where there is a diffuse abnormality of myocytes, occurring in the clinical context of a maternally inherited disorder in which there is cardiac hypertrophy or a dilated cardiomyopathy [75, 80]. Rhabdomyoma may also occur as multiple nodules, but careful consideration of histological features should enable the pathologist to distinguish between the two entities.

Primary Cardiac Sarcoma

The vast majority of primary malignant tumors of the heart are sarcomas (Fig. 12.21). However, overall malignant tumors as a group are rare and account for only 10% of primary cardiac tumors [81]. The commonest of the classifiable sarcomas is angiosarcoma, which accounts for 33% of cases [82]. Rhabdomyosarcoma is the commonest primary cardiac sarcoma of childhood [83]. The following soft tissue tumors have also been documented as primary cardiac tumors, although the individual tumor incidence varies between different series: fibrosarcoma, osteosarcoma and chondrosarcoma, malignant peripheral nerve sheath tumor, leiomyosarcoma (Fig. 12.22), liposarcoma, synovial sarcoma, fibromyxosarcoma, myxofibrosarcoma, and undifferentiated sarcoma [81–85].

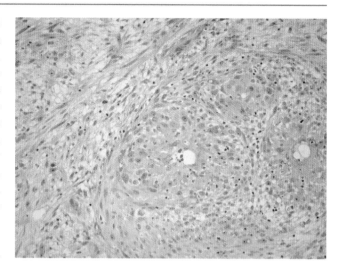

Fig. 12.22 Leiomyosarcoma of the heart with epithelioid and pleomorphic sarcomatous elements (Hematoxylin and eosin)

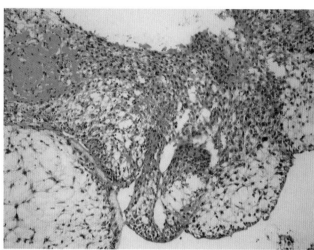

Fig. 12.23 Myxoid cardiac sarcoma with variable cell density and moderate pleomorphism (Hematoxylin and eosin)

Many sarcomas of the heart tend to have a variable amount of myxoid stroma (Fig. 12.23), which can lead to a misdiagnosis of the common cardiac myxoma. Careful attention to morphology is therefore required. Both angiosarcoma and synovial sarcoma may be confused with mesothelioma, which again is a more common entity at this site. Negative cytokeratin and calretinin staining, with strong positivity for endothelial markers, favors angiosarcoma. Genetic studies for the X:18 translocation may be required to confirm a diagnosis of synovial sarcoma.

The commonest classifiable sarcomas of adults and children, angiosarcoma and rhabdomyosarcoma, will be specifically considered. The remainder are relatively rare, and only very occasional case reports exist for each entity. All the sarcomas parallel their extracardiac counterparts.

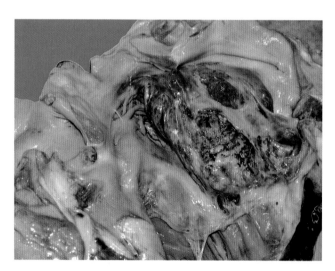

Fig. 12.21 Macroscopic view of a right atrial angiosarcoma showing infiltration of the right atrial wall and projection into the cavity (Courtesy of Dr. A Bell)

Primary Cardiac Angiosarcoma

This malignant neoplasm arises from the endothelial lining of blood vessels and shows endothelial differentiation. It is the commonest cardiac sarcoma, accounting for 33% of cases [82]. Angiosarcoma of the heart occurs over a wide age range (3–80 years), but it is extremely rare in childhood. It is commonest in the fourth decade and there is a male predominance [81, 86, 87]. The tumor may present with sudden death or signs and symptoms associated with a mass lesion within the heart. Hemopericardium may feature [81, 86–88] and patients may present with metastatic disease. Older reviews tend to quote a metastatic rate of greater than 60%. However, with improved imaging techniques, patients now tend to be diagnosed relatively early, potentially before metastases have occurred.

Despite earlier presentation than in the past, the prognosis for cardiac angiosarcoma is very poor. Patients die either from localized effects of the tumor, which may include cardiac rupture, or metastatic disease, commonly to the lungs or brain. There is an increased incidence in brain metastases following surgical intervention. This is postulated to be due to dissemination of tumor cells occurring at the time of surgery [87]. Patients who do not undergo surgical resection have a mean survival of 3.8 months, whereas the mean postoperative survival for those who undergo cardiac transplantation or total or partial resection is 10.6 months. Occasional "long-term" (up to 53 months) survivors have been documented [87].

Angiosarcomas tend to occur on the right side, most commonly the right atrium [86, 87]. The tumors are large, hemorrhagic, and infiltrative. They involve the myocardium and pericardium and may also infiltrate the cardiac valves, caval and pulmonary vessels, and ascending aorta [87]. The histological appearance of cardiac angiosarcoma does not differ from that of angiosarcoma found elsewhere. Histological grade is not an independent prognostic indicator in cardiac angiosarcomas and is not statistically correlated with survival [87]. Cytology of pericardial effusions generally has a poor diagnostic yield [87, 88], and cardiac biopsy is the diagnostic modality of choice.

Endothelial markers CD31 and factor VIII are helpful in establishing the diagnosis of a malignant vascular tumor, as many sarcomas in the heart may have poorly differentiated phenotypes (Fig. 12.24). However, factor VIII in particular lacks sensitivity and is reported to be negative in the majority of cases [87]. CD34 is another marker of endothelial cells, but its relative lack of specificity limits its value.

The differential diagnosis includes benign or malignant mesothelial proliferations, hemangioma, and primary pericardial angiosarcoma. On biopsy specimens, angiosarcomas may be difficult to differentiate from reactive mesothelial

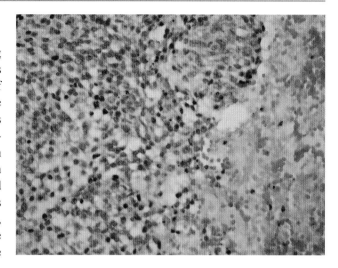

Fig. 12.24 High magnification view of a cardiac angiosarcoma. There may be little evidence of endothelial differentiation, requiring CD34, CD31, or factor VIII immunohistology for positive identification (Hematoxylin and eosin)

hyperplasia or mesothelioma, particularly if the tumor is pericardial [81, 87]. Cytokeratin combined with endothelial markers may be useful in such cases. Cytokeratins are generally negative, although weak focal staining of conventional angiosarcomas has been reported, and positive staining in epithelioid variants also occurs [87]. However, strong diffuse staining with cytokeratin should alert the pathologist to the alternative diagnosis of mesothelioma or carcinoma. Synovial sarcoma should also be considered in cases of cytokeratin-positive primary cardiac tumors, although this too is rare. If the tumor is well differentiated, a benign hemangioma should be considered. In addition to histological features, macroscopic appearances and imaging studies may be helpful. Primary pericardial angiosarcoma may also occur, although much less commonly than myocardial angiosarcoma. It should be suspected if the tumor presents with marked diffuse thickening of the pericardium rather than a mass lesion within the myocardium [87].

Rhabdomyosarcoma

This sarcoma shows differentiation towards striated muscle. Rhabdomyosarcoma is the commonest malignant primary cardiac tumor in the pediatric age group [82, 89, 90], but can occasionally occur in adults. It should be noted that the rarity of rhabdomyosarcomas, as a primary cardiac tumor, means that epidemiological and other data are based on relatively few cases. Current evidence shows that rhabdomyosarcoma occurs equally in both sexes, and 75% occur in children less than 1 year old [82]. The prognosis is poor, with recurrence and/or metastases leading to death within one year [90], even with aggressive intervention, although there is a report of long-term survival following cardiac transplantation [91] for a primary cardiac rhabdomyosarcoma in an adult.

Rhabdomyosarcoma may originate anywhere in the heart [90], and 60% of cases appear multicentric [82]. They tend to arise within the myocardium, with no chamber bias, rather than as intraluminal masses [90]. However, they can be large and expand to fill the cardiac chambers. They are also infiltrative, with the pericardium usually involved at presentation [82]. Involvement of the cardiac valves may occur [82]. The tumors are often macroscopically mucoid or gelatinous and variably necrotic [90].

Primary cardiac rhabdomyosarcomas are usually embryonal in histological type, although sarcoma botryoides has been described. Alveolar rhabdomyosarcomas are only described in cases of metastasis to the heart [90]. As for rhabdomyosarcomas at other sites, stains for desmin, myogenin, and Myo D1 are positive in tumor cells.

Primary Sarcoma of the Major Pulmonary Vessels

There are several types of sarcoma, which may be characteristically encountered in the large vessels in close proximity to the heart. These may be classified as discrete entities [92, 93]:

- Pulmonary artery sarcoma – sometimes split into intimal and mural types
- Sarcoma of the aorta
- Sarcoma of the pulmonary veins
- Sarcoma of the inferior vena cava

All are exceptionally rare, but sarcoma of the pulmonary artery, intimal type, is the commonest and will be considered here. It is thought to arise from intimal pluripotential mesenchymal cells [93, 94]. Most texts do not differentiate between intimal and mural types [93].

Pulmonary artery sarcoma occurs over an age range of 21–80 years with an equal sex distribution. Clinical presentation is with symptoms and signs secondary to pulmonary outflow tract obstruction. Imaging studies are often misinterpreted as showing pulmonary thromboembolism [92, 95]. The tumor is very rare, and the true incidence was hidden [93] until recently when the pulmonary thromboendarterectomy procedure was introduced. Prior to this, the diagnosis was usually made at postmortem, and many cases were probably misdiagnosed as pulmonary thromboembolism on imaging. In recent years these cases have sometimes been first diagnosed in surgical material obtained during thromboendarterectomy [96, 97]. In the authors' center, over a six-year period, four cases out of a total of 235 pulmonary thromboendarterectomy specimens were found to be pulmonary artery sarcomas. In these cases (all intimal), the possibility of malignancy was suspected, either radiologically or in view of intraoperative appearances.

Pulmonary endarterectomy has recently been heralded as a successful, palliative treatment for pulmonary artery sarcoma [96, 98], which previously had a uniformly dire prognosis, even if correctly diagnosed antemortem.

The tumor usually arises from the intimal surface of the pulmonary trunk as a gelatinous polypoid mass, associated with thrombus, which grows intraluminally, often extending into the main pulmonary arteries. Retrograde extension, with involvement of the pulmonary valve and sometimes the right heart chamber, may also occur [93, 95]. Tumor emboli to the more distal intrapulmonary vessels may be difficult to distinguish from multifocal disease or metastases.

Intimal pulmonary sarcomas grow along the vessel lumen. On microscopy they can be seen to extend along the vessel wall, splitting apart the layers of intima and media [92], but tend to remain superficial and are confined within the vessel. The tumors are usually myxoid spindle cell lesions, with varying degrees of atypia between cases (Fig. 12.25). Many documented cases show at least focal differentiation, leading to classification as one of the following tumor types: leiomyosarcoma, osteosarcoma, chondrosarcoma, rhabdomyosarcoma, fibromyxosarcoma, mesenchymoma, myxosarcoma, or angiosarcoma [95].

Intimal pulmonary artery sarcoma shows immunohistochemical evidence of myofibroblastic differentiation, with positivity for vimentin and variable staining for actin [93]. Those tumors showing differentiation towards another specific sarcoma phenotype show immunostaining accordingly [93]. The differential diagnosis includes thromboembolic material and cardiac myxoma.

Primary Cardiac Lymphoma

Primary cardiac lymphoma is defined as a lymphoma confined to the heart and pericardium, with no or minimal evidence of concurrent or previous extracardiac involvement [99]. Cardiac involvement by systemic lymphoma occurs relatively frequently, but primary cardiac lymphoma is very rare and accounts for only 1% of primary cardiac tumors [99]. However, in the setting of cardiac transplantation, posttransplant lymphoproliferative (PTLPD) disorder occurs much more frequently, with a prevalence of 14% at 5 years and 32% at 10 years [100] (see Chap. 10).

For primary cardiac lymphoma (Fig. 12.26), the mean age at presentation is 60 years with a male predominance [99], although other ages of presentation do occur. Other risk factors for lymphoma, such as HIV, may be present. The patient may present with signs and symptoms secondary to the mass and/or an intractable pericardial effusion, which can be massive [99]. Pulmonary embolus or systemic symptoms may

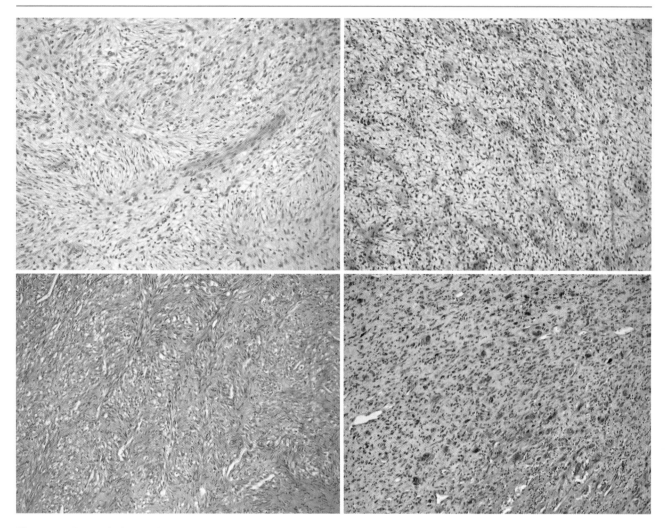

Fig. 12.25 Composite image of varying microscopic appearances of primary pulmonary artery sarcomas. Some appear relatively bland and low grade, with others showing pleomorphic polynucleate cells (Hematoxylin and eosin)

occur [99]. The prognosis is poor, with a mean survival of only 7 months, despite modern lymphoma chemotherapy.

The tumors are predominantly right sided and commonly involve more than one cardiac chamber [99]. Usually there is diffuse infiltration of the cardiac tissues (Fig. 12.27), or alternatively, multiple tumor nodules can be present [99]. Some tumors encase the heart with contiguous involvement of the pericardium.

Primary cardiac lymphomas are almost invariably non-Hodgkin lymphomas of B-cell type. The commonest primary cardiac lymphoma is diffuse large B-cell lymphoma, which accounts for 80% of cases [101]. Where a pericardial effusion is present, in such cases the lymphoma may be detected in cytology samples in up to 88% of cases [101]. The immunohistochemical antibody panel may reflect the lymphoma morphology.

The differential diagnosis, in transplant cases, includes posttransplant lymphoproliferative disorder and benign reactive lymphocytosis. In the setting of cardiac transplantation,

there should be a high index of suspicion for posttransplant lymphoproliferative disorder, and ancillary tests for the detection of Epstein–Barr virus should be performed in addition to other studies. Pericardial fluid samples may be misinterpreted as "inflammatory," and flow cytometry studies may be required to confirm lymphoma.

Tumors of the Pericardium

Tumors common to the pleura, namely, mesothelioma (Fig. 12.28) and solitary fibrous tumor, may also occur in the pericardium, albeit rarely [102, 103]. In addition, primary germ cell tumors can occur at this site. It is believed that germ cell tumors are derived from ectopic primordial germ cells, which have undergone migration arrest on their journey from yolk sac to the gonads during embryogenesis. Benign teratomas are the commonest tumor of this group in the heart and usually occur prenatally or in infancy. Pericardial

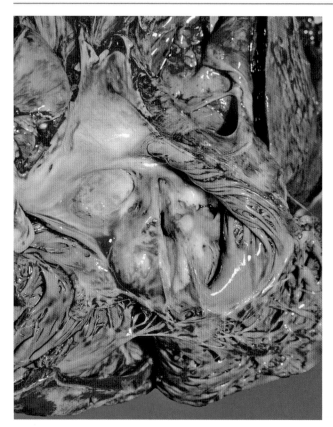

Fig. 12.26 Primary cardiac lymphoma in a teenage male who died suddenly and with no antecedent history. There are irregular lobulated masses of tumor interfering with chamber alignment and blood flow

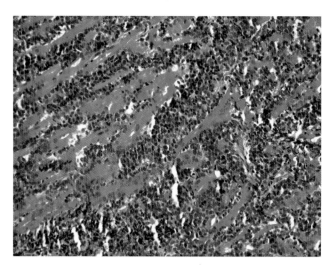

Fig. 12.27 Cardiac lymphoma showing separation and destruction of myocytes by infiltrating lymphoid cells (Hematoxylin and eosin)

germ cell tumors in adults are vanishingly rare but, when they do occur, are more often malignant [104]. As with cardiac tumors themselves, pericardial metastases are more common than primary neoplasia (Fig. 12.29).

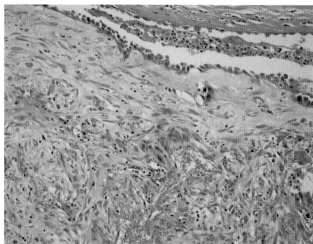

Fig. 12.28 Pericardial histology showing epicardial primary mesothelioma (Hematoxylin and eosin)

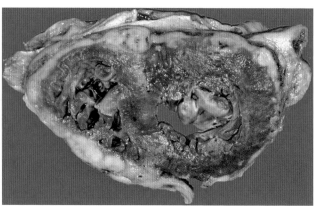

Fig. 12.29 Cross section of autopsy heart with pericardial encasement by metastatic lung carcinoma

References

1. Yu K, Liu Y, Wang H, et al. Epidemiological and pathological characteristics of cardiac tumours: a clinical study of 242 cases. Interact Cardiovasc Thorac Surg. 2007;6:636–9.
2. Suvarna SK, Royd JA. The nature of cardiac myxoma. Int J Cardiol. 1996;57:211–6.
3. Krikler DM, Rode J, Davies MJ, Woolf N, Moss E. Atrial myxoma: a tumour in search of its origins. Br Heart J. 1992;67:89–91.
4. Thomas-de-Montpreville V, Nottin R, Dulmet E, Serraf A. Heart tumours in children and adults: clinicopathological study of 59 patients from a surgical centre. Cardiovasc Pathol. 2007;16:22–8.
5. Yu K, Liu Y, Wang H, Hu S, et al. Epidemiological and pathological characteristics of cardiac tumours: a clinical study of 242 cases. Interact Cardiovasc Thorac Surg. 2007;6:636–9.
6. Bjessmo S, Ivert T. Cardiac myxoma: 40 years experience in 63 patients. Ann Thorac Surg. 1997;63:697–700.
7. Pucci A, Gagliardotto P, Zanini C. Histopathologic and clinical characterisation of cardiac myxoma: Review of 53 cases from a single institution. Am Heart J. 2000;140(1):134–8.
8. Fletcher C. Diagnostic histopathology of tumours. 2nd ed. New York: Churchill Livingstone; 2000. p. 17.

9. Reyen K. Cardiac myxomas. NEJM. 1995;333(24):1610–7.

10. McCarthy PM, Piehler JM, Carney JA, et al. The significance of multiple, recurrent and 'complex' cardiac myxomas. J Thorac Cardiovasc Surg. 1986;91:389–96.

11. Edwards A, Bermudez G, Maiers E, et al. Carney's syndrome: complex myxomas. Report of four cases and review of the literature. Cardiovasc Surg. 2002;10(3):264–75.

12. Gattuso P, Reddy VB, David O, Spitz DJ, Haber MH. Differential diagnosis in surgical pathology. Philadelphia: WB Saunders; 2002.

13. Travis WD, Brambilla E, Muller-Hermelink HK, Harris CC, editors. World Health Organization classification of tumours. Pathology and genetics of tumours of the lung, pleura, thymus and heart. Lyon: IARC Press; 2004. p. 284.

14. Sheppard M, Davies M. Practical cardiovascular pathology. London: Arnold; 1998. p. 150.

15. Keeling IM, Oberwalder P, Rigler B, et al. Cardiac myxomas: 24 years of experience in 49 patients. Eur J Cardiothorac Surg. 2002;22:971–7.

16. Burke A, Virmani R. More on cardiac myxomas. NEJM. 1996;335:1462–4.

17. Kusumi T, Minakawa M, Fukui K, et al. Cardiac tumour comprising two components, including typical myxoma and atypical hypercellularity suggesting malignant change. Cardiovasc Pathol. 2009;18:369–74.

18. Travis WD, Brambilla E, Muller-Hermelink HK, Harris CC, editors. World Health Organization classification of tumours. Pathology and genetics of tumours of the lung, pleura, thymus and heart. Lyon: IARC Press; 2004. p. 263–5.

19. Mariscalco G, Bruno VD, Sala A, et al. Papillary fibroelastoma: insight into a primary cardiac valve tumour. J Card Surg. 2010;25:198–205.

20. Fletcher CDM. Diagnostic histopathology of tumors. 2nd ed. London: Churchill Livingstone; 2001. p. 26–8.

21. Sheppard M, Davies MJ. Practical cardiovascular pathology. 1st ed. London: Arnold; 1998. p. 155–6.

22. Kumar TK, Kuehl K, Jonas RA, et al. Multiple papillary fibroelastomas of the heart. Ann Thorac Surg. 2009;88:66–7.

23. Sydow K, Willems S, Meinertz T, et al. Papillary fibroelastomas of the heart. Thorac Cardiovasc Surg. 2008;56:9–13.

24. Akay MH, Seiffert BS, Ott DA. Papillary fibroelastoma of the aortic valve as a cause of transient ischaemic attack. Tex Heart Inst J. 2009;36(2):158–9.

25. Kuwashiro T, Toyoda K, Minematsu K, et al. Cardiac papillary fibroelastoma as a cause of embolic stroke: ultrasound and histopathological characteristics. Int Med. 2009;48:77–80.

26. Hirose H, Matsunaga I, Strong MD. Left atrial fibroelastoma. Ann Thorac Cardiovasc Surg. 2009;15(6):412–4.

27. Ibrahim CPH, Thakker P, Miller PA, Barron D. Cardiac rhabdomyoma presenting as left ventricular outflow tract obstruction in a neonate. Interact Cardiovasc Thorac Surg. 2003;2:572–4.

28. Karsuski RA, Hesselson AB, Landolfo KP, et al. Cardiac rhabdomyoma in an adult patient presenting with ventricular arrhythmia. Chest. 2000;118(4):1217–21.

29. Kawada H, Kawada J, Iwahara K, et al. Multiple cutaneous rhabdomyomas in a child. Eur J Dematol. 2004;14(6):418–20.

30. Chao AS, Chao A, Wang TH, et al. Outcome of antenatally diagnosed cardiac rhabdomyoma: case series and a meta-analysis. Ultrasound Obstet Gynaecol. 2008;31:289–95.

31. Uzun O, Wilson DG, Vujanic GM, et al. Cardiac tumours in children. Orphanet J Rare Dis. 2007;2:11. Review.

32. Ramirez-Marrero MA, Cuenca-Peiro V, Zabala-Arguelles JI, Conejo-Munoz L. Early complete regression of multiple cardiac tumours suggestive of cardiac rhabdomyomas. Rev Esp Cardiol. 2009;62(6):708–9.

33. Travis WD, Brambilla E, Muller-Hermelink HK, Harris CC, editors. World Health Organization classification of tumours. Pathology and genetics of tumours of the lung, pleura, thymus and heart. Lyon: IARC Press; 2004. p. 254–6.

34. Atik E. Late spontaneous regression of obstructive tumour in the mitral valve. Arq Bras Cardiol. 2009;93(4):48–50.

35. Amonkar GP, Kandalkar BM, Balasubramanian M. Cardiac rhabdomyoma. Cardiovasc Pathol. 2009;18:313–4.

36. Fletcher CDM. Diagnostic histopathology of tumors. 2nd ed. Edinburgh: Churchill-Livingstone; 2001. p. 21–3.

37. Travis WD, Brambilla E, Muller-Hermelink HK, Harris CC, editors. World Health Organization classification of tumours. Pathology and genetics of tumours of the lung, pleura, thymus and heart. Lyon: IARC Press; 2004. p. 268–9.

38. Parmley LF, Salley RK, Head B, et al. The clinical spectrum of cardiac fibroma with diagnostic and surgical considerations: noninvasive imaging enhances management. Ann Thorac Surg. 1988;45:455–65.

39. Sheppard M, Davies MJ. Practical cardiovascular pathology. 1st ed. London: Arnold; 1998. p. 154–5.

40. Krane M, Bauernschmitt R, Lange R, et al. Right ventricular fibroma in a 61 year old man. Thorac Cardiovasc Surg. 2009;57:232–42.

41. Agrawal SKB, Rakhit DJ, Harden SP, et al. Large intra-cardiac benign fibrous tumour presenting in an adult patient identified using MRI. Clin Radiol. 2009;64:637–40.

42. Gasparovic H, Coric V, Jelic I, et al. Left ventricular fibroma mimicking an acute coronary syndrome. Ann Thorac Surg. 2006;82(5):1891–2.

43. Cameselle-Tejieiro J, Abdulkader I, Soares P, et al. Cystic tumour of the atrioventricular node of the heart appears to be the heart equivalent of the solid cell nests (ultimobranchial rests) of the thyroid. Am J Clin Pathol. 2005;123(3):369–75.

44. Evans CA, Suvarna SK. Cystic atrioventricular node tumour: not a mesothelioma. J Clin Pathol. 2005;58(11):1232.

45. Travis WD, Brambilla E, Muller-Hermelink HK, Harris CC, editors. World Health Organization classification of tumours. Pathology and genetics of tumours of the lung, pleura, thymus and heart. Lyon: IARC Press; 2004. p. 272.

46. Saito S, Kobayashi J, Tagusari O, et al. Successful excision of a cystic tumour of the atrioventricular nodal region. Circ J. 2005;69:1293–4.

47. Paniagua JR, Sadaba JR, Davidson LA, Munsch CM. Cystic tumour of the atrioventricular nodal region: report of a case successfully treated with surgery. Heart. 2000;83:e6.

48. Tran TT, Starnes V, Wang X, Getzen J, Ross BD. Cardiovascular magnetics resonance diagnosis of cystic tumour of the atrioventricular node. J Cardiovasc Magn Reson. 2009;11:13.

49. Ruggiero NJ, Doherty JU, Ferrari VA, Hansen CL. Myocardial perfusion defect caused by intramyocardial lipoma. J Nucl Cardiol. 2008;15(2):286–9.

50. Gulmez O, Pehlivanoglu S, Turkoz R, et al. Lipoma of the right atrium. J Clin Ultrasound. 2009;37(3):185–8.

51. Riva L, Banfi C, Gaeta R, Vigano M. Lipomatous hypertrophy of the interatrial septum. Minerva Cardioangiol. 2006;54(6):789–92.

52. Sheppard M, Davies MJ. Practical cardiovascular pathology. 1st ed. London: Arnold; 1998. p. 158–9.

53. Travis WD, Brambilla E, Muller-Hermelink HK, Harris CC, editors. World Health Organisation classification of tumours. Pathology and genetics of tumours of the lung, pleura, thymus and heart. Lyon: IARC Press; 2004. p. 271.

54. Arena V, Valerio L, Capelli A. Lipomatous hypertrophy vs cardiac hibernoma. What criteria differentiate them? Cardiovasc Pathol. 2009;18:250–1. [Correspondence].

55. Zhang J, Chong E, Chai P, Poh KK. Contrasting fatty involvement of the right ventricle: lipoma versus lipomatous hypertrophy. Singapore Med J. 2009;50(10):342–5.

56. Dettrick AJ. Lipomatous hypertrophy of the interatrial septum: a report of an unusual case. Histopathology. 2009;54:777–9.

57. Ganame J, Wright J, Bogaert J. Cardiac lipoma diagnosed by cardiac magnetic resonance imaging. Eur Heart J. 2008;29(6):697.

58. Ucak A, Inan K, Onan B, Yilmaz AT. Resection of intrapericardial hibernoma associated with constrictive pericarditis. Interact Cardiovasc Thorac Surg. 2009;9:717–9.

59. Brodwater B, Erasmus J, McAdams HP, Dodd L. Pericardial haemangioma. J Comput Assist Tomogr. 1996;20(6):954–6.

60. Mongal LS, Salat R, Anis A, et al. Enormous right atrial haemangioma in an asymptomatic patient: a case report and literature review. Echocardiography. 2009;26(8):973–6.

61. Eftychiou C, Antoniades L. Cardiac haemangioma in the left ventricle and brief review of the literature. J Cardiovasc Med. 2009;10(7):565–7.

62. Kojima S, Sumiyoshi M, Suwa S, et al. Cardiac haemangioma: a report of two cases and review of the literature. Heart Vessels. 2003;18:153–6.

63. Yaganti V, Patel S, Yaganti S, Victor M. Cavernous haemangioma of the mitral valve: a case report and review of the literature. J Cardiovasc Med. 2009;10(5):420–2.

64. Kasmani R, Holt R, Narwal-Chadha R, et al. An incidental right atrial mass: cavernous haemangioma. Am J Med Sci. 2009;338(4):328–9.

65. Travis WD, Brambilla E, Muller-Hermelink HK, Harris CC, editors. World Health Organization classification of tumours. Pathology and genetics of tumours of the lung, pleura, thymus and heart. Lyon: IARC Press; 2004. p. 266–7.

66. Abad C, de Varona S, Limeres MA, et al. Resection of a left atrial haemangioma. Report of a case and overview of the literature on resected cardiac haemangiomas. Tex Heart Inst J. 2008;35(1):69–72.

67. Pucci A, Valori A, Muscio M, et al. Asymptomatic inflammatory myofibroblastic tumour of the heart: immunohistochemical profile, differential diagnosis, and review of the literature. Cardiovasc Pathol. 2009;18:187–90.

68. Di Maria MV, Campbell DN, Mitchell MB, et al. Successful orthotopic heart transplant in an infant with an inflammatory myofibroblastic tumour of the left ventricle. J Heart Lung Transplant. 2008;27(7):792–6.

69. Sebire NJ, Ramsay A, Sheppard M, et al. Intravascular inflammatory myofibroblastic tumours in infancy. Paediatr Dev Pathol. 2002;5(4):400–4.

70. Burke A, Li L, Kling E, et al. Cardiac inflammatory myofibroblastic tumour: a "benign" neoplasm that may result in syncope, myocardial infarction, and sudden death. Am J Surg Pathol. 2007;31(7):1115–22.

71. Li L, Cerilli LA, Wick MR. Inflammatory pseudotumour (myofibroblastic tumour) of the heart. Ann Diagn Pathol. 2002;6(2):116–21.

72. Miller DV, Tazelaar HD. Cardiovascular pseudoneoplasms. Arch Pathol Lab Med. 2010;134:362–8.

73. Travis WD, Brambilla E, Muller-Hermelink HK, Harris CC, editors. World Health Organization classification of tumours. Pathology and genetics of tumours of the lung, pleura, thymus and heart. Lyon: IARC Press; 2004. p. 270.

74. Sheppard M, Davies MJ. Practical cardiovascular pathology. 1st ed. London: Arnold; 1998. p. 157–8.

75. Travis WD, Brambilla E, Muller-Hermelink HK, Harris CC, editors. World Health Organization classification of tumours. Pathology and genetics of tumours of the lung, pleura, thymus and heart. Lyon: IARC Press; 2004. p. 256–8.

76. Becker AE. Tumors of the heart and pericardium in diagnostic histopathology of tumors. Edinburgh: Churchill Livingstone; 2000.

77. Shehata BM, Patterson K, Thomas JE, et al. Histiocytoid cardiomyopathy: three new cases and a review of the literature. Pediatr Dev Pathol. 1998;1:56–69.

78. Finsterer J. Histiocytoid cardiomyopathy: a mitochondrial disorder. Clin Cardiol. 2008;31:225–7.

79. Prahlow JA, Teot LA. Histiocytoid cardiomyopathy: case report and literature review. J Forensic Sci. 1993;38:1427–35.

80. Gallo P, d'Amati G. Cardiomyopathies. In: Silver MD, Gotlieb AI, Schoen FJ, editors. Cardiovascular pathology. Philadelphia: Churchill Livingstone; 2001. p. 315–6.

81. Burke A. Primary malignant cardiac tumors. Semin Diagn Pathol. 2008;25:39–46.

82. Neragi-Miandoab S, Kim J, Vlahakes GJ. Malignant tumours of the heart: a review of tumour type, diagnosis and therapy. Clin Oncol. 2007;19:748–56.

83. Burke AP, Virmani R. Atlas of tumour pathology. 3rd ed. Washington (DC): Armed Forces Institute of Pathology; 1995.

84. Donsbeck AV, Ranchere D, Loire R, et al. Primary cardiac sarcomas: an immunohistochemical and grading study with long-term follow-up of 24 cases. Histopathology. 1999;34:295–304.

85. Simpson L, Kumar SK, Moynihan TJ, et al. Malignant primary cardiac tumors. Review of a single institution experience. Cancer. 2008;112(11):2440–6.

86. Carpino F, Pezzoli F, Gaudio C, et al. Angiosarcoma of the heart: structural and ultrastructural study. Eur Rev Med Pharmacol Sci. 2005;9:231–40.

87. Butany J, Weiming Y. Cardiac angiosarcoma: two cases and a review of the literature. Can J Cardiol. 2000;16(2):197–205.

88. El-Osta HE, Yammine YS, Mattar BI, et al. Unexplained hemopericardium as a presenting feature of primary cardiac angiosarcoma: a case report and a review of the diagnostic dilemma. J Thorac Oncol. 2008;3(7):800–2.

89. Becker AE. Primary heart tumours in the paediatric age group: a review of salient pathologic features relevant for clinicians. Paediatr Cardiol. 2000;21(4):317–23.

90. Travis WD, Brambilla E, Muller-Hermelink HK, Harris CC, editors. World Health Organization classification of tumours. Pathology and genetics of tumours of the lung, pleura, thymus and heart. Lyon: IARC Press; 2004. p. 279.

91. Grandmougin D, Fayad G, Warembourg H, et al. Total orthotopic heart transplantation for primary cardiac rhabdomyosarcoma: factors influencing long-term survival. Ann Thorac Surg. 2001;71:1438–41.

92. Weiss SW, Goldblum JR. Enzinger and Weiss soft tissue tumors. 5th ed. Philadelphia: Mosby Elsevier; 2008. p. 557–9.

93. Travis WD, Brambilla E, Muller-Hermelink HK, Harris CC, editors. World Health Organization classification of tumours. Pathology and genetics of tumours of the lung, pleura, thymus and heart. Lyon: IARC Press; 2004. p. 109–10.

94. Johansson L, Carlen B. Sarcoma of the pulmonary artery: a report of four cases with electron microscopic and immunohistochemical examinations, and review of the literature. Virchows Arch. 1994;424:217–24.

95. Corrin B, Nicholson AG. Pathology of the lungs. 2nd ed. London: Churchill Livingstone Elsevier; 2006. p. 627–9.

96. Kerr KM. Pulmonary artery sarcoma masquerading as chronic thromboembolic pulmonary hypertension. Nat Clin Pract Cardiovasc Med. 2005;2(2):108–12.

97. Maruo A, Okita Y, Tanimura N, et al. Surgical experience for the pulmonary artery sarcoma. Ann Thorac Surg. 2006;82:2014–6.

98. Thakrar MV, Hirani N, Helmersen D. Recurrent pulmonary artery sarcoma treated with repeat pulmonary endarterectomy. Am J Respir Crit Care Med. 2010;181:A1587.

99. Gowda RM, Khan IA. Clinical perspectives of primary cardiac lymphoma. Angiology. 2003;54(5):599–604.

100. Manlhiot C, Pollock-BarZiv SM, Dipchand AI, et al. Post-transplant lymphoproliferative disorder in pediatric heart transplant recipients. J Heart Lung Transpl. 2010;29(6): 648–57.

101. Travis WD, Brambilla E, Muller-Hermelink HK, Harris CC, editors. World Health Organization classification of tumours. Pathology and genetics of tumours of the lung, pleura, thymus and heart. Lyon: IARC Press; 2004. p. 282–3.

102. Thomason R, Schlegel W, Lee S. Primary malignant mesothelioma of the pericardium. Case report and review of the literature. Tex Heart Inst J. 1994;21(2):170–4.

103. Andreani SM, Tavecchio L, Bedini AV. Extrapericardial solitary fibrous tumour of the pericardium. Eur J Cardiothorac Surg. 1998;14:98–100.

104. Travis WD, Brambilla E, Muller-Hermelink HK, Harris CC, editors. World Health Organization classification of tumours. Pathology and genetics of tumours of the lung, pleura, thymus and heart. Lyon: IARC Press; 2004. p. 285–8.

Congenital Heart Disease

13

Michael T. Ashworth

Abstract

All congenital heart disease can be understood by systematic examination of their component parts and how they relate one to the other – sequential segmental analysis. Secondary changes such as muscular hypertrophy or fibrosis may obscure some features, but the basic abnormalities are usually discernible beneath this secondary overlay. A small number of rather straightforward entities make up the bulk of cases of congenital heart disease seen in autopsy practice. In essence, these comprise abnormal communications between the systemic and pulmonary components of the circulation and physical impediments to systemic or pulmonary blood flow. These common entities are described in some detail and illustrated in this chapter together with some rarer, but archetypal, lesions.

Keywords

Ventricular septal defect • Atrial septal defect • Coarctation • Pulmonary atresia • Aortic stenosis • Ebstein's malformation • Common arterial trunk • Anomalous pulmonary venous connection • Hypoplastic left heart

Introduction

Congenital heart disease has developed a reputation among many pathologists as a difficult subject. In fact, examination of the structurally malformed heart is usually straightforward and, provided that basic principles are followed, should hold no terrors for the pathologist. The heart is examined in the logical fashion of "sequential segmental analysis" [1], in which the segments of the heart are identified and their connections established and associated abnormalities noted. Standard tables of appropriate heart weights and dimensions at varying ages are available [2, 3]. A working knowledge of the commoner forms of surgery for congenital heart disease is necessary [4] since most cases coming to the attention of the general pathologist will have undergone some form of

M.T. Ashworth, M.D., FRCPath
Department of Histopathology,
Great Ormond Street Hospital for Children,
London WC1N 3JN, UK
e-mail: michael.ashworth@gosh.nhs.uk

surgical procedure. If in doubt, it is always safer to refer to the heart for specialist examination [5].

There are eight lesions that together account for about 80% of all cases of structural congenital heart disease [6]. These are:
1. Ventricular septal defect
2. Patent arterial duct
3. Atrial septal defect
4. Tetralogy of Fallot
5. Pulmonary stenosis
6. Coarctation of the aorta
7. Aortic stenosis
8. Transposition of the great arteries

The basic anatomy of these conditions is straightforward. They are described below, together with other distinct, albeit rarer and more complex, entities. The mainstay of the cardiologist in examining the congenitally malformed heart is echocardiography, although cardiac MR is increasingly used. There are several standard echocardiographic views of the heart [7], of which the three most common are the four-chamber view (Fig. 13.1), the long-axis view (Fig. 13.2), and

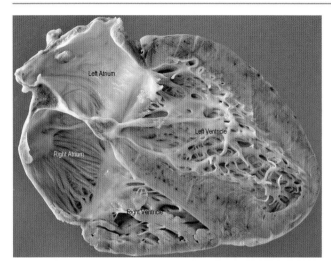

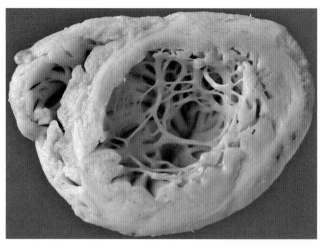

Fig. 13.1 Heart cut in a simulated echocardiographic four-chamber view. This heart actually shows dilated cardiomyopathy. Nevertheless, it demonstrates the normal anatomy very well. Note the muscular trabeculations in the right atrium that extend all the way around the atrioventricular junction – the left atrium, by contrast, is smooth. The muscular trabeculations at the apex of the right ventricle are coarse and parallel, and at the apex of the left ventricle, they are small and have a crisscross arrangement. Note also that the tricuspid valve has chordal attachments to the interventricular septum; the mitral valve does not. The mitral valve is attached to the interventricular septum at a higher level than the attachment of the tricuspid valve, so-called offsetting. This view of the heart is especially good for demonstrating relative chamber sizes

Fig. 13.3 Heart cut in a simulated echocardiographic short-axis view. This view is very familiar to pathologists since it forms part of the standard assessment of the heart. It includes both right and left ventricular walls and interventricular septum and, depending on the height of the cut, can include the tension apparatus of the atrioventricular valves

Ventricular Septal Defect

Ventricular septal defect (VSD), a communication between the right and left ventricular cavities can occur in isolation but also occurs as a part of many complex cardiac abnormalities (including tetralogy of Fallot, common arterial trunk, and atrioventricular septal defect). Its clinical effect depends on its size, location, and the presence of associated lesions. The defect is usually round or oval and varies in size from a few millimeters in the fetus to several centimeters postnatally [8].

Two basic forms are described depending on their relation to the membranous interventricular septum (Fig. 13.4): those involving the membranous septum, the so-called perimembranous VSD (Fig. 13.5) and those in which muscle is interposed between the defect and the membranous septum, the so-called muscular VSD (Fig. 13.6) [9]. In the normal heart, the septal leaflet of the tricuspid valve is attached to the membranous septum, and the mitral valve attachment on the left side is also related to the membranous septum. Thus, a perimembranous defect will, by definition, have fibrous continuity between the tricuspid and mitral valves through the defect. Muscular VSD may occur at any part of the interventricular septum and may be multiple. They may be located in the ventricular inlet, at the apex, or in the ventricular outlet. Due to associated ventricular hypertrophy, those occurring in the lower parts of the septum can be easily missed, even on close inspection of the heart, being hidden among the hypertrophied muscular trabeculations. Perimembranous and muscular VSD can coexist in the same heart. In the setting of a double-outlet ventricle, the outflow from the smaller ventricle will be dependent on the size of the VSD, and, if too small, the VSD is said to be restrictive.

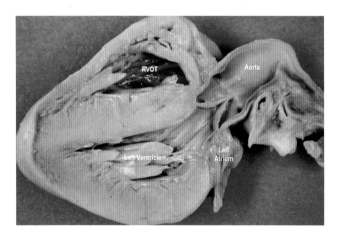

Fig. 13.2 Normal heart cut in a simulated echocardiographic long-axis view. By convention, the apex is presented on the *left* of the picture. This view of the heart demonstrates very well the left-sided structures – left atrium, mitral valve, left ventricle, left ventricular outflow tract, aortic valve, and aorta. The only part of the right heart seen in this view is the right ventricular outflow tract (*RVOT*) which is a complete muscular ring forming the pulmonary infundibulum – the pulmonary valve is anterior to the plane of section

the short-axis view (Fig. 13.3). These standard echocardiographic views can be simulated in dissection of the heart. It is possible to examine the heart perfectly adequately without employing them, but they do provide images of the heart that can be readily understood by the cardiologist or surgeon, and they are used extensively in this chapter.

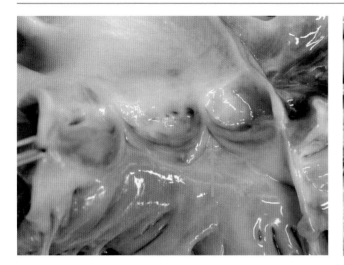

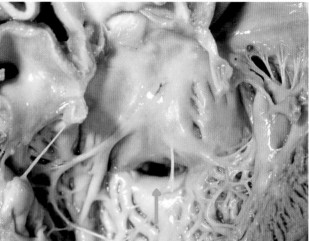

Fig. 13.4 Interventricular membranous septum. A photograph of the opened left ventricular outflow tract to demonstrate the aortic valve. The anterior leaflet of the mitral valve has been divided, and its cut edges are visible at the extreme *right* and *left sides* of the *mid part* of the picture. The three cusps of the aortic valve are visible: the left cusp on the *left* of the picture, the right cusp in the *center*, and the noncoronary cusp on the *right side*. There are two small accessory vessels arising from the right coronary sinus – a common variant of normal. The membranous septum is visible as a triangle of *gray* tissue interposed between the ventricular attachments of the right and noncoronary cusps (*arrow*)

Fig. 13.6 Muscular ventricular septal defect. A heart opened in a similar fashion to that in Figs. 13.4 and 13.5 to demonstrate the left ventricular outflow tract and interventricular septum. There is a ventricular septal defect in the mid part of the interventricular septum (*arrow*). The edges of the defect are smooth. The membranous septum (*asterisk*) is intact. Muscular defects are less common than perimembranous defects. Those near the ventricular apex may be very difficult to see because of hypertrophy of the muscular trabeculations at this location

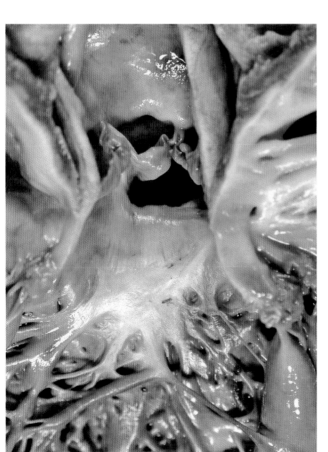

The significance of the distinction of perimembranous and muscular VSD lies in the intimate relation of the atrioventricular conduction tissue to the membranous septum (Fig. 13.7) and its susceptibility to damage during surgical closure of the defect [10]. At postmortem, small perimembranous VSDs are usually better appreciated from the left ventricular outflow tract. On the right side, these VSDs may be obscured by the chordal and leaflet tissue of the tricuspid valve.

A VSD occurring in the right ventricular outflow tract may permit fibrous continuity between the aortic and pulmonary valves. Such defects (which may be either muscular or perimembranous) are said to be doubly committed and juxta-arterial [11].

Blood will tend to flow through the VSD from left to right ventricle because of the pressure gradient between the two ventricles (unless there is restricted outflow through the pulmonary valve), and the right ventricle will suffer volume overload. Ventricular septal defects, if small, may close

Fig. 13.5 Perimembranous ventricular septal defect. A photograph of the left ventricular outflow tract opened in a similar fashion to that in Fig. 13.4. There is a perimembranous ventricular septal defect that is roughly triangular in shape and that occupies the position of the membranous septum. The defect also extends a short distance beneath the right coronary cusp of the aortic valve. Note the smooth edges of the defect. Such defects are much easier to appreciate from the left side of the heart; on the right side, they may be obscured by the septal leaflet of the tricuspid valve

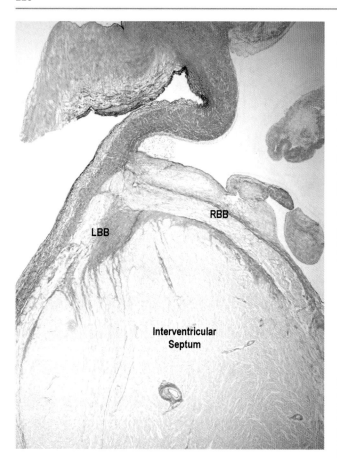

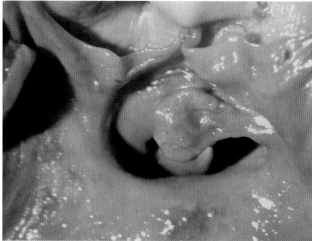

Fig. 13.8 Closing perimembranous VSD. A close-up *view* of a small perimembranous VSD viewed from the left ventricular outflow tract. The defect is largely closed by fibrous tissue related to the tricuspid valve on the right side of the defect. Such a defect would have been expected to seal spontaneously

Fig. 13.7 Membranous septum. A photomicrograph of a section through the crest of the interventricular septum to include the membranous septum (*asterisk*). Clearly visible are the right (*RBB*) and left (*LBB*) bundle branches of the atrioventricular conduction axis. The attachments of the septal leaflet of the tricuspid valve are visible on the *right* of the picture. The superficial location and potential vulnerability of the conduction tissue to surgical trauma is easily appreciated (elastic van Gieson stain)

spontaneously by fibrosis (Fig. 13.8), but tissue tags associated with VSD may cause subvalvar obstruction in the left ventricular outflow tract. Frequently, a surgical patch (usually Dacron) (Fig. 13.9) is required to close the defect. VSDs are also a potential site for infective endocarditis (Fig. 13.10).

Development of VSDs is related to defective growth of the interventricular septum and its fusion with the endocardial cushions.

Patent Arterial Duct (Ductus Arteriosus)

The arterial duct is a muscular artery interposed between the aorta and pulmonary trunk, both of which are elastic arteries [12]. It develops from the embryonic sixth aortic arch. It becomes redundant at birth and closes by muscular contraction in the first postnatal day (Fig. 13.11). This contraction

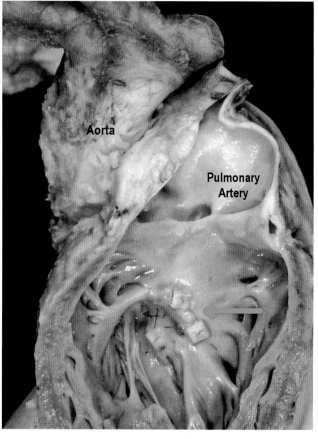

Fig. 13.9 Patched perimembranous ventricular septal defect. A view into the opened right ventricular outflow tract. The pulmonary valve is visible in the *center* of the field. Beneath it and separated from it by a wide muscle bar is a ring of pledgeted sutures around the VSD patch (*arrow*). The endocardium has grown over the pledgets and partly incorporated them

Fig. 13.10 Infective endocarditis affecting a ventricular septal defect. Photomicrograph of a section through the interventricular septum of a heart with a VSD. The defect is visible running vertically through the center of the field. The vegetations are visible as roughened areas on its margins (*arrow*)

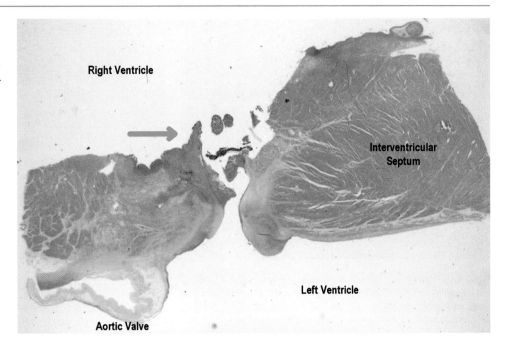

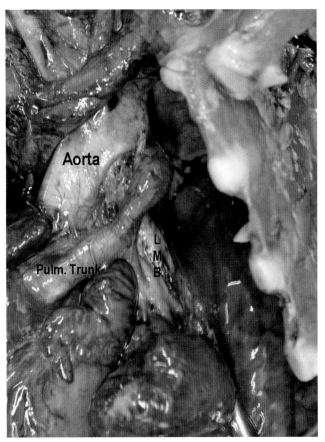

Fig. 13.11 Normal arterial duct at term. The chest has been opened and the pericardium removed. The heart has been retracted to the right and the left lung pulled down to expose the arterial duct. This structure runs posteriorly and upward from the pulmonary trunk to the inner aspect of the descending arch of the aorta. Note the constriction associated with early closure. The left main bronchus (*LMB*) is just visible posterior to the left pulmonary artery

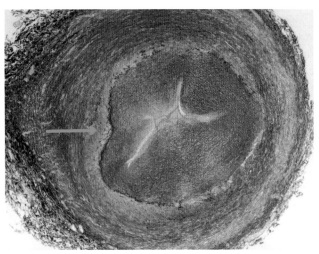

Fig. 13.12 Closure of the arterial duct. Histological cross section of the arterial duct of a term infant dying at 1-month of age of unrelated disease. The lumen of the duct is obliterated and is still visible as a stellate outline in the *center* of the field. Intimal cushions are visible internal to the internal elastic lamina (*arrow*). The pale tissue in the media is the muscular and myxoid tissue that is very characteristic of the structure of the arterial duct (elastic van Gieson stain)

approximates the intimal cushions that form in late fetal life and causes ischemia of the smooth muscle of the wall of the duct leading to fibrosis of the tunica media. Over the following weeks, permanent closure is achieved by fibrosis (Fig. 13.12), and the duct becomes a thick fibrous cord – the ligamentum arteriosum – that frequently calcifies in later life. Closure is usually complete and permanent by 3–4 weeks of age.

The duct remains functionally patent [13] for the first few days of life in most premature infants (Fig. 13.13).

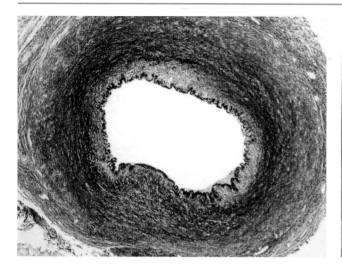

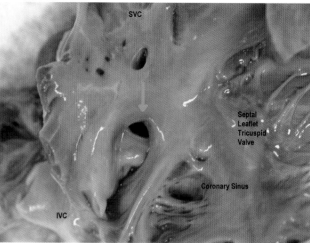

Fig. 13.13 Patent arterial duct. Histological cross section of the arterial duct of an infant born at 36 weeks' gestation who died suddenly and unexpectedly at 3 weeks of age. The duct is patent and there is little or no intimal cushion development. There is a small amount of intimal fibrosis at the four o'clock position. The characteristic normal pallor of the media is evident (elastic van Gieson stain)

Fig. 13.14 Atrial septal defect of secundum type. The opened right atrium with the right ventricle to the *right* of the picture. The oval fossa is visible in the *center* of the picture as an oval depression with raised edges. Its floor is covered by a flap valve that is deficient superiorly to give a triangular atrial septal defect (*arrow*). Any defect in the oval fossa is of secundum type. This child had trisomy 21

Administration of the prostaglandin synthesis inhibitor, indomethacin, causes closure of the duct in most, but not all, cases, and a closed duct may reopen by poorly understood mechanisms. Persistently patent duct is associated with the development of chronic lung disease in premature infants. Persistent patency of the duct also occurs in association with structural heart disease and its patency in some being essential to life (e.g., in pulmonary atresia). Patent arterial duct and peripheral pulmonary artery stenosis are the commonest cardiac manifestation of maternal rubella infection. Infective endocarditis may develop in a persistently patent arterial duct, usually at the pulmonary arterial end.

Atrial Septal Defect

The majority of atrial septal defects occur within the oval fossa. Such defects are, by definition, of secundum type. In about 10–20% of the general population, there is probe patency of the interatrial septum at the anterosuperior part of the oval fossa [14]. It is sometimes referred to as persistent foramen ovale (PFO). As the pressure of blood in the left atrium is normally higher than in the right, the flap remains closed. Deficiency of the anterosuperior aspect of the flap valve of the oval fossa is responsible for true secundum atrial septal defects (Fig. 13.14). The defects may involve merely a tiny part of the oval fossa or, when extreme, the entire oval fossa. The defect may be fenestrated with multiple small holes within the flap valve (Fig. 13.15). There may be slight surrounding endocardial fibroelastosis but usually no other consequence. ASD may, of course, occur in combination with

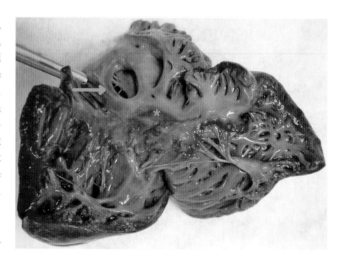

Fig. 13.15 Fenestrated atrial septal defect of secundum type. A child with trisomy 21 who died of a viral respiratory infection. The right heart has been opened to expose the right atrium and right ventricle. The oval fossa of the right atrium shows a fenestrated septal defect, two thin fibrous strands dividing the defect into smaller divisions (*arrow*). This heart also shows an abnormally large membranous septum – a feature of trisomy 21 – evident in this picture as an area of discontinuity at the commissure between the septal and anterior leaflets of the tricuspid valve (*asterisk*)

any other cardiac defect and, in some, is essential for the continued well-being of the child (Fig. 13.16).

The other types of atrial septal defect, with the exception of the ostium primum defect (discussed below under AVSD), are very rare. They are:

1. Coronary sinus defect where the interatrial communication is at the level of the coronary sinus, that is, inferior and posterior to the oval fossa [15]

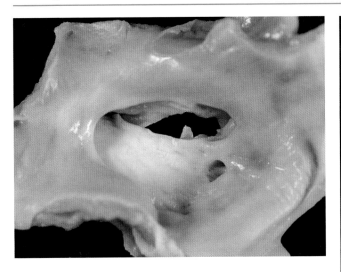

Fig. 13.16 Balloon septostomy. A 10 year-old girl on with severe viral myocarditis placed on extracorporeal membrane oxygenation (ECMO). She required atrial septostomy to maintain ECMO but died within a few days from myocarditis. This close-up view of the right side of the oval fossa shows a defect with ragged margins in the upper part of the oval fossa, caused by pulling the catheter balloon through the septum

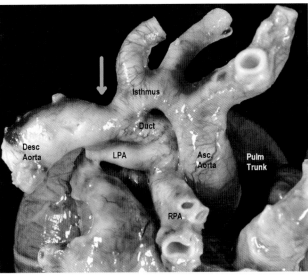

Fig. 13.17 Coarctation aorta. Eight-week-old male infant who died of cardiac failure. The great vessels in this example are viewed from behind and from the right. There is a notch (*arrow*) in the aorta at the level of insertion of the arterial duct where the lumen is narrowed

2. Sinus venosus defect which is usually associated with anomalous drainage of the right pulmonary veins through the defect into the right atrium [16]

Coarctation of the Aorta

Coarctation is a narrowing of the aorta at the site of insertion of the arterial duct. The narrowing may be discrete, or it may be accompanied by tubular hypoplasia of the aorta. The discrete lesion is usually evident externally as a notch in the aortic arch wall [17], most prominently on its convex aspect opposite the ductal insertion (Fig. 13.17). Internally, there is a shelf of tissue protruding into the lumen from the side of aortic wall opposite the site of insertion of the arterial duct (Fig. 13.18). A degree of post-stenotic dilatation may be visible, but in infants, it is usually not marked. The normal aortic isthmus (that segment of the aortic arch between the left subclavian artery and the arterial duct) is normally narrower than the remainder of the aorta, and it is important not to mistake this normal appearance for tubular hypoplasia. Coarctation of the aorta may occur as an isolated lesion, or it may accompany other cardiovascular malformations, most notably ventricular septal defect and left-sided obstructive lesions [18]. Histologically, a sling of ductal tissue extends around the aortic wall causing the narrowing (Fig. 13.19). Secondary intimal fibrous proliferation further narrows the lumen [19]. Those infants with severe coarctation present in the first weeks of life with evidence of cardiac failure [20].

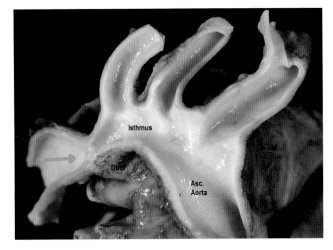

Fig. 13.18 Coarctation aorta. Same case as Fig. 13.17 opened to show the hour-glass constriction (*arrow*) of the internal diameter of the aorta at the level of the insertion of the arterial duct

Atrioventricular Septal Defect

Atrioventricular septal defect (AVSD) results from failure of fusion of the endocardial cushions, and the alternative nomenclature of this defect is endocardial cushion defect. This causes a cluster of abnormalities of the structures at the center of the heart [21], involving the contiguous parts of the interatrial and interventricular septa, the aortic outflow, and the atrioventricular valves. In the fully developed lesion, there is a common atrioventricular junction (Fig. 13.20). The junction is guarded by a common valve (Fig. 13.21), and,

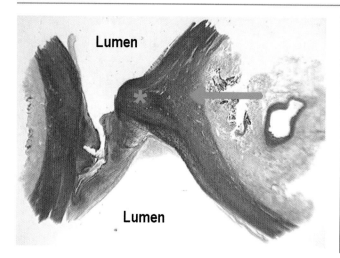

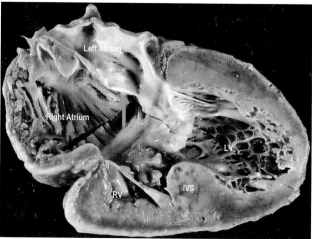

Fig. 13.19 Coarctation aorta. Longitudinal histological section of a resected segment coarctation of the aorta stained with elastic van Gieson. A shelf of ductal tissue (*asterisk*) projects into the lumen. A notch is visible (*arrow*) on the external surface. There is secondary intimal fibroelastic tissue deposition

Fig. 13.21 AVSD. Common atrioventricular valve. Same cases as Fig. 13.20 cut in a simulated four-chamber view. The right ventricle is small. The crest of the interventricular septum (*IVS*) lies well below the plane of the atrioventricular junction and has no valvar tissue attached to it. The inferior bridging leaflet (*asterisk*) extends from chordal attachments in the right ventricle (*RV*) to the left ventricle (*LV*). There is free interventricular communication beneath the leaflet. There is a large interatrial communication between the atrioventricular valve and the lower border of the interatrial septum (*arrow*)

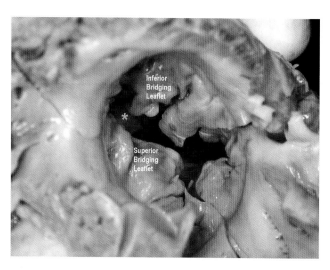

Fig. 13.20 AVSD. Common atrioventricular junction. A 9-month-old girl with trisomy 21 and complete AVSD. AVSD is the characteristic cardiac anomaly in trisomy 21. This is a view from the atria into the ventricular cavity. The interatrial septum has been removed. The common atrioventricular junction is readily apparent as are the bridging leaflets. The crest of the interventricular septum is just visible beneath the valve leaflets. The right ventricle was small and the septum is, thus, more to the right than usual

septum and which have papillary muscle attachments in both ventricles (Fig. 13.23). On the left side, there is a (usually) small mural leaflet and on the right side, anterior and inferior leaflets. The valvar tissue may be dysplastic and there is commonly valvar regurgitation. After surgical closure of the defect, this valvar regurgitation may be clinically significant. AVSD is termed complete when the bridging leaflets float freely and are attached to neither interatrial septum, the interventricular septum, nor to each other. There is free communication of blood between both ventricles beneath the valvar leaflets and between both atria above.

Where there is attachment of the bridging leaflet tissue to the crest of the interventricular septum, or where a tongue of leaflet tissue joins the two bridging leaflets over the interventricular septum (in effect creating two valvar orifices, albeit there is still a common junction), the defect is called a partial AVSD (Fig. 13.24). In this case, there is some restriction in the mixing of blood at the ventricular level.

Where the bridging leaflets are attached to the crest of the interventricular septum so as to obliterate the interventricular communication the defect becomes, in effect, an interatrial communication and is the so-called ostium primum atrial septal defect (Fig. 13.25). That the ostium primum defect is, in all essentials, an atrioventricular septal defect is reflected in the features it shares with other forms of AVSD – the common AV junction (despite separate orifices), the anteriorly displaced aorta, the scooped-out crest of the interventricular septum, and the vestige of the fused bridging leaflets in the

because of the common junction, the aorta is displaced from its normal position to lie anterior to the common atrioventricular junction (Fig. 13.22). The lower border of the interatrial septum is not connected to the ventricular septum and is a freestanding structure. The upper border of the interventricular septum has a scooped-out appearance and lies beneath the plane of the atrioventricular junction.

The common atrioventricular valve has superior and inferior bridging leaflets that cross (bridge) the interventricular

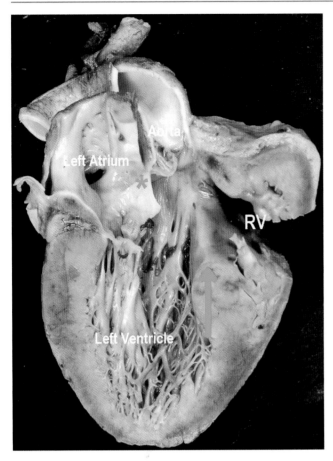

Fig. 13.22 AVSD. Anterior displacement of aorta. The heart is viewed from behind, looking anteriorly. The superior bridging leaflet has been removed to show the left ventricular outflow tract (LVOT). The LVOT, instead of lying in its usual position in the normal heart – at the side of the interventricular septum (*arrow*) – has been displaced anteriorly to the front of the interventricular septum

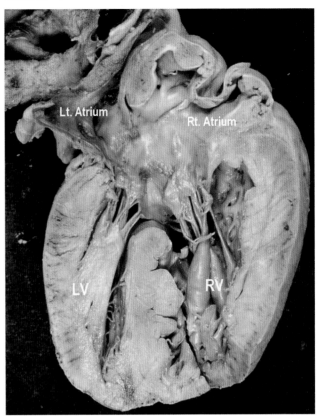

Fig. 13.23 AVSD. Bridging atrioventricular leaflets. A simulated four-chamber view of a heart with complete AVSD viewed from posteriorly looking forward. The interventricular septum (*asterisk*) lies vertically in the center of the picture, and the superior bridging leaflet is readily apparent with obvious attachments to papillary muscles in both right (*RV*) and left ventricles (*LV*). Note also how the crest of the interventricular septum lies well below the plane of the atrioventricular junction

abnormal anterior leaflet of the mitral valve that is attached to the interventricular septum.

In AVSD, the relative sizes of both ventricles can vary, and there is often disproportion (Fig. 13.26). AVSD can coexist with other forms of congenital heart disease such as arterial valve obstruction and is an almost universal finding in cases of right atrial isomerism. AVSD is also the characteristic cardiac defect occurring with trisomy 21. Given the anterior displacement of the aorta in this defect, the aortic outflow tract is lengthened and narrowed. While this does not cause significant obstruction, it takes little additional obstruction, for example, by valvar tissue tags, to cause clinical symptoms. As the structures of the membranous septum are absent, the atrioventricular conduction tissue is abnormally sited. The atrioventricular node is located more inferiorly than usual in the so-called nodal triangle whose borders are the atrioventricular junction, the mouth of the coronary sinus, and the posteroinferior leading edge of the atrial septum. The bundle of His is unusually long and

travels on the crest of the interventricular septum before dividing [22].

The defect tends to present with cardiac failure in the first few weeks rather than the first days of life. Cyanosis is usually not present. The defect is treated [23] by early operation with a two-patch repair (Fig. 13.27). In untreated cases, unless there is associated pulmonary stenosis, pulmonary hypertension develops rapidly even in the first year of life.

Pulmonary Stenosis and Atresia (Including Tetralogy of Fallot)

Congenital atresia of the pulmonary valve may occur with, or without, a ventricular septal defect. The two entities are distinct clinically and have separate pathological associations. There may be severe stenosis of the pulmonary valve instead of atresia, and there is evidence from ultrasound scanning that some cases of pulmonary atresia develop from pulmonary stenosis.

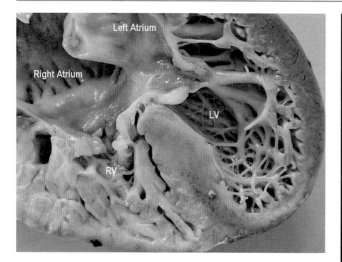

Fig. 13.24 AVSD. Partial AVSD. A heart cut in a simulated four-chamber view to demonstrate a partial AVSD. This heart shares all the features of the other hearts with AVSD above, with the exception that the inferior bridging leaflet is attached by fibrous cords to the crest of the interventricular septum (*asterisk*), creating two valvar orifices (but still with a common atrioventricular junction). There is still an interventricular component to the defect, but the greater part lies above the atrioventricular valve and below the lower border of the interatrial septum (*arrow*)

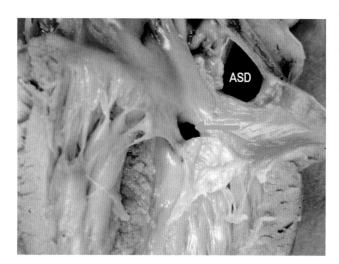

Fig. 13.25 AVSD. Ostium primum AVSD (*arrow*). The specimen is viewed from the left side and shows the left atrium, with a secundum atrial septal defect (*ASD*) and the left ventricle. There is an atrioventricular septal defect. The defect lies above the atrioventricular valve but outside the oval fossa. The defect has the features of an AVSD: scooped-out interventricular septum, displaced LVOT (in the normal heart, the LVOT would be at the site of attachment of the atrioventricular valve to the septum), and the remains of bridging leaflets. The mitral valve leaflet is composed of two parts – the vestiges of the superior and inferior bridging leaflets in the normal heart and the anterior leaflet of the mitral valve would not be attached to the septum at all and would be rectangular in outline, not "cleft" as here

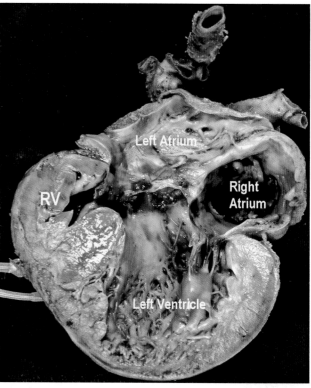

Fig. 13.26 AVSD. Ventricular disproportion. Four-chamber view of the heart looked at from behind, looking forward. There is a complete AVSD with as superior bridging leaflet that crosses from right to left ventricles. The interventricular septum (*asterisk*) is displaced, and the right ventricle correspondingly reduced in size. There is, thus, malalignment of the interatrial and interventricular septa, such that both atria open for the most part into the left ventricle (double-inlet left ventricle). The ventriculo-arterial connections are discordant.

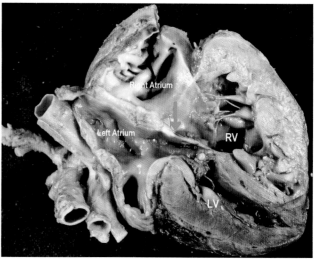

Fig. 13.27 AVSD. Repair. Four-chamber view of heart with repaired AVSD. Four-month-old girl. The heart is viewed from behind, looking forward. There is a partial AVSD with a large atrial component. The atrial component has been closed with a patch (*arrow*) between the inferior border of the interatrial septum and the upper border of the interventricular septum (*asterisk*). The atrioventricular valvar tissue is sutured to the patch

Pulmonary Atresia with Intact Interventricular Septum

There is usually a patent oval foramen and arterial duct. The right atrium is dilated. The right ventricle is usually small with a hypertrophied wall. The degree of ventricular hypertrophy may be so great as to obliterate the outlet and apical trabecular components [24], leaving only an inlet component (Fig. 13.28). The tricuspid valve is small, and in about 10% of cases, there is associated Ebstein's malformation. The pulmonary trunk is small – but rarely atretic – and the valve annulus is narrow. The pulmonary valve is imperforate (Fig. 13.29). The branch pulmonary arteries are thin-walled. The left ventricle may also be hypertrophied. Right ventricular-coronary artery sinusoids are a characteristic feature of pulmonary atresia with intact septum. These arise from persistence of the normal ventricular-coronary communications in the embryo,

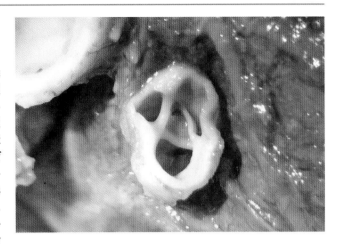

Fig. 13.29 Pulmonary atresia with intact interventricular septum. A view of the pulmonary valve from above. The pulmonary trunk has been transected above the valve. The vessel is tiny – compare it to the size of the left coronary artery that skirts its *left side* and to the aorta in the *top left hand* corner of the field. Three valve leaflets are present, but the orifice is sealed by a central plug of fibrous tissue. This suggests that the valve may once have been patent – a situation that is sometimes detected on echocardiography

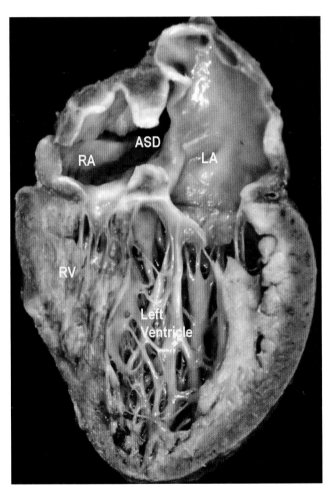

Fig. 13.28 Pulmonary atresia with intact interventricular septum. A simulated four-chamber view of the heart. The right ventricle is small, and there is marked muscular thickening of its wall with obliteration of the apex of the ventricle. Compared to the mitral valve, the tricuspid valve is small. There is a large atrial secundum septal defect that has permitted survival

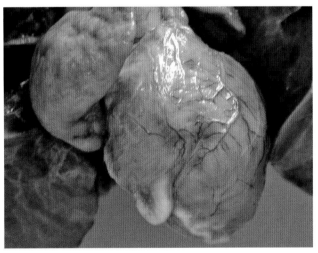

Fig. 13.30 Pulmonary atresia with intact interventricular septum. Thickened epicardial right coronary artery. The external surface of the heart is viewed from the front. The right ventricle is small and does not contribute to formation of the ventricular apex. A large caliber, thick, white coronary artery can be seen that has a tortuous course running along the right free margin of the heart. This appearance is characteristic of the arteries with connections with the ventricular lumen in pulmonary atresia with intact septum

supposedly due to persistently elevated right ventricular pressure, although they may precede the onset of pulmonary valve obstruction [25]. The sinusoids are readily seen on echocardiography but are almost impossible to demonstrate pathologically. However, their presence can be inferred from dramatic secondary changes in the affected coronary arteries (Fig. 13.30). These vessels are thick-walled – sometimes up to two to three times their normal size (Fig. 13.31).

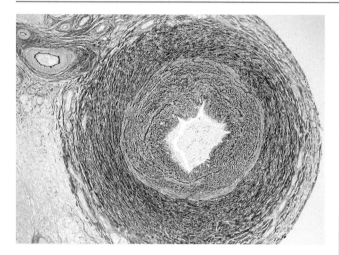

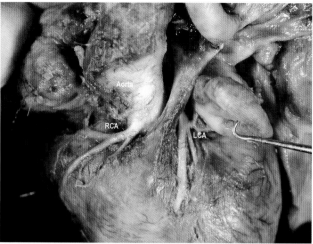

Fig. 13.31 Pulmonary atresia with intact interventricular septum. A transverse histological section of the coronary artery from the preceding figure stained with elastic van Gieson. The wall of the vessels is thickened and the lumen narrowed. There is increased elastic tissue in all three layers of the vessel wall – adventitia, media, and intima. There is an increase in collagenous fibrous tissue and a corresponding decrease in smooth muscle. There is concentric intimal thickening

Fig. 13.32 Pulmonary atresia with ventricular septal defect. A heart from a child with pulmonary atresia and VSD. The pulmonary trunk (*asterisk*) is atretic, consisting of no more than a thin fibrous thread between the ventricular mass at the base of the heart and the confluence of the pulmonary arteries. The trunk is embraced by the origins of the right (*RCA*) and left (*LCA*) coronary arteries. Just visible at the top of the field is a Blalock-Taussig shunt anastomosed to the left pulmonary artery

The affected coronary artery may lose its communication with the aorta because of the intimal proliferation. The perfusion of the myocardium supplied by that artery may then be crucially dependent on the elevated right ventricular pressure for retrograde perfusion.

Pulmonary Atresia with Ventricular Septal Defect

This is a quite distinct abnormality from pulmonary atresia with intact septum. This lesion does not show the diminutive and hypertrophied ventricle of pulmonary atresia with intact septum. The pulmonary trunk is usually atretic, being represented only by a thin tread-like cord (Figs. 13.32 and 13.33). The branch pulmonary arteries may be of normal size and supplied by an arterial duct. The duct may be absent, in which case the lungs derive their blood supply from major aortopulmonary collateral arteries (MAPCA). These vessels [26], some of which are hypertrophied bronchial arteries, arise from the aortic arch and descending aorta (Fig. 13.34). Many cases represent tetralogy of Fallot with pulmonary valvar atresia.

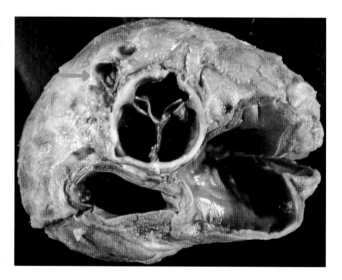

Fig. 13.33 Pulmonary atresia with ventricular septal defect. The base of the heart viewed from above. The roofs of both atria and all but the most proximal parts of the great arteries have been removed. The aortic valve occupies the center of the base of the heart with its characteristic three cusps. Slightly above it and to its left, the atretic pulmonary trunk is visible (*arrow*). The arterial lumen is patent, albeit very narrow, and the valve tissue comprises no more than nodular fibrous tissue. There was no communication with the underlying ventricle

Pulmonary Stenosis with VSD – Including Tetralogy of Fallot

Tetralogy of Fallot refers to a group of four abnormalities occurring together: pulmonary stenosis, VSD, overriding aorta, and right ventricular hypertrophy [27]. The basic defect is abnormal anterior insertion of the ventriculo-infundibular fold into the anterior limb of the septomarginal trabeculation

(Fig. 13.35). Normally, the ventriculo-infundibular fold inserts between the limbs of the septomarginal trabeculation (Fig. 13.36). The abnormal anterior insertion leaves a VSD posteriorly and causes narrowing of the right ventricular outflow tract anteriorly. The aorta overrides the VSD, and the presence of pulmonary stenosis leads eventually to right

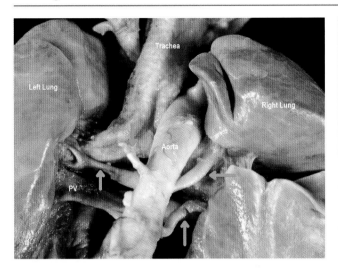

Fig. 13.34 Pulmonary atresia with ventricular septal defect. The specimen is viewed from behind. The posterior aspect of the trachea is visible at the *top center* and clearly gives rise to the left main bronchus. A right-sided aortic arch crosses over the right main bronchus to descend medial to the right lung. Arising from the descending aorta, there are major aortopulmonary collateral arteries (*arrows*) – that supply the lungs, entering the pulmonary hilum posterior to the bronchi and pulmonary veins (*PV*)

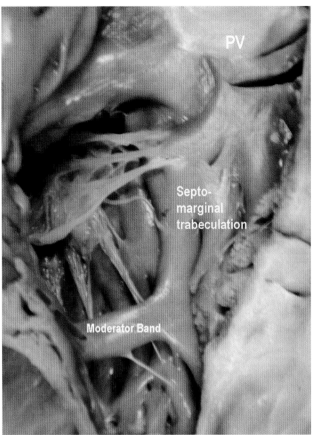

Fig. 13.36 A normal heart exposing the same structures as in Fig. 13.35. The apex is slightly more inferiorly situated in this picture. However, the septomarginal trabeculation is well seen as an inverted Y-shaped structure on the septum, its lowermost part giving origin to the moderator band. Its anterior limb runs forward to the pulmonary valve, and its posterior limb runs backward and anchors the medial commissure of the tricuspid valve. The supraventricular crest (*asterisk*) which forms the posterior aspect of the pulmonary infundibulum is inserted into the septum between the two limbs of the septomarginal trabeculation. Anterior displacement of this structure creates the characteristic anatomy of tetralogy of Fallot

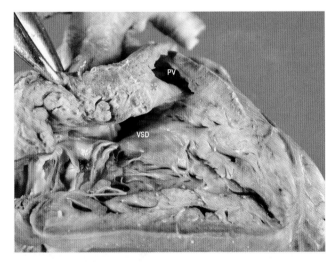

Fig. 13.35 Tetralogy of Fallot. The right ventricle of a case of tetralogy of Fallot opened to show the characteristic anatomy. The apex is to the *right* of the picture, and the septal aspect of the right ventricle is exposed by removal of the right free wall and part of the right ventricular outflow tract. The ventricular wall is thick and muscular. There is a *VSD* visible, lying between the two limbs of the septomarginal trabeculation. The posterior limb of the septomarginal trabeculation shows attachment of the medial commissure of the tricuspid valve. The supraventricular crest (*asterisk*) is inserted abnormally anteriorly into the anterior limb of the septomarginal trabeculation, thus narrowing the pulmonary outflow tract. The fourth feature of tetralogy of Fallot – overriding aorta – is not seen in this view

ventricular hypertrophy. About one quarter of cases have a right-sided aortic arch. The arterial duct may be absent. The aorta is usually large and the pulmonary artery small and thin-walled. The VSD is usually large and may extend to the membranous septum (Fig. 13.37). The degree of aortic override is

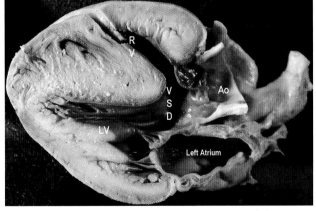

Fig. 13.37 Tetralogy of Fallot. Heart cut in a simulated long-axis view to show clearly the ventricular septal defect (*VSD*) and overriding aorta (*Ao*) of tetralogy of Fallot. The right ventricular (*RV*) hypertrophy is well seen also, but the subpulmonary obstruction cannot be well appreciated in this view

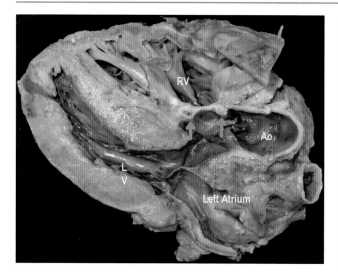

Fig. 13.38 Tetralogy of Fallot. Long-axis view of an operated heart from a case of tetralogy of Fallot. The heart is cut in a simulated long-axis view. As in the immediately preceding figure, the overriding aorta can be seen. However, the lower part of the aorta has been connected to the right side of the interventricular septum by a patch (*arrows*), thus ensuring that the aorta receives blood only from the left ventricle (*LV*). There has been improvement in the hemodynamics in that the right ventricle (*RV*) does not show significant myocardial hypertrophy

also variable. If the override is greater than 50%, the case is then, arbitrarily, classified as double-outlet right ventricle. Infundibular stenosis is present in all cases, but there is variable valvar stenosis. Approximately 20% of cases have pulmonary atresia. The condition presents with cyanosis, usually in the first few months of life. Operative treatment [28] involves patching the VSD so as to commit the aorta fully to the left ventricle (Fig. 13.38), with relief of the pulmonary stenosis, either by resection of muscle beneath the valve or insertion of a valved conduit between the right ventricle and the pulmonary artery (Fig. 13.39). Sudden death may occur, even in operated cases [29].

Aortic Stenosis

Aortic stenosis is classified into three forms: valvar stenosis, subvalvar stenosis, and supravalvar stenosis [30]. Valvar stenosis is the commonest form.

Valvar Stenosis

This may occur as an isolated lesion or may be associated with other abnormalities such as mitral stenosis, aortic coarctation, or VSD. The valve orifice is usually narrow, and there is fusion and dysplasia [31] of the valve leaflets (Fig. 13.40).

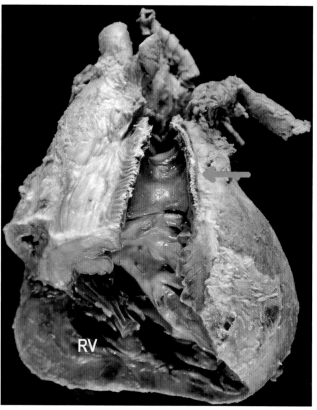

Fig. 13.39 Tetralogy of Fallot. Operated case with a valved conduit inserted between the anterior right ventricle and the pulmonary arteries. Much of the right ventricular free wall has been removed, and the conduit has been opened anteriorly and part of its anterior wall removed. The ribbed wall of the conduit is visible (*arrow*). The wide attachment to the ventricular mass can be appreciated, and the remains of a rather thin valve can be seen in the conduit lumen just distal to the level of the *arrow*

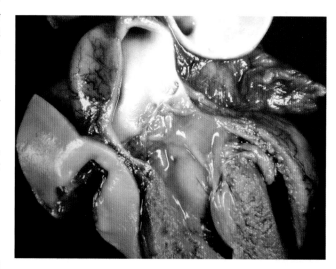

Fig. 13.40 Valvar aortic stenosis. The left ventricular outflow tract has been opened to demonstrate the dysplastic aortic valve. The leaflets, although not very much thickened, are nodular and are adherent, one to the other, causing narrowing of the valvar orifice. This was an isolated finding in this heart

Subvalvar Stenosis

Subvalvar stenosis may be caused by muscular obstruction, as, for example, in hypertrophic cardiomyopathy (Fig. 13.41), by hypertrophy of an anomalous muscle bar, or by hypertrophied outlet septum in cases of double-outlet ventricle. The obstruction may be caused by a subvalvar fibrous shelf (Fig. 13.42) or may be caused by fibrous tissue tags or atrioventricular valvar tissue associated with a VSD.

Supravalvar Stenosis

Supravalvar aortic stenosis is caused by irregular thickening of the aortic wall some 1–2 cm above the aortic valve [33]. It is usually associated with Williams syndrome due to mutations in the elastin gene on chromosome 7. The stenosis, viewed externally, has a characteristic hour-glass appearance (Fig. 13.43). There is usually thickening and fibrosis of the coronary arteries [34]. The left ventricle is hypertrophied.

Hypoplastic Left Heart

This is a group of abnormalities characterized by a small left ventricle unable to support the systemic circulation [35]. The usual case has a thread-like ascending aorta (Fig. 13.44) that is patent and supplies blood to the coronary arteries in a retrograde fashion. The mitral valve is usually small and dysplastic, in which case the ventricle shows marked endocardial fibroelastosis (Fig. 13.45). If the mitral valve is atretic, there is no endocardial fibroelastosis. The left atrium is small. The aortic valve is more usually atretic (Fig. 13.46) but may be severely stenotic and dysplastic, in which case the ascending

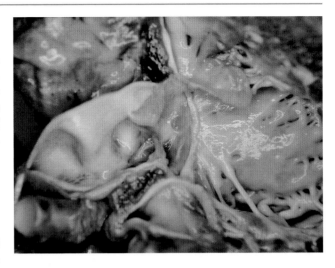

Fig. 13.42 Subvalvar aortic stenosis. A view of the left ventricular outflow of this heart shows a mildly thickened aortic valve. A short distance beneath it, there is a fibrous ridge that projects into the lumen of the outflow tract causing narrowing. Note the endocardial fibrosis (From: Ashworth [32]. Reprinted with permission)

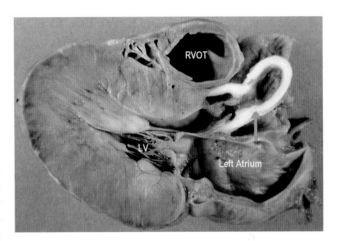

Fig. 13.43 Supravalvar aortic stenosis. Long-axis view of a heart from a child with Williams syndrome. There is a thick white hour-glass constriction (*arrow*) of the aorta above the aortic valve. The left ventricular myocardium is greatly thickened (From: Ashworth [32]. Reprinted with permission)

aorta is correspondingly larger (Fig. 13.47). The interventricular septum is usually intact, but there may be a VSD if there is mitral atresia (Fig. 13.48). Externally, the coronary arteries delimit the hypoplastic left ventricle. The left ventricular myocardium is hypertrophic, and up to 80% of cases show myofiber disarray histologically (Fig. 13.49). The appearances are analogous to the right heart in pulmonary atresia with intact septum, and, in some cases, ventriculo-coronary artery communications can also be demonstrated [36]. About two-thirds of cases show coarctation of the aorta [37]. Repair is by Norwood operation (Fig. 13.50). This is a staged procedure, the three stages being separated by months to years. The first stage involves removal of the interatrial septum and

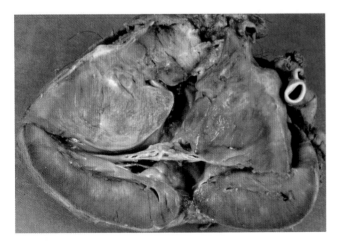

Fig. 13.41 Subvalvar aortic stenosis. A case of hypertrophic cardiomyopathy opened to show the greatly hypertrophied interventricular septum bulging into the left ventricular outflow to cause subaortic stenosis

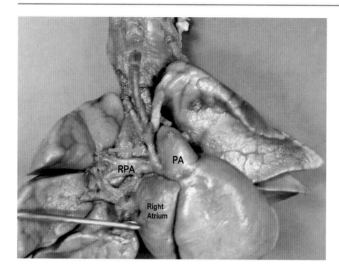

Fig. 13.44 Hypoplastic left heart. The heart and lungs from a fetus with hypoplastic left heart. The thread-like ascending aorta is readily visible between the pulmonary trunk (*PA*) and the right pulmonary artery (*RPA*). The great vessels are supplied by the arterial duct (*asterisk*) with retrograde flow in the ascending aorta to supply the coronary arteries

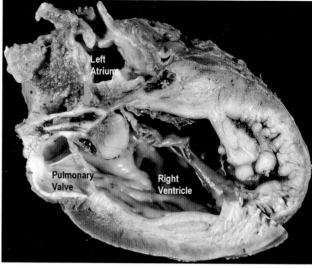

Fig. 13.46 Hypoplastic left heart. A semi-long-axis view of the heart. The left atrium is small and the mitral valve tiny and imperforate. The left ventricular cavity (*asterisk*) is tiny and filled with blood. A thin fibrous strand connects it to the diminutive aorta, but there is no luminal communication. There is hypertrophy of the left ventricular muscle. The right ventricle is dilated

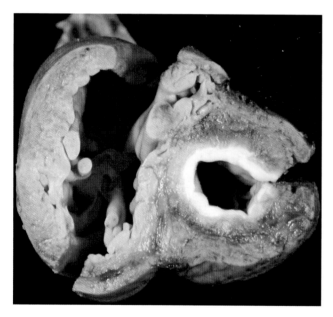

Fig. 13.45 Hypoplastic left heart. Short-axis view of the heart to demonstrate severe thickening of the endocardium of the small left ventricle

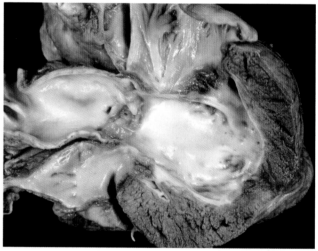

Fig. 13.47 Hypoplastic left heart. The aortic valve is stenotic and dysplastic. The left ventricular cavity is small and thick-walled and shows dense fibroelastosis of its endocardium. The ventricle does not form the apex of the heart, which can be seen further to the *right* of the picture. The mitral valve is slightly smaller than normal. This case illustrates that hypoplastic left heart forms a spectrum of abnormality from a ventricle that is scarcely recognizable to the naked eye to a ventricle that is marginally smaller than normal. This latter group can be particularly problematical in deciding whether to opt for a two-ventricle repair

closure of the arterial duct. The pulmonary arteries are disconnected from the pulmonary trunk which is anastomosed to the aorta, the anastomosis usually augmented by a patch (Damus-Kaye-Stansel anastomosis). To provide blood to the pulmonary arteries, a modified Blalock-Taussig shunt (a Gore-Tex conduit) is inserted between the (usually) brachiocephalic artery and the confluence of the pulmonary arteries. In the stage 2 procedure, the Blalock-Taussig shunt is taken down, and the superior caval vein is detached from the right atrium

and anastomosed directly to the pulmonary arteries. The third and final stage involves directing the inferior caval blood to the pulmonary arteries, either by a conduit within the right atrium (lateral conduit) or by an extracardiac conduit (Sano modification). The connection of the entire venous return to

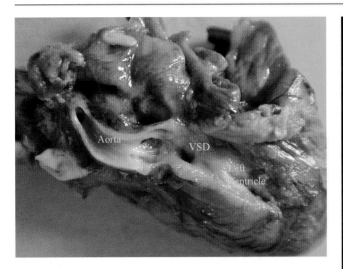

Fig. 13.48 Hypoplastic left heart. There is mitral atresia with a small but patent aortic valve. The left ventricle is small and there is a *VSD*

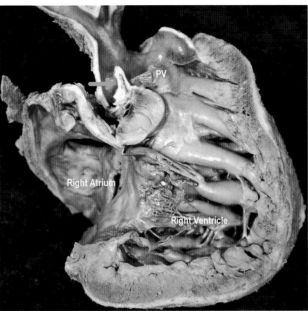

Fig. 13.50 Hypoplastic left heart. A heart following a stage 1 Norwood operation, opened to show the Damus-Kaye-Stansel anastomosis. In this operation, the pulmonary trunk is transected and anastomosed in an end-to-side fashion to the atretic aorta, the anastomosis being augmented by a patch. The heart shows the opened right atrium and ventricle with the pulmonary trunk arising above the pulmonary valve (*PV*). The pulmonary trunk and aorta have been joined (*arrow*)

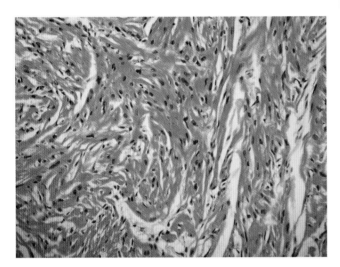

Fig. 13.49 Hypoplastic left heart. Photomicrograph of left ventricular myocardium from a heart with hypoplastic left heart. There is myocyte hypertrophy and disarray, indistinguishable from that seen in hypertrophic cardiomyopathy. As many as 90% of these hearts show myocyte disarray

the pulmonary arteries without involvement of the heart is also referred to as the Fontan circulation [38]. There is still considerable morbidity and mortality associated with the operation [39], and heart transplantation may be preferred.

Transposition of the Great Arteries

In transposition, there is discordance of the ventriculoarterial connections, with the aorta arising from the right ventricle and the pulmonary artery from the left (Fig. 13.51). In the usual situation (complete transposition), there are concordant atrioventricular connections [40]. In the majority of cases, the

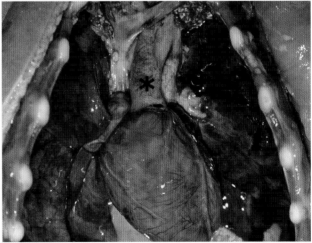

Fig. 13.51 Transposition. A fatal case of transposition in the neonatal period. The baby appeared unremarkable at delivery but collapsed and died on the first day of life, presumably as the arterial duct began to close. The diagnosis was only made at autopsy. The opened pericardium displays the heart with a parallel configuration of the great vessels. The aorta (*asterisk*) arises anteriorly – the origin of the left coronary artery can just be discerned. The pulmonary trunk arises posteriorly. There was no VSD. The arterial duct and oval fossa were closed. Children with unsuspected congenital heart disease who collapse and die in the first days of life are likely to have either transposition or hypoplastic left heart

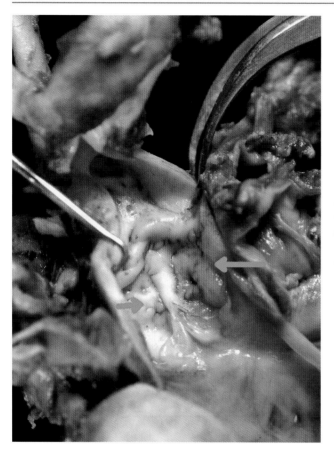

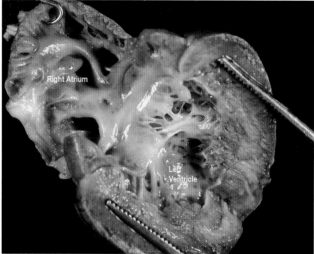

Fig. 13.53 Congenitally corrected transposition. A heart with discordant atrioventricular and ventriculoarterial connection – so-called congenitally corrected transposition. In this view, the heart has been opened to show a normal right atrium connected to a left ventricle – note the mitral valve. Not visible in this picture is the pulmonary artery arising from the right-sided, morphologically left ventricle

atrioventricular with discordant ventriculoarterial connections [42]. The vast majority of these hearts have associated cardiac malformations, most having abnormalities of the tricuspid valve and a VSD.

Fig. 13.52 Transposition – neonatal arterial switch operation. The aorta has been opened anteriorly. A circumferential suture line (*asterisk*) is visible at the level of the forceps. Also visible are two circular patches (*arrows*) each with a surrounding suture line and each lying in a sinus of Valsalva. These are the coronary arteries with a surrounding button of arterial wall that are transplanted to the neo-aorta as part of the switch procedure. Meticulous surgical technique is required to prevent kinking

Common Arterial Trunk (Truncus Arteriosus)

This lesion is uncommon, accounting for about only 0.5% of all cases of structural congenital heart disease. A single arterial trunk arises from the base of the heart that gives rise to the pulmonary arteries, the systemic arteries, and the coronary arteries (Fig. 13.54). There is, of necessity, a subarterial VSD. The truncal valve may have three, two, four, or even five leaflets and may be dysplastic. The origin of the pulmonary arteries from the trunk is the basis of subclassification of this lesion [43]. The arterial duct is usually absent. The coronary artery origins and course are abnormal [44]. If the truncal valve is competent, there are few or no symptoms in the first couple of weeks of life. Falling pulmonary vascular resistance with consequent increased pulmonary blood flow leads to the development of breathlessness and heart failure. If the valve is incompetent, symptoms occur in the first days of life. The lesion develops on the basis of failure of septation of the ventricular outflows.

aorta arises anterior and to the right of the pulmonary artery. The aorta has a complete muscular infundibulum, and the pulmonary valve is in fibrous continuity with the mitral valve. The aorta and pulmonary trunk lack the usual spiral relation to each other. Instead, they arise parallel within the pericardial sac. The coronary artery origins from the aorta are more variable than usual [41]. There may be an atrial septal defect which allows some mixing of systemic and pulmonary circulations. If this does not exist, it must be created artificially to permit survival until an arterial switch operation can be performed. Complete transposition may be complicated by VSD (~20% of cases), coarctation (~7% cases), or pulmonary stenosis (~7% cases). In the absence of a VSD, the baby appears normal at birth but becomes cyanosed on the first day of life and quickly becomes acidotic. In those cases with VSD, breathlessness and cardiac failure develop within the first week of life, and cyanosis is minimal.

Treatment of complete transposition is by neonatal arterial switch operation (Fig. 13.52). The term congenitally corrected transposition (Fig. 13.53) refers to discordant

Anomalous Pulmonary Venous Connection

This may be partial or total. Although the pulmonary veins may connect separately to an anomalous site, it is usual for them to join to form a single channel that then connects

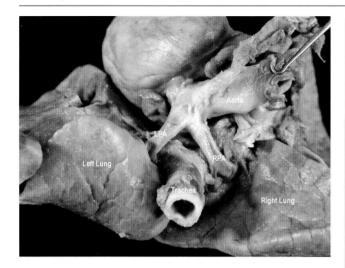

Fig. 13.54 Common arterial trunk (truncus arteriosus). A heart showing a common arterial trunk arising from the ventricular mass and giving rise to aorta and right (*RPA*) and left (*LPA*) pulmonary arteries

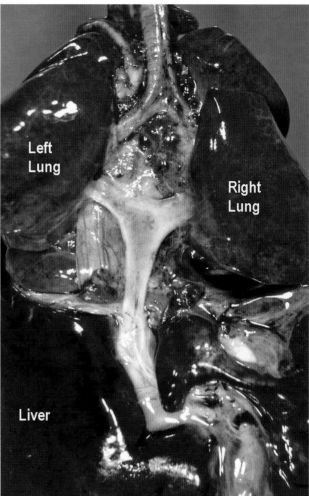

Fig. 13.55 Infradiaphragmatic total anomalous pulmonary venous connection. The thoracic organs and liver viewed from behind. The pulmonary veins come to a confluence (*asterisk*) behind the heart, and the common veins descend through the diaphragm to insert into the portal vein behind the liver. There was no connection to the left atrium. Such anomalous venous pathways are prone to obstruction

anomalously [45]. The anomalous connection may be to the heart itself (cardiac) or to the veins draining to the superior caval vein (supracardiac) or to those draining to the inferior caval vein (infracardiac). The sites of infracardiac connection include portal vein (Fig. 13.55), hepatic vein, and ductus venosus. Connection is rarely directly to the inferior caval vein. Supracardiac connection is more common and may be to superior caval vein (on either side), azygos vein, or innominate vein. Cardiac connection is almost always to the coronary sinus. There is frequently an element of obstruction to flow in the anomalous pathway. Obstruction is much more likely with infracardiac connection. The lesion may occur as an isolated abnormality but also occurs as part of a more complex malformation. As a consequence of the lack of pulmonary venous inflow, the left atrium is small. Pulmonary hypertension often develops early. If obstruction is present, the infant presents in the first few days of life with cyanosis and respiratory difficulty, but with nonobstructive connection, the infant will not present with symptoms for the first few months of life. Respiratory difficulty and failure to thrive are then the commonest features.

Partial anomalous pulmonary venous connection may involve one or more veins and may involve the drainage from a whole lung. Partial anomalous connection is an integral part of the sinus venosus atrial septal defect.

Ebstein's Malformation

The essential defect in this malformation is an abnormally low attachment of the tricuspid valve leaflets. The attachment, instead of being at the atrioventricular junction, is in the inlet part of the right ventricle [46]. The septal and infe-

rior leaflets show the abnormal attachment, and the septal leaflet is sometimes no more that a row of nodular excrescences descending in an oblique line on the right aspect of the interventricular septum (Fig. 13.56). The anterosuperior leaflet is also abnormal, being large and rectangular and attached to the papillary muscles in such a way as to obstruct the ventricular inflow. The valve tissue is frequently dysplastic with excess of redundant valvar tissue. The area of ventricular myocardium incorporated into the right atrium by the abnormally low attachment of the valve becomes thin and "atrialized." The valve is incompetent and there is often massive dilatation of the right atrium. Pulmonary stenosis (or atresia) is a frequent association. The condition may present in utero with cardiac failure and hydrops.

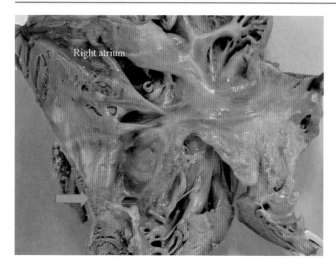

Fig. 13.56 Ebstein's malformation. A heart opened to demonstrate the abnormal attachment of the tricuspid valve to the septum. Instead of at the atrioventricular junction (*fine arrows*), the septal leaflet of the tricuspid valve is attached on an oblique line along the septum (*large arrow*). The remaining leaflet tissue of the tricuspid valve is also rather thin and nodular and shows abnormal attachments of the papillary muscles and chordae

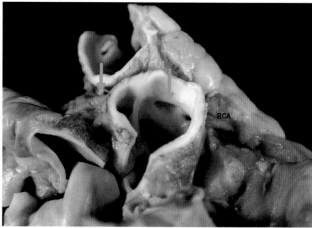

Fig. 13.57 Intramural course of left coronary artery. The aorta opened to demonstrate both coronary arteries arising from the right sinus. The right coronary artery leaves the aorta perpendicular to the wall. The left coronary artery exits the wall obliquely (*arrow*) to emerge anterior to the aorta (*second arrow*). This oblique intramural course corresponds to the line of apposition of aorta and pulmonary trunk

Anomalous Origin of the Coronary Arteries

Anomalous Origin of the Coronary Arteries from the Aorta

In the normal heart, the coronary arteries arise from the right and left facing sinuses of the aortic valve close to the sino-tubular junction. The right coronary artery is dominant in about 90% of cases, that is, it supplies the posterior interventricular artery. The coronary arteries arise at right angles to the aortic wall, and both main vessels skirt the pulmonary trunk but are not compressed between it and any other structure. In about 50% the normal population, two, sometimes even three, right coronary arteries arise from the right facing sinus [47]. The extra vessel is usually tiny, supplying only a small part of the pulmonary infundibulum (Fig. 13.4). There are numerous variations on one or other artery arising anomalously from the opposite coronary sinus [48]. Although there are cases reports of all being associated with an increased incidence of sudden death, it is likely that only two patterns are associated with a significant risk of vascular occlusion: an oblique course of the anomalous artery through the wall of the aorta such that the expansion of the aorta in systole acts to close the vessel lumen (Fig. 13.57) and an epicardial course of an anomalous artery between the aorta and the pulmonary trunk with potential for compression of the coronary artery between the two great vessels [49], particularly with exercise when the pulmonary trunk dilates. A single coronary artery arising from the aorta and supplying both right and left coronary circulations is extremely uncommon

in an otherwise normal heart [50] (incidence less than 1:7,000). It is much commoner in association with transposition of the great arteries.

An abnormally high take-off of the coronary arteries from the aorta, arbitrarily defined as greater than 1 cm above the sino-tubular junction, is associated with increased cardiac morbidity possibly because of an oblique course through the aortic wall.

The situation of disconnection of the coronary arteries from their aortic attachment has already been mentioned in the context of pulmonary atresia with intact ventricular septum.

Anomalous Origin of the Coronary Arteries from the Pulmonary Trunk

Where two coronary arteries arise normally from the aorta, it is possible, occasionally, to see a small supernumerary artery arising from the anterior pulmonary trunk. This vessel is very small, supplies usually only a small part of the anterior right ventricular wall, and is of no consequence.

Origin of the left coronary artery from the pulmonary trunk is of much greater significance [51]. This anomaly presents no problem in utero, but in the first weeks of life, as the pulmonary artery pressure falls, perfusion of the affected coronary artery territory is seriously compromised. The child presents with signs of myocardial ischemia, infarction, and cardiac failure or shock. Sudden death may occur. If the child survives, because of well-developed collateral circulation, presentation may be at a later age. Collateral vessel development may be so extensive as to result in steal to the

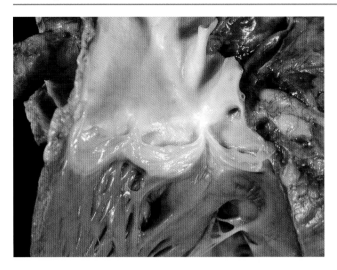

Fig. 13.58 Anomalous origin of the left coronary artery from the aorta. A 13-year-old who collapsed and died suddenly. At postmortem, the only abnormality was origin of the left coronary artery from the pulmonary artery. The *picture* shows the pulmonary artery (complete muscular infundibulum) and the widely patent left coronary artery arising from one of the sinuses of the pulmonary valve

pulmonary circulation. The artery usually arises from the posterior, leftward pulmonary sinus (Fig. 13.58). Over time, the left coronary artery becomes thin-walled. Ischemic fibrosis develops in the left ventricular myocardium, in association with endocardial fibrosis. There may be mitral regurgitation because of ischemic papillary muscle damage.

References

1. Anderson RH, Ho SY. Sequential segmental analysis – description and categorization for the millennium. Cardiol Young. 1997;7:98–116.
2. Rowlatt UF, Rimoldi HJA, Lev M. The quantitative anatomy of the normal child's heart. Pediatr Clin N Am. 1963;10:499–588.
3. Eckner FAO, Brown BW, Davidson DL, Glagov S. Dimensions of normal human hearts. Arch Pathol Lab Med. 1969;88:497–507.
4. Ashworth M. Cardiovascular pathology. In: Sebire NJ, Malone M, Ashworth M, Jacques TS, editors. Diagnostic paediatric surgical pathology. New York: Elsevier Ltd; 2010. p. 503–10.
5. Gallagher PJ, Sheppard M. Cardiac pathology Network. Bull R Coll Pathologists. 2010. p. 150,
6. Jordan SC, Scott O. Incidence, aetiology and recurrence of congenital heart disease. In: Jordan SC, Scott O, editors. Heart disease in paediatrics. 3rd ed. Oxford: Butterworth Heinemann; 1989. p. 3–9.
7. Skinner J, Alverson D, Hunter S. Echocardiography for the neonatologist. Churchill Livingstone; 2000,
8. Arey JB. Malformations of the ventricular septum. In: Arey JB, editor. Cardiovascular pathology in infants and children. Philadelphia: WB Saunders Company; 1984. p. 77–111.
9. Minette MS, Sahn DJ. Ventricular septal defects. Circulation. 2006;114:2190–7.
10. Milo S, Ho SY, Wilkinson JL, Anderson RH. The surgical anatomy and atrioventricular conduction tissues of hearts with isolated ventricular septal defects. J Thorac Cardiovasc Surg. 1980;79:244–55.
11. Anderson RH, Lennox CC, Zuberbuhler JR. The morphology of ventricular septal defects. Perspect Pediatr Pathol. 1984;8:235–68.
12. Silver MM, Freedom RM, Silver MD, et al. The morphology of the human newborn ductus arteriosus: a reappraisal of its structure and closure with special reference to prostaglandin E1. Hum Pathol. 1981;12:1123–36.
13. Tynan M. The ductus arteriosus and its closure. N Eng J Med. 1993;329:1570–2.
14. Fisher DC, Fisher EA, Budd JH, et al. The incidence of patent foramen ovale in 1,000 consecutive patients. A contrast transesophageal echocardiography study. Chest. 1995;107:1504–9.
15. Lee ME, Sade RM. Coronary sinus septal defect. Surgical considerations. J Thorac Cardiovasc Surg. 1979;78:563–9.
16. Al Zaghal AM, Li J, Anderson RH. Anatomic criteria for the diagnosis of sinus venosus defects. Heart. 1997;78:298–304.
17. Pellegrino A, Deverall PB, Anderson RH. Aortic coarctation in the first three months of life. Anatomopathological study with respect to treatment. J Thorac Cardiovasc Surg. 1985;89:121–7.
18. Becker AE, Becker MJ, Edwards JE. Anomalies associated with coarctation of the aorta. Particular reference to infancy. Circulation. 1970;41:1067–75.
19. Russell GA, Berry PJ, Watterson K, et al. Patterns of ductal tissue in coarctation of the aorta in the first three months of life. J Thorac Cardiovasc Surg. 1991;102:368–9.
20. Elzenga NJ, de Groot Gittenberger AC. Localised coarctation of the aorta. An age dependent spectrum. Br Heart J. 1983;49:317–23.
21. Anderson RH, Ho SY, Falcao S. The diagnostic features of atrioventricular septal defect with common atrioventricular orifice. Cardiol Young. 1998;8:33–49.
22. Thiene G, Wenink ACG, Frescura C, et al. The surgical anatomy of the conduction tissues in atrioventricular defects. J Thorac Cadiovasc Surg. 1981;82:928–37.
23. Weintraub RG, Brawn WJ, Venables Aw. Two patch repair of complete atrioventricular septal defect in the first year of life: results and sequential assessment of atrioventricular valve function. J Thorac Cardiovas Surg. 1990;99:320–6.
24. Daubeney PE, Delaney DJ, Anderson RH, et al. Pulmonary atresia with intact ventricular septum: range of morphology in a population based study. J Am Coll Cardiol. 2002;39:1670–9.
25. de Groot Gittenberger AC, Erlap I, Lie-Venema H, et al. Development of the coronary vasculature and its implications for coronary abnormalities in general and specifically in pulmonary atresia without ventricular septal defect. Acta Pediatr Suppl. 2004; 93:13–9.
26. Liao PK, Edwards WD, Julsrud PR, et al. Pulmonary blood supply in patients with pulmonary atresia and ventricular septal defect. J Am Coll Cardiol. 1985;6:1343–50.
27. Anderson RH, Allwork SP, Ho SY, et al. Surgical anatomy of tetralogy of Fallot. J Thorac Cardiovasc Surg. 1981;81:887–96.
28. Cobaanoglu A, Schultz JM. Total correction of tetralogy of Fallot in the first year of life: late results. Ann Thorac Surg. 2002;74: 133–8.
29. Zhao HX, Miller DC, Reitz BA. Surgical repair of tetralogy of Fallot. Long term follow up with particular emphasis on late death and reoperation. J Thorac Cardiovasc Surg. 1985;89:204–20.
30. Edwards JE. Pathology of left ventricular outflow tract obstruction. Circulation. 1965;31:586–99.
31. McKay R, Smith A, Leung MP, et al. Morphology of the ventriculoaortic junction in critical aortic stenosis. Implications for hemodynamic function and clinical management. J Thorac Cardiovasc Surg. 1992;104:434–42.
32. Ashworth MT. The cardiovascular system. In: Keeling JW, Khong TY, editors. Fetal and neonatal pathology. 4th ed. Berlin: Springer; 2007. p. 571–621.
33. Peterson TA, Todd DB, Edwards JE. Supravalvular aortic stenosis. J Thorac Cardiovasc Surg. 1965;50:734–41.

34. Van Son JAM, Edwards WD, Danielson GK. Pathology of coronary arteries, myocardium and great arteries in supravalvular aortic stenosis. Report of five cases with implications for surgical treatment. J Thorac Cardiovasc Surg. 1994;108:21–8.

35. Salmon AP. Hypoplastic left heart syndrome – outcome and management. Arch Dis Child. 2001;85:450–1.

36. O'Connor WN, Cash JB, Cottrill CM. Ventriculocoronary connections in hypoplastic left hearts: an autopsy microscopic study. Circulation. 1992;66:1078–86.

37. Elzenga NJ, de Groot Gittenberger AC. Coarctation and related aortic arch anomalies in hypoplastic left heart syndrome. Int J Cardiol. 1985;8:379–93.

38. D'Udekem Y, Iyengar AJ, Cochran AD. The Fontan procedure. Contemporary techniques have improved long-term outcomes. Circulation. 2007;116(11 Suppl):I 157–64.

39. Bartram U, Grunenfelder J, van Praagh R. Causes of death after modified Norwood procedure: a study of 122 postmortem cases. Ann Thorac Surg. 1997;63:1795–802.

40. Anderson RH, Henry GW, Becker AE. Morphologic aspects of complete transposition. Cardiol Young. 1991;1:41–53.

41. Yacoub MH, Radley Smith R. Anatomy of the coronary arteries in transposition of the great arteries and methods of their transfer in anatomical correction. Thorax. 1978;33:418–24.

42. Allwork SP, Bentall HH, Becker AE, et al. Congenitally corrected transposition of the great arteries: morphologic study of 32 cases. Am J Cardiol. 1976;38:910–23.

43. Collett RW, Edwards JE. Persistent truncus arteriosus: a classification according to anatomic types. Surg Clin N Am. 1949;29:1245–70.

44. de la Cruz MV, Cayre R, Angelini P, et al. Coronary arteries in truncus arteriosus. Am J Cardiol. 1990;66:1482–6.

45. DeLisle G, Ando M, Calder AL, et al. Total anomalous pulmonary venous connection: report of 93 autopsied cases with emphasis on diagnostic and surgical considerations. Am Heart J. 1976;91:99–122.

46. Anderson RK, Lie JT. Pathologic anatomy of Ebstein's anomaly of the heart revisited. Am J Cardiol. 1978;41:739–45.

47. Becker AE. Variations of the main coronary arteries. In: Becker AE, Losekoot TG, Marcellettti C, Anderson RH, editors. Paediatric cardiology. 3rd ed. Edinburgh: Churchill Livingstone; 1981. p. 263–77.

48. Neufeld HN, Schneeweiss A. Congenital variations of coronary arteries. In: Neufeld HN, Schneeweiss A, editors. Coronary artery diseases in infants and children. Philadelphia: Lea & Febiger; 1983. p. 65–78.

49. Ness MJ, McManus BM. Anomalous right coronary origin in otherwise unexplained infant death. Arch Pathol Lab Med. 1988;112:626–9.

50. Kimbiris D, Iskandrian AS, Segal BL, et al. Anomalous aortic origin of coronary arteries. Circulation. 1978;58:606–15.

51. Arey JB. Malformations of the coronary vessels. In: Arey JB, editor. Cardiovascular pathology in infants and children. Philadelphia: WB Saunders Company; 1984. p. 204–17.

Sudden Cardiac Death

14

S. Kim Suvarna

Abstract

Sudden death from cardiac disease is common, and this section deals with how to confirm the cardiac disease as the cause of the death. It also considers other (noncardiac) conditions that may masquerade as cardiac disease. A pragmatic approach to the common disorders of ischemic heart disease, valvular pathology, cardiomyopathy, and myocarditis is given. An analysis of channelopathies is provided together with consideration of abnormal conduction pathways. Issues regarding deaths following stressful events are debated, particularly from a medicolegal perspective, and aspects of postoperative deaths are also described. The role of obesity in sudden cardiac death is presented along with rarer causes of sudden death (thrombotic thrombocytopenic purpura, commotio cordis, and muscular dystrophy). A simple tabular analysis of the likelihood of cardiac pathology being implicated in the cause of death is provided.

Keywords

Sudden death • Ischemic heart disease • Valve disease • Cardiomyopathy • Myocarditis • Channelopathy • Muscular dystrophy • Cardiac surgery • Congenital heart disease • Obesity Stress • Microangiopathy • Commotio cordis

Introduction and General Considerations

This section follows the previous chapters and aims to assist consideration of cases of sudden, possibly cardiac, death. Even with a fairly good understanding of cardiac disease, this is probably one of the most difficult areas to define in terms of pathology substrate [1–6]. Sudden cardiac death is also a term misunderstood and variably misused by medical practitioners and the public.

What Is Sudden Cardiac Death?

From study data, sudden cardiac death appears to apply both to men and women, from the young to the old. It is difficult to define prevalence of this condition since the quality of autopsy practice, range and usage of diagnostic tests, and death certification statements vary even within a single country and significantly across the world [1, 2, 7–9].

One can consider the concept of sudden cardiac death from a variety of standpoints. However, starting from preliminary aspects of case analysis, it should be understood that the 'sudden' quality is related to an unexpected death or one that occurs within a short time frame. The period of time under consideration varies, according to those who have considered this subject [1, 2], from being almost immediate through to 24 h. Pragmatically, it is reasonable to consider a case as possible sudden cardiac death where symptoms (syncope, palpitations, chest pain, etc.) start and progress to death over a matter of minutes or possibly up to 2 h. Two to six

S.K. Suvarna, MBBS, B.Sc., FRCP, FRCPath
Histopathology, Northern General Hospital, Sheffield Teaching Hospitals NHS Foundation Trust,
Sheffield S5 7AU, UK
e-mail: s.k.suvarna@sheffield.ac.uk

Fig. 14.1 Part of a bedroom scene of death photograph from a young student found dead unexpectedly. There is clearly a syringe and lighter visible along with citric acid sachets (often used to assist dissolving heroin). Clearly, this evidence points to illicit drug use (later confirmed by toxicology) and indicates this is not likely to revolve around cardiac pathology

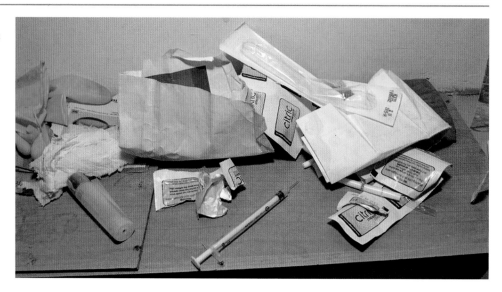

hours, as a time frame being called sudden, is debatable. However, it could well be argued that it is excessive to suggest that anything over 6 h is sudden!

The term sudden cardiac death often implies that the diagnosis is, at that point of consideration, still undefined – although suspected as cardiac. Therefore, one should perhaps not use this designation in cases of previously known and well-defined cardiac disease (e.g., hypertrophic cardiomyopathy, ischemic heart disease) as these deaths are better classified according to the underlying pathology – in this author's opinion. For example, one could simply consider a case of death (45 min after symptoms started) in a case of coronary atheroma and acute myocardial infarction as simply that of death due to ischemic heart disease. Whether one chooses to call it *ischemic heart disease*, *myocardial infarction due to coronary artery disease*, or another formulation covering this situation is a matter of local practice/preference.

The sudden cardiac death designation alternatively may be used to imply an occult cardiac pathology, potentially of an inheritable or subtle type. In this regard, caution in the use of this descriptive/diagnostic phrase is advocated. Irrespective of whether any genetic influences may be suspected, pushing this diagnostic concept forwards at any early stage of the death investigation can prompt undue alarm to relatives and unnecessary family investigations.

Within the broad group of sudden deaths, many have no (or only limited) antemortem clinical data at the outset of the investigation. Rapid progress to an autopsy may be the wrong approach. Rather, the key pathology may be suggested by history, provided from relatives and background medical sources – if one takes the time to request and review this information stream before the autopsy. The background circumstances,

medical history, drug (therapeutic/illicit) history, and home circumstances (such as photographic evidence from the scene) (Fig. 14.1) can guide the approach to the autopsy examination and the diagnostic tests to be used [3, 10, 11].

Although the focus will often be on the heart/cardiovascular disease, one must diligently exclude noncardiac disease. Sudden cardiac death is a tempting title to bestow on cases of death, lacking instant cause and effect data – particularly in the young. Thus, overzealous use of this phrase is a problem if it misdirects attention falsely onto the heart and if it ignores other potential pathology. An example might be deaths where some coronary atheroma is found and ascribed as the cause of death but where the cranial content tissues are not examined – thereby missing the diagnosis of an intracranial catastrophe.

Thus, given these realities and considerations, one may see "sudden cardiac death" as a concept diagnosis, occurring within a short time frame and one that may reflect cardiac disease. The key task is to define the underlying cardiac pathology substrate.

Before the Autopsy

As has already been discussed, the background history is pivotal to any case. Lifestyle realities are pertinent and it is recommended that detailed data is required in terms of smoking history, therapeutic drug prescriptions, previous and ongoing illegal drug usage, gender, age, and exercise/background health realities. In addition, information with regard to where and when the death occurred (sleeping, waking, activity-based) should be sought.

Fig. 14.2 Two ECGs (**a**, **b**), taken 4 h apart, of a single person in a case of Brugada syndrome. The recordings show some electrical variability and an abnormal ECG complex. These recordings antedated the sudden death in this young adult 9 months later

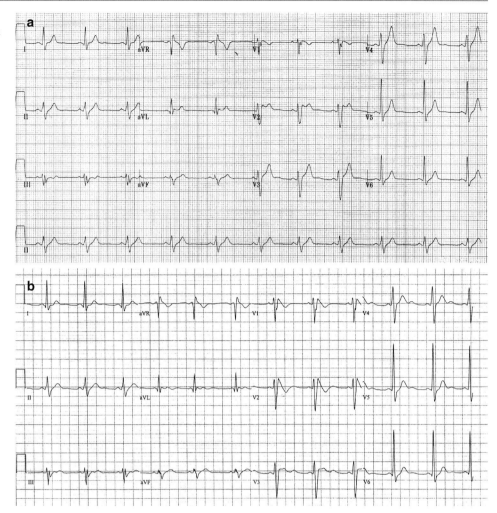

The previous medical and family history of the individual are vital together with knowledge of previous investigations, particularly around the time of death [3, 10]. The opportunity to review any antemortem ECG (Fig. 14.2) evidence should not be missed. Commentary from any clinicians attending the deceased is also particularly valuable, and an attempt should be made to access the family physician data.

Practical Considerations in Cases of Sudden (Unexpected) Death

It goes without saying that a full and thorough examination of the body is needed. Furthermore, an experienced autopsy practitioner should perform the case study. In cases of high probability of inherited cardiac disease, one can argue that cases should be referred to specialist practitioners and/or units with experience in cardiac disease.

The external appearances of the body as a whole must be considered before the autopsy knife is put to skin. Features of significance include petechial hemorrhages (Fig. 14.3), splinter hemorrhages, congestive qualities around the face, positional lividity, clubbing (Fig. 14.4), features of intravenous drug use (Fig. 14.5), signs of prior thoracic surgery/ intervention, sepsis (Fig. 14.6), peripheral edema, and so on. Most good texts on autopsy practice will deal with these issues [11]. Without this inspection, vital clues of underlying disease may be missed or lost, whether they reflect heart disease or other issues.

Of particular value in cases of sudden death is the opportunity to access a colleague with similar interests/skills. The potential to have a separate independent pair of eyes looking at cardiac/other tissues is of particular benefit in cases of legal scrutiny. As an adjunct, photography of tissues/lesions is of value for later review – even if the tissues appear normal.

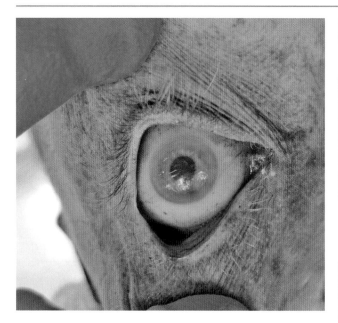

Fig. 14.3 Macroscopic photograph of small scleral and conjunctival petechial hemorrhages. This case involved acute complete airway obstruction

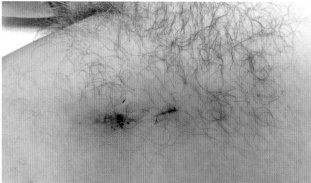

Fig. 14.5 The groin of an intravenous drug abuser with numerous needle marks, bruising, and the suggestion of local sepsis/scarring

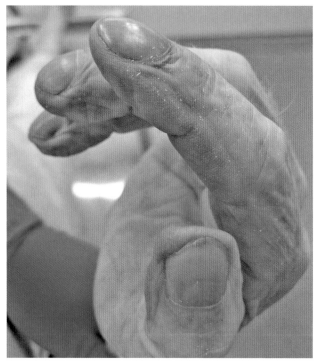

Fig. 14.4 Finger clubbing. This can be seen in a variety of systemic illnesses, some of which may reflect cardiac phenomena

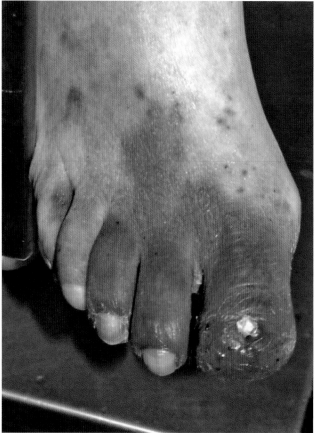

Fig. 14.6 Peripheral zonal ischemic changes reflecting septic emboli from a case of infective endocarditis

One of the common questions attached to such cases is whether one has personally/examined and fully dissected the case. It is recognized that many autopsy practitioners work closely with mortuary technicians who will open the bodies and dissect tissues in a busy public mortuary, on behalf of the pathologist. It is realistic to understand that this process is efficient. However, cases of sudden (potentially cardiac) death, especially in the young, deserve particular scrutiny and close inspection by the autopsy practitioner personally at all stages. In these circumstances, the entire dissection should be performed by the pathologist or, at the very least, with the pathologist watching the early dissection process by the technician and with him/her proceeding with the rest of the examination. The concept of "bucket autopsies" – wherein organs are removed *en-bloc* and placed into a bucket by a technician before the pathologist even arrives in the mortuary – should never occur! The pathologist should perform the examination, covering all major systems with reservation of histology, toxicology, and other samples [3, 11] – as described in the autopsy chapter earlier.

Hopefully, macroscopic pathology will guide the pathologist towards the diagnosis. Nevertheless, many cases are, even after careful examination in effect, a "negative" initial autopsy, with no macroscopic clues. Cases lacking overt naked eye pathology may include a variety of disorders. These include cardiomyopathy, abnormal cardiac conduction pathways, genetic abnormalities (storage disorders, channelopathies, etc.), and a variety of metabolic defects, as will be discussed later in this chapter.

It is recommended that when a case of sudden death, without macroscopic findings is encountered, one should ensure that all aspects of the clinical record are revisited. Ideally, one should be searching for additional clinical data – perhaps by triangulating data from other family members and those who saw the deceased before death. There must, of course, be complete review of the macroscopic findings in their entirety. It is easily possible, even for those practiced in this arena, to miss a very small focal occlusive coronary lesion such as focal vasculitis. Diligent reexamination of the tissues, sometimes with a colleague assisting, can often be helpful. Widespread histology sampling of the tissues involving all noncardiac systems is also required. Detailed cardiac histology must be taken, as described in the earlier autopsy chapter. If samples have been taken for toxicology, then these should be analyzed. Similarly, samples for microbiology (ideally taken as one progresses throughout the autopsy to avoid contamination) are recommended for identification of standard/atypical bacteria, fungi, and viral agents [11].

Perhaps one of the most surprising aspects of this work is the reality that there are still a significant number of sudden death cases that are examined minimally and/or with limited tests. Surprisingly, there are even cases with no ancillary laboratory investigations to support the macroscopy! From a pragmatic perspective there exist published and readily available checklists of possible interpretations that can be considered against the possible/likely causes of sudden death [3, 11]. It is recommended that the Royal College of Pathologists' cardiac/sudden death scenario [10] is available (and consulted) to permit exclusion of the various pathological disorders. Other standard sets of guidelines will also assist the pathologist [3, 4]. This approach will enhance the likelihood of a diagnosis and should also prevent criticism if the case is reviewed by relatives and others. It is certainly apparent that the diligent autopsy for cardiac disease is increasingly held to be of significance by society. Regrettably, adverse comment by the legal profession and some medical

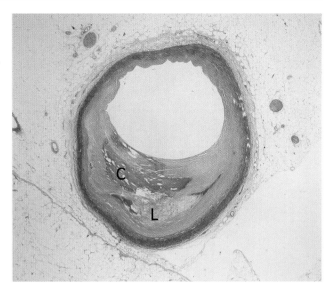

Fig. 14.7 Microscopic view of moderate atheromatous disease, with areas of calcification (C) and lipid-rich necrotic material (L), commonly present in many individuals of middle age and above in the "westernized" world. Such lesions are relatively common in the autopsy room but do not necessarily indicate death from coronary disease (hematoxylin and eosin)

professional bodies has been made of autopsy practitioners within recent decades who have failed to consider appropriately cases of sudden cardiac death. Certainly, poor practice will no longer be accepted by the courts, the relatives, or the press!

Starting with Noncardiac Sudden Death

It may seem perverse to start any sudden death investigation with noncardiac disease at the front of one's mind, but the practitioner is advised to initially focus upon noncardiac disorders and disease before considering the heart itself. Furthermore, some awareness of background (expected) pathology is needed. Given that many adults in the "westernized" world have some coronary atheroma (Fig. 14.7), often in the range 20–50% and/or a degree of cardiac hypertrophy (reflecting lifestyle issues), one must avoid simply jumping at this, as a disease, if one is to avoid missing another significant disorder. As has already been indicated, the diagnosis of the relevant pathology is one of careful consideration, with exclusion of lesser pathologies.

It must be appreciated that some sudden deaths with noncardiac pathology can mimic cardiac disease with rapidly fatal outcomes – often with symptoms that suggest a primary cardiac disorder. The best example of this is pulmonary embolism (Fig. 14.8), wherein significant thrombus matter travels from a deep vein (usually from the pelvis or leg) to impact in the proximal pulmonary artery circulation causing sudden cardiac overload and cardiac arrest. This is clearly

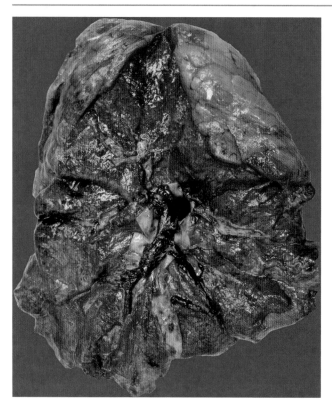

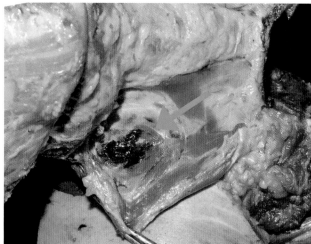

Fig. 14.9 Soft tissues from the neck in a homicide case of strangulation. The neck is seen running transversely across the *top part* of the photograph, with the thorax to the *right side*. The right sternocleidomastoid muscle has been reflected outwards to show the irregular bruising (*arrowed*) associated with pathological neck compression

Fig. 14.8 A large pulmonary embolism completely occluding the major branches of a pulmonary artery. The other lung was also affected with smaller fragments in segmental bronchi, thereby explaining the sudden death of this individual

not a primary cardiac pathology but one that produces features that can be easily misinterpreted by family members, or even the clinician, as cardiac disease. The presence of an abnormal ECG and raised/potentially false-positive serum troponin levels may further complicate matters in some cases who survive for a period of time after the embolism. Despite this, any competent autopsy examination should be able to identify the pulmonary embolism and furthermore point to the source of the thrombosis/embolus.

Particular attention upon the larynx and adjacent neck structures with local soft tissue bruising (Fig. 14.9) and/or petechial hemorrhage should be made in cases of sudden death, so as to not miss the opportunity to diagnose airway obstruction in cases of asphyxia/homicide. In a similar manner, respiratory disease such as acute obstruction of the major airways or severe asthma can cause sudden death. The careful and thorough autopsy will permit diagnosis of the type of airway obstruction. Awareness of asthma should allow macroscopic diagnosis of many of the features (gas trapping/overinflated lungs, mucus plugs, etc.). On occasion, histology (Fig. 14.10) can be of value in supporting pathological considerations. It should also be remembered that alterations to the gases inspired may cause apparent sudden death, whether the gases are introduced in an accidental or suicidal manner.

Consideration of all the circumstances of the death, supported by scene of death images, will be of particular value. Indeed, some situations (such as carbon monoxide poisoning) can be easily overlooked if due autopsy diligence is not taken.

Pathology in the cranial cavity and primary disease of the brain, such as skull fracture (often with local or contrecoup brain parenchymal trauma), spontaneous intracranial hemorrhage, and epilepsy, may also create the situation of apparent sudden cardiac death. Some of these pathologies can be revealed by a full autopsy. It cannot be overstated that the appropriate medical history and toxicology is also paramount in such cases. It is further emphasized that the opening of the cranial cavity is mandatory in all cases of putative sudden cardiac death to exclude noncardiac disease.

Another disorder commonly overlooked is that of acute bacteremia/septicemia. Such cases involving the young without anatomical cause of death can be perplexing. Clues regarding septicemia can be seen in the brown discoloration of arterial intimal and endocardial surfaces (Fig. 14.11), due to intravascular hemolysis terminally. The spleen (Fig. 14.12) in these cases is often enlarged and congested and shows a softened (almost fluid) parenchyma. Histological evidence is often seen in the form of blood vessels with significant bacterial overgrowth widely affecting many organ systems. This often suggests that numerous bacteria were present in the blood stream at the point of death and, when blood has ceased flowing, after death, these bacteria can proliferate further within the tissues for a short period of time. Clearly, appropriate microbiology [11] (sampling not only for standard bacteria but also atypical agents) needs to be undertaken if such a diagnosis is to be secured.

There are other rarer causes of sudden death that can mimic cardiac disease. These include, to name a few, acute

Fig. 14.10 A sudden death case explained by consideration of the histology. The findings of pronounced eosinophilia, inflammation, and mucus plugging within the airways indicated asthma as the likely cause of the collapse and death of this individual. It was later determined that there was a background history of asthma, but interestingly, the individual has no asthmatic medications on him at the time of death (hematoxylin and eosin)

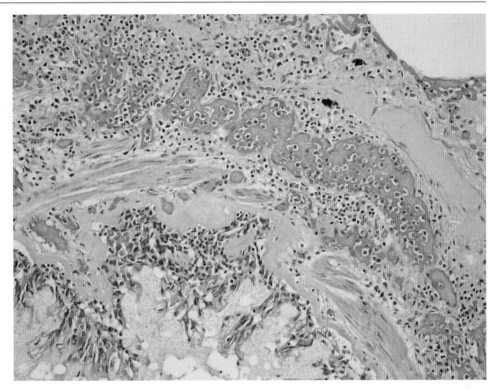

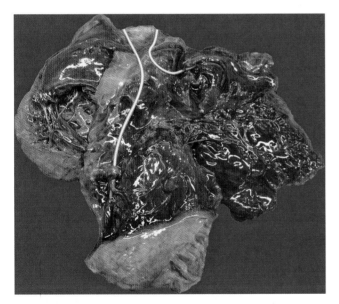

Fig. 14.11 The surface of the endocardium shows a brown discoloration. This may also be seen involving the intimal surfaces of major vessels. This was a case of streptococcal sepsis with hemolysis and heavy bacteremia (septicemia)

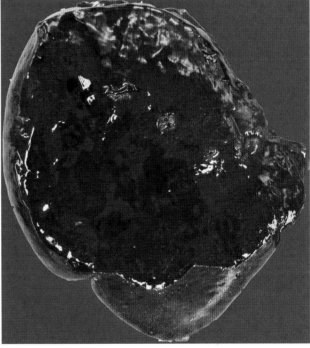

Fig. 14.12 A softened spleen is seen in some case of systemic sepsis. The cut surface is semiliquified

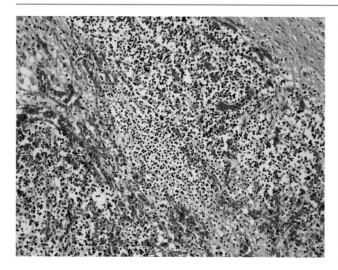

Fig. 14.13 The adrenal tissues in a case of sudden death were noted to have pronounced lymphoid destruction of the cortical tissues, as seen in this high-magnification image. No normal cortical cells are seen. By contrast, there was preservation of the medullary parenchyma. This was an acute Addisonian crisis. There was some family history of autoimmune disease (hematoxylin and eosin)

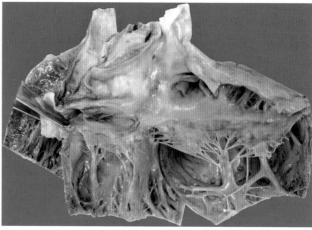

Fig. 14.14 This case of a sudden death in a young adult female was referred as a possible inherited cardiomyopathy. The histology and toxicology was reported as negative. Only after one family member raised some queries did further questioning of the relatives allow the history of suicidal intent to come forward. The deceased had apparently taken the cardiac therapy medications from another family member. The routine toxicology assay did not identify this drug initially

anaphylaxis, Addison-type crisis (Fig. 14.13), various drug reactions, and so on. This chapter does not have the luxury to explore all of these realities, but securing blood and other body fluids for toxicology [11] (e.g., drugs of abuse and therapeutic agents) and serology (serum tryptase, serum electrolytes, vitreous glucose, etc.) often aids the identification of the pathology in these cases.

Nonnatural death (i.e., such as homicide) can be suggested in terms of individuals with features of compressive contusions (see Fig. 14.9) or other significant trauma. Suicidal intent may be suggested by notes that are left behind. It should be noted that their absence does not exclude the possibility of suicide, and their presence does not automatically exclude homicide!

One should also have considered the possibility that relatives, and indeed medical staff, will try to "tidy up" bodies following death. The opportunity to identify illegal drugs of abuse [11] and suicidal intent may be impeded by such activities, and one needs to have an open and, to a degree, a suspicious mind. Indeed, sudden deaths with an apparent normal phenotype and a negative toxicology screen may be problematical when considered, and obscure toxins may only be identified if one is prepared to consider all possibilities (Fig. 14.14). Ultimately, there is no substitute for having a suspicious and wide-ranging mind!

Deaths due to Cardiac Disease

The main cardiac pathologies, in the western world, liable to cause sudden death include ischemic heart disease, cardiomyopathy, valvular heart disease, and myocarditis. These

are covered in detail in the earlier chapters, but these, and some other conditions, are now reviewed within this chapter to assist case analysis of potential sudden cardiac death cases.

However, when defining a case a cardiac in nature, one question often given cursory attention by the pathologist is "why did the heart fail and cause death at that point in time?" This is pertinent when so many of the population have some degree of cardiac abnormality/pathology. This is clearly stable one day and yet fatal later! Understanding the likely pathophysiology will ideally reassure one in terms of defining the cause of death.

For those dying suddenly, it is possible to consider the cause of cardiac disease-related death within two broad categories. The first broad cause of death is that of "pump failure." This implies that whatever disease is present, it has adversely affected the ability of the heart to contract and deliver blood in a unidirectional flow pattern into the systemic and pulmonary artery systems. The underlying causes for this process are often blatant and structural, including valvular disease, acute myocardial infarction, cardiac tamponade, etc. Nevertheless, one may need to consider other occult subtle toxicological/toxemic events which diminish overall cardiac performance.

The second broad cause of cardiac dysfunction involves the electrophysiological disorders (often seen in cases of cardiac dysrhythmia). Accepting that cardiac contraction requires coordinated and sequential cell depolarization, with muscle contraction followed subsequently by repolarization, means that any factors interfering with this mechanism can readily culminate with sudden death. These processes can also be overt, in cases of myocardial infarction involving

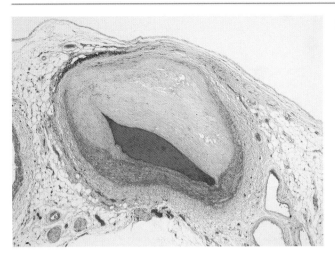

Fig. 14.15 Coronary artery with high-grade fibro-lipid atheroma narrowing the vascular lumen eccentrically. There is some coagulum in the lumen, not to be confused with thrombus (hematoxylin and eosin)

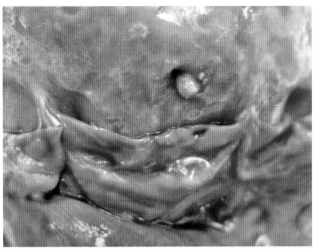

Fig. 14.16 The coronary ostium can occasionally be occluded by an irregular atheromatous plaque with lesser changes of atheroma in the downstream vasculature. Careful consideration of the ostia is required in all cases of sudden death, and it should be noted that opening flat the aortic root may apparently show less ostial stenosis than when intact as a ring

important tracts of conducting tissue, although more subtle disorders such as histology infiltrates, drugs, and inherited conditions (e.g., channelopathies) need to be considered. Many of these cases of sudden death are underpinned by acute tachy/bradyarrhythmias, with perhaps the best recognized being ventricular fibrillation.

Ischemic Heart Disease as a Cause of Sudden Death

Coronary artery disease is very common, as discussed in the earlier chapter, and mostly reflects atheroma. However, one common reality within the United Kingdom and other similar countries is that many adults in adult and later life have a degree of coronary atheroma (see Fig. 14.7). This is clearly not normal, but rather it is a predictable reality of "westernized" diets and lifestyles for much of the population. Several questions arise from this reality:

- How much atheroma is needed to invoke this pathology as the cause of death?
- Is another pathology (e.g., scarring fibrosis/acute infarction/other) required to validate or substantiate the diagnosis?

It is generally accepted that sudden death is associated with coronary stenosis of 70%, or more, narrowing (Fig. 14.15). This level of disease can usually be readily assessed in the autopsy room and is a realistic naked eye threshold – even allowing for some interobserver variability [12, 13]. Furthermore, one can easily understand how having two or more affected vessels will magnify the risks of cardiac ischemic death, even if only one artery is at the 70%, or more, level.

Likewise, one can appreciate that moderate atheromatous disease (e.g., at about 40–50%) can be complicated by endol-

umenal thrombosis on top of an erosion or ruptured plaque. Such thrombosis can precipitously raise the degree of stenosis, create sudden cardiac tissue hypoxia, and thereby lead to sudden death. Many of these cases terminate as sudden cardiac dysrhythmia-associated death, and the key investigation needed is to identify the culprit thrombus. One classic catch, when only moderate atheroma is found, is the presence of high-grade atheroma at the coronary ostium (Fig. 14.16). This can be associated with a high-grade obstruction and yet have lesser atheroma downstream within the coronary vessels.

When faced with sudden death in coronary artery cases, one can debate whether it is required to block and histologically examine the entirety or parts of these vascular tissues. Sampling protocols and permissions vary across the world. The UK practice, defined by HM Coroner, is that such examination is not needed [14] *if the diagnosis has been made.* However, this is not an ideal reality within which to work. Histology is valuable, and practiced pathologists, including this author, are regularly surprised by the degree of atheroma being somewhat different from the macroscopic evaluation. The possibility of combined pathology such as associated dissection and vasculitis can, of course, be missed without histology.

Cases in the autopsy room with myocardial infarction are known clinically to be associated with sudden death. Clearly, septal or lateral wall rupture creating cardiac tamponade (Figs. 14.17 and 14.18) cause sudden "pump" decompensation and death. However, the diagnosis of early infarction is not always an easy task – even with modern, and/or histological, techniques. Nevertheless, the diagnosis of a well-defined, acute infarction (Fig. 14.19) allows considerable comfort in defining this as the likely cause of sudden death.

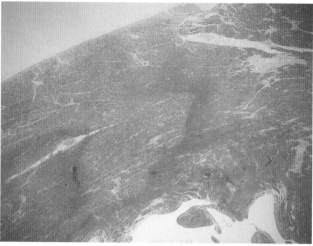

Fig. 14.19 Acute infarction changes in a case of untreated community-based coronary thrombosis. Well-defined infarction of tissues is seen with in inflammatory border (mainly polymorphs and macrophages) at the edge. The infarcted tissues show coagulative necrosis (hematoxylin and eosin)

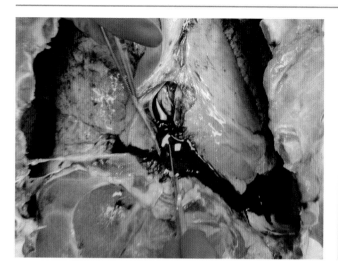

Fig. 14.17 Sudden death in a case of cardiac tamponade following myocardial rupture. The pericardial sac has been opened anteriorly to demonstrate the fresh blood in the sac

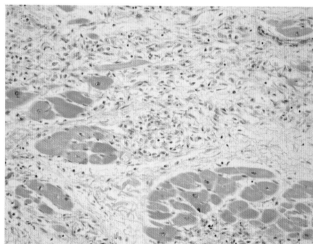

Fig. 14.20 Subacute ischemic changes are seen with some preserved myocytes, edematous fibrous connective tissue, scattered mixed inflammatory cells, and minor hemosiderin deposits. Small capillaries are present focally (hematoxylin and eosin)

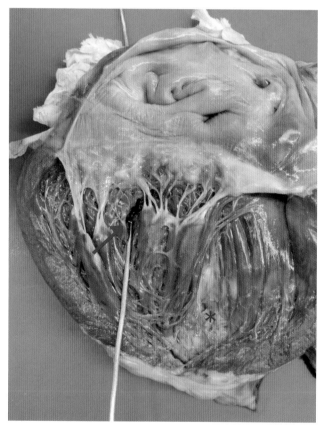

Fig. 14.18 A case of cardiac tamponade with an area of old infarction scarring (*) towards the apex and a fresh infarction, through which blood has flowed causing cardiac tamponade and death. The rupture is *arrowed* and a probe is in place to indicate the track of the blood

Subacute changes and/or patchy infarction can be a problem. Such changes often reflect infarction processes that have occurred sometime previously (Fig. 14.20). They can be difficult to date – particularly if revascularization treatments

have been provided to the patient. Subacute infarction and tissue regeneration/repair is also often the consequence of tissue rescue by modern therapeutic revascularization regimens. Similar changes that can be easily misinterpreted are foci of microinfarction from inotrope-treated individuals from the intensive care unit (Fig. 14.21) as well as hibernating or stunned myocardium – following myocardial infarction (Figs. 14.22 and 14.23). The latter are characterized by foci of myocyte loss with local young fibroblastic tissue, with vacuolated and/or shrunken myocytes. However, all of these changes are potential drivers for sudden dysrhythmic death.

The matter of established prior infarction and fibrosis can also be problematical. Aside from the fact that scarring can be

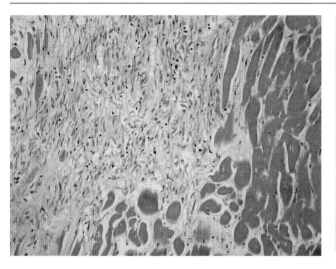

Fig. 14.21 Inotrope-related damage is seen as microinfarction changes akin to subacute ischemic phenomena (hematoxylin and eosin)

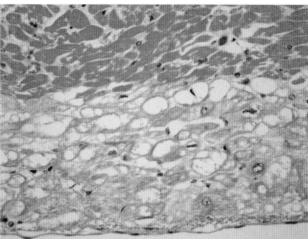

Fig. 14.23 Stunned myocardium is noted with vacuolar change involving cardiac myocytes and local edema (hematoxylin and eosin)

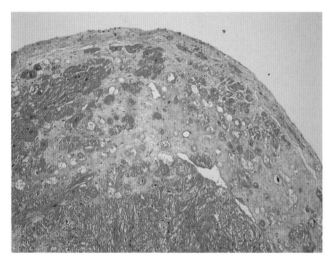

Fig. 14.22 Hibernating myocardium is seen with large vacuolated cardiac myocytes with some local fibrosis (hematoxylin and eosin)

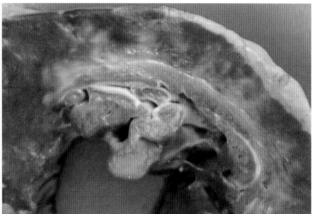

Fig. 14.24 Close up macroscopic view of old infarction damage (showing fibrosis and some lipoatrophy) in the left ventricle. This elderly female had suffered uncomplicated myocardial infarction 10 years previously and had been otherwise well. She was found dead at home, with no other significant illness or pathology

seen in cases of noncardiac death, one may take the view that scarring can be associated with dysrhythmias and thereby the sudden death. Thus, one faces the question, "how much fibrosis is needed to invoke this link, and why did it cause the death on that day and not in the week beforehand, and so on?"

Many autopsy cases have some cardiac scarring, although the pattern and extent varies. In the face of an acute dysrhythmic event, it may not be unreasonable to "blame" the old infarction (Figs. 14.24 and 14.25) – *if all else is negative.* These fibrosis-associated sudden deaths should have associated background, significant atheromatous disease. Unfortunately, as stated, many cases at autopsy have some mild/patchy myocardial scarring in the context of only mild-moderate coronary disease. The coronary stenosis seen is often in the region of 50% or less. This provides a ready source of consternation for many autopsy practitioners, and it is clear that some pathologists opt for the easy option of a quick

(potentially incorrect) diagnosis, rather than considering that there might be an alternative noncardiac pathology (e.g., in the cranial cavity or another, yet to be shown, by histology).

In the situation of focal scarring and mild coronary disease (<40% stenosis), one could be dogmatic and state that the criteria for ischemic disease have not been met. However, one must remember that such atheromatous plaque disease can be altered radically with surface thrombus and can create a sudden increase in the degree of stenosis and thereby focal ischemia/infarction. Nevertheless, proving the thrombus link may be a problem. In the era of "clot-busting" therapy and/or natural thrombolysis, there is a finite chance that the moderate grade stenosis with added significant thrombus may have resolved days (Fig. 14.26), months, or years previously – but still leave some myocardial damage acutely or chronically. In these circumstances, if all else is negative (toxicology, histology, microbiology, etc.), then one might conclude that

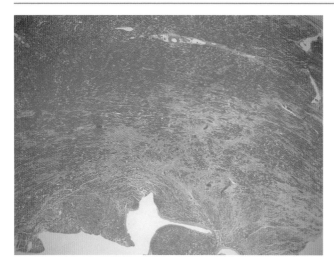

Fig. 14.25 Established patchy fibrosis is seen in a case of sudden death. This elderly individual had significant triple vessel atheroma. He was found dead at home with no warning symptoms (hematoxylin and eosin)

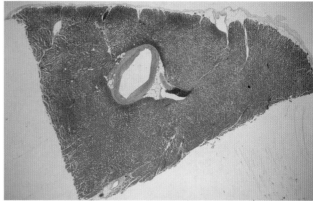

Fig. 14.27 The coronary vessel in this case is seen to be below the level of the epicardial aspect of the ventricular wall. This measured less than 1 cm length and was only within the myocardium focally. Caution must be taken not to overinterpret such phenomena as a myocardial bridge (hematoxylin and eosin)

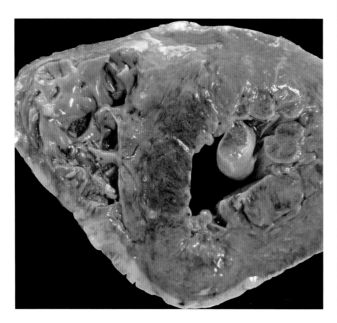

Fig. 14.26 Moderate hemorrhagic changes, mainly in the septum, are present in this case of myocardial ischemia successfully treated with clot lysis therapy 3 days beforehand. These changes are clearly seen when acute, but myocardial fibrosis/scarring would have been the chronic consequence, had the patient survived. In fact, the patient developed acute cardiac failure despite the treatments and died from a dysrhythmia

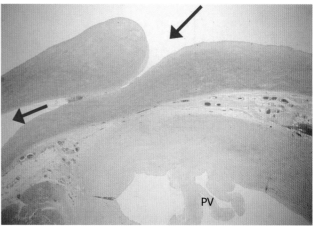

Fig. 14.28 An anomalous coronary artery is noted to be running obliquely through the aortic wall and to pass between the aorta and pulmonary artery. The lumen has a narrowing, impeding the path of blood flow (*arrowed*). Some reactive intimal changes are present at the origin where repetitive compression of the arterial origin caused downstream ischemic change. Part of the pulmonary valve is marked (PV) (hematoxylin and eosin)

death was possibly due to cardiac dysrhythmia in the context of ischemic fibrosis. However, this has to be an endpoint diagnosis of exclusion, and it should be not entered into without detailed consideration to exclude other realities. It should also be supported by relevant clinical history.

Of course, other nonatheromatous vascular disorders can be associated with ischemic damage. Myocardial bridging is an easily abused issue/diagnosis. The concept, put simply, is

that of myocardial tissue running over the top of a segment of coronary artery, causing partial/complete occlusion during systole. This diagnosis, as a specific pathology, should only be invoked when all other investigations are judged negative and when there is a significant length of coronary artery (i.e., 10 mm or more) artery positioned at least 3 mm below the myocardial surface. A minor degree of coronary artery depression into the myocardial tissues is commonly encountered in cardiac examinations of those dying of other (noncardiac) disorders (Fig. 14.27). Indeed, due stringency must be applied to avoid an over-call of minor anatomical coronary artery variations.

It is recognized that anomalous coronary arteries (Fig. 14.28) and arteries with "high takeoff" may be involved

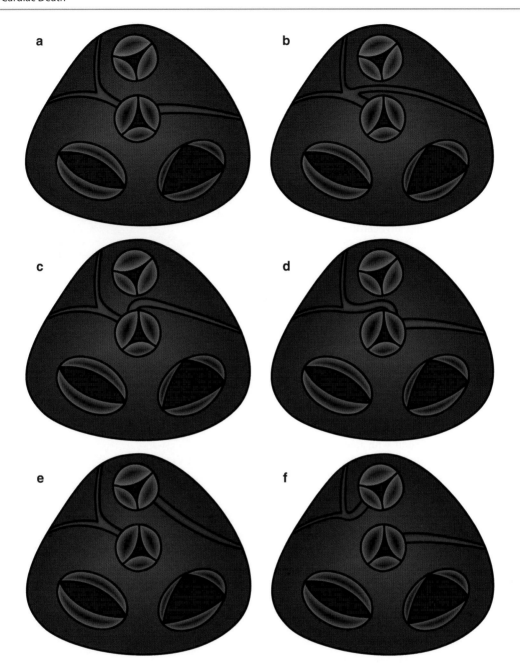

Fig. 14.29 Diagrammatic representations of coronary artery geography. (**a**) Viewed from above, the normal cardiac silhouette pattern shows the central aorta with tricuspid and mitral valves behind and the pulmonary artery anteriorly. One notes the right and left coronary systems, passing to their respective sides of the heart from the ostia sited at the base of the aorta. (**b**) Very rarely coronaries with a common origin may be linked to sudden death perhaps reflecting compression of the branch that runs between the pulmonary artery and aorta. (**c**, **d**) Those with coronary vessels coming from the wrong side of the aorta and passing between the aorta and pulmonary artery appear to be associated with sudden deaths, again probably reflecting artery compression between the aorta and pulmonary artery. (**e**, **f**) Those with a coronary artery originating from the pulmonary artery are linked to sudden deaths

in terms of sudden cardiac death. The main pathology liable to cause sudden cardiac death involves those coronary arteries running between the aorta and pulmonary artery, wherein compression of the coronary vessel occurs during systole with subsequent downstream ischemic consequences. There are various (Fig. 14.29) permutations in terms of coronary artery anatomy, but not all variations predispose to sudden death. Specifically, a coronary origin from the pulmonary

artery and those with coronary arteries running between the great vessels appear most liable to cause sudden cardiac dysrhythmia/death. A similar issue arises in the coronary arteries with a high origin/takeoff on the aorta. These arteries may have an oblique, long, poorly supported, and flexible coronary courses. They are potentially able to twist partially or fully obstruct the coronary vessel, with associated sudden cardiac ischemic consequences. Pragmatically, this author only cites the abnormal coronary anatomy as a specific pathology if all other (cardiac and noncardiac) causes of sudden death have been deemed to have been excluded. In addition, there should ideally be some evidence of myocardial ischemic damage present for these infrequent causes of cardiac ischemia.

The competent autopsy will also search for areas of coronary vasculitis or dissection. These can mimic standard atheromatous disease in terms of end result, but may be localized and relatively small in volume.

Finally, within the context of nonatheromatous disease, for cases of young adults with mild-moderate atheroma and irregular patchy scarring in the myocardium, one should consider illicit drugs. Cocaine, amphetamine, and mephedrone, to name just a few, can cause progressive and significant myocardial damage in this format (probably acting via localized ischemia and microinfarction). They are also often associated with some degree of cardiac hypertrophy – suggesting a chronicity in drug usage. Toxicology is paramount in the exclusion of such possibilities.

Cardiomyopathies and Sudden Death

Cardiomyopathies, as discussed in detail earlier in the book, are fully accepted to be associated with familial/individual sudden deaths, usually from dysrhythmias. In many cases, a good antemortem family/individual history will be accessible, even before examining any case. As with all quality autopsy examination, the appropriate analysis of tissue and widespread (including DNA) sampling is advised. This should permit the accurate diagnosis or confirmation of the following disorders. This is vital given the potential consequences for surviving relatives.

The possibility of *hypertrophic cardiomyopathy* (*HCM*) needs careful consideration of the macroscopic findings (Fig. 14.30) (e.g., asymmetric hypertrophy, valve impact lesions) as well as with examination of multiple histology blocks to examine for myocardial disarray. Gross cases of hypertension can be readily misdiagnosed by the unwary (Fig. 14.31). While the classical HCM case may be overt, the features of disarray can be relatively subtle and patchy. Consequently, it is unrealistic to expect an absolute diagnosis with only a few blocks. Nevertheless, from the histology perspective, it is not unreasonable to expect there to be 5–10% of the myocardial substrate affected, in order for the diagnosis of HCM to be entertained. These histology and macroscopic changes should be supported by other data (family history, genetic analysis, etc.). Pragmatically, it must also be remembered that some cardiac disarray can occur at the interface between the left and right ventricles both anteriorly and posteriorly. This is a natural consequence of ventricular development. Thus, one needs more than just a

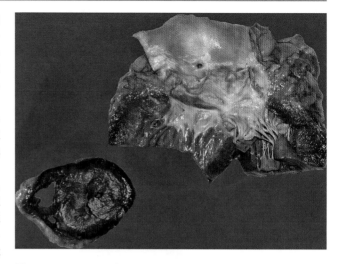

Fig. 14.30 A case of hypertrophic cardiomyopathy (HCM) is seen with slightly asymmetric ventricular hypertrophy which can be easily misinterpreted as hypertensive phenomena. The presence of a septal mitral valve impact lesion is an important clue, although histology and consideration of family history is necessary

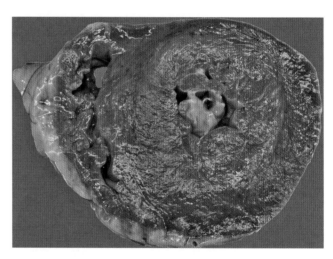

Fig. 14.31 The heart in a case of an adult hypertensive male with poor compliance with his medications. He died suddenly, most probably from a sudden tachyarrhythmia. The hypertrophy should not be confused with hypertrophic cardiomyopathy (HCM)

suspicious phenotype and limited histology (i.e., only one or two blocks) for diagnosis.

Turning to *arrhythmogenic right ventricular cardiomyopathy* (*ARVC*), sometimes designated arrhythmogenic cardiomyopathy (as it is not solely right-sided in layout), one must be balanced in considering the pathology and autopsy evidence. Many cases have been overdiagnosed by the unwary [15]. One appreciates that the degree of fat within the right ventricle may be of variable level, reflecting gender and age [16]. Gross examples of markedly fatty right ventricular tissues are strongly suggestive of ARVC (Fig. 14.32). However, some fat in the right ventricle is normal. Furthermore, prominent fat alone is insufficient for the diagnosis of ARVC

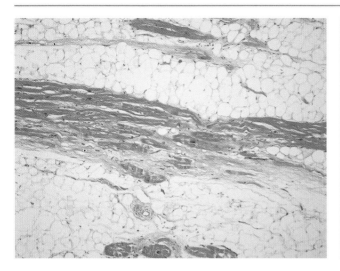

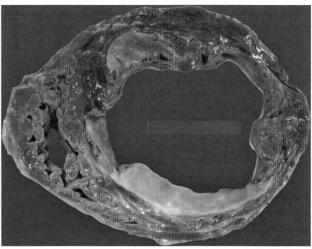

Fig. 14.32 A section from the right ventricle free wall of a young adult female who died suddenly. The fatty tissue replacement is marked, and the associated fibrous element points clearly towards ARVC

Fig. 14.34 A grossly dilated heart (bar marker 40 mm) from a case of ischemic heart disease, with associated cardiac failure. Despite careful macroscopic, histological, and other investigation, many cases of dilated cardiomyopathy (DCM) have no etiological clues – being designated DCM, not otherwise specified

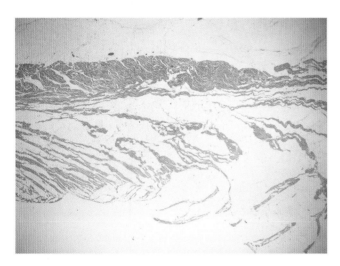

Fig. 14.33 Right ventricle view with fatty parenchyma in an elderly female who died from noncardiac disease. This moderately fatty architecture, without fibrosis, should not be misinterpreted as arrhythmogenic right ventricular cardiomyopathy (ARVC)

(Fig. 14.33). One should also be aware of patchy subendocardial-biased fat seen in the ventricular tissues of the very frail elderly patient, the so-called "tabby cat" heart [17]. Ideally, one must search out the centripetal myocyte replacement pattern by fat with associated fibrosis (with variable lymphoid infiltrates) to confirm true cases of ARVC.

Dilated cardiomyopathy (DCM) is often an endpoint [18] for many different inflammatory, degenerative, genetic, and toxic processes (Fig. 14.34). It is clearly a common substrate for terminal cardiac "pump" failure as well as a potent source of cardiac dysrhythmia and thereby sudden cardiac death. In

most cases, the dilated pathology is readily appreciated and confirmed at autopsy. However, beyond this stage, diagnostically specific macroscopic, microscopic, or electron microscopic features may be absent. However, due diligence must be applied to avoid missing a diagnosis of significance, since about 30–40% of dilated cardiomyopathy cases can have some degree of genetic linkage [18, 19]. The possibility of family inheritance with ongoing realities affecting the surviving family must always be considered. So, for cases of DCM in the young (i.e., those less than 40 years) and in those with no apparent etiology, the full range of autopsy investigations (see cardiomyopathy and autopsy sections) is recommended.

Other rare cardiomyopathies [20–22] may be picked up with due diligence in a similar manner. Cases of anthracycline/chemotherapy toxicity, glycogen storage disorders, and so on may be identified by schematic macroscopic, histological, and associated tests – although history and antemortem clinical tests are pertinent. Cases of Fabry's disease (Fig. 14.35), mitochondrial myopathy (Fig. 14.36), can be identified by some pathology tests. Those cases with patchy disease such as amyloidosis and sarcoid (Fig. 14.37) should either have many foci of the disorder evident, or they should have focal pathology involving a vital structure, such as the His bundle [23].

Peripartum cardiomyopathy [24] is a rare condition that, as its name implies, occurs during pregnancy or immediately after delivery. This progressive cardiac debility is poorly understood, but it can have a significant effect. It can be managed medically but unfortunately some cases do present with sudden cardiac death. There are no specific pathological features, but clearly, the pregnancy and antemortem data will provide the diagnostic setting, thereby permitting the diagnosis.

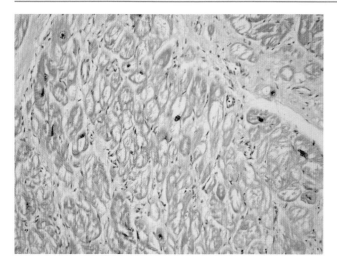

Fig. 14.35 A case of Fabry's disease is demonstrated with the characteristic vacuolated myocytes (hematoxylin and eosin)

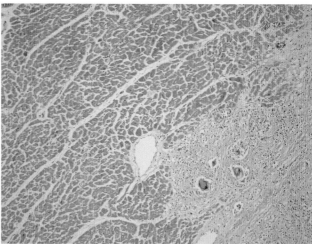

Fig. 14.37 A case of sudden death with foci of granulomatous inflammation containing giant cells in a patient, subsequently designated sarcoid (hematoxylin and eosin)

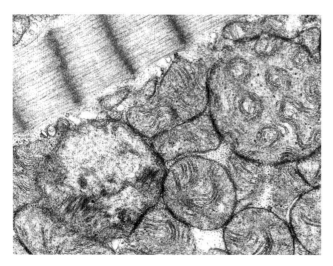

Fig. 14.36 Ultrastructural evidence of a mitochondrial myopathy is seen with atypical forms of mitochondria. This diagnosis should serve to prompt genetic testing in affected families

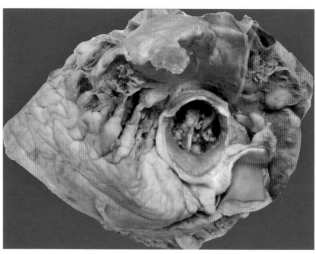

Fig. 14.38 A case of sudden death in an unrecognized bicuspid aortic valve disease. The nodular calcification of the valve is seen from above

Sudden Death due to Valve Disease

Valvular disease, in variable format and degree, is a common finding in the autopsy room when considering sudden death cases. The valve disorders are discussed in detail earlier in this book. However, some basic considerations must exist, if one is not to overinterpret valvular findings in the context of sudden death. As previously discussed, it is prudent to take advantage of any antemortem clinical or imaging data as a support for valve pathology being of significance.

Aortic stenosis (Fig. 14.38) is well known to be associated with sudden death. It also is closely linked to significant coronary artery atheroma, indicating a similar underlying pathophysiology. To accept the diagnosis of aortic stenosis

as relevant to sudden death, one should need to see tight stenosis (crudely, the inability to permit passage of a small finger through the valve orifice). This is generally associated with left ventricle hypertrophy. The valve stenosis strains the heart and also limits coronary artery blood delivery. Associated coronary atheroma heightens the likelihood of association with sudden death, as a consequence of myocardial ischemia.

Aortic valve regurgitation/incompetence may also be related to sudden deaths, although chamber dilatation and muscle wall remodeling would be reasonable additional requirements for this pathology to be invoked. Likewise, mitral valve stenosis or mixed mitral valve disease needs to have associated cardiac chamber remodeling or other

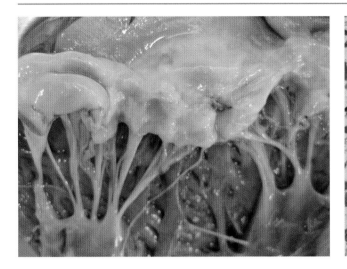

Fig. 14.39 A floppy myocardial valve seen in opened format. Ideally, if this is suspected, then opening the ventricular chamber and trying to inflate the ventricle to confirm regurgitation can be of benefit, although this is a fiddly process. Histology is of use in cases highlighting the mucoid/myxoid matrix changes to the fibrosa

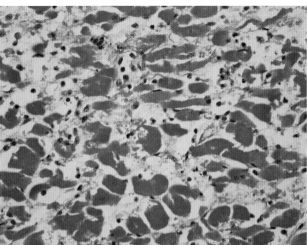

Fig. 14.40 A case of myocarditis is seen with patchy myocyte destruction with associated edema and an inflammatory reaction. Moderate numbers of eosinophils are noted (hematoxylin and eosin)

alterations to allow the valve pathology to be seen as significant. Correlation against antemortem clinical and imaging data is advised.

The diagnosis of sudden death due to mitral valve prolapse (Fig. 14.39) is a diagnosis of exclusion. This is mostly in the form of "floppy" valve tissues and is statistically associated with sudden death. A thorough cardiac and general autopsy is required along with exclusion of alternate realities. Evidence of prolapsing tissue (e.g., balloon change, jet lesions) may support the diagnosis of mitral valve prolapse. However, since this valvular prolapse is a chronic condition, it is unclear what provokes the sudden death on the day in question. Presumably this reflects a tachyarrhythmia, but there may be other factors acting in combination for such individuals. A pragmatic approach to diagnosing this condition requires the good general autopsy, thorough heart examination, and very careful consideration of the valvular tissue substrate. In young persons, the possibility of underlying inherited connective tissue disorders needs to be considered. Photography of the tissues and review of any clinical record data is of particular value when reviewing these cases.

Triscuspid and pulmonary valve pathologies are relatively rare in terms of sudden deaths. They are also not usually seen as the sole drivers of adult sudden death, unless they are part of a multivalve process (e.g., rheumatic valve disease). In children and adolescents, the pathology affecting these valves is more commonly congenital in nature. Consequently, attention to autopsy valve architecture is always important. Subtle congenital valvular heart disease can be readily overlooked and/or may also be part of a more complex heart disease complex.

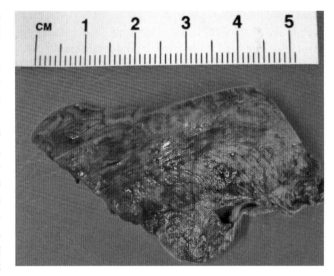

Fig. 14.41 Even though only a small piece of left ventricle was photographed, the myocardial tissue is clearly abnormal with edema, fibrosis, and variable congestion. This was a case of florid viral myocarditis

Myocarditis and Sudden Death

Myocarditis is a potent cause of sudden death, as has been described in an earlier chapter. The key issue in these cases of sudden death involves the pathological confirmation of the disorder, ideally with the cause being defined (Fig. 14.40).

Careful case dissection and appropriate sampling for microbiology, polymerase chain reaction (PCR) testing, and other related tests is necessary as discussed in the myocarditis chapter. The blatant case (Fig. 14.41) is often easy to identify, even if only a few blocks are taken, and analysis of

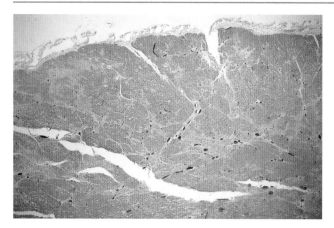

Fig. 14.42 The left ventricle in a case of previous myocarditis can be seen to have marked fibrosis (*green stained matrix*) mapping to the antemortem data of progressive cardiac failure (Masson's trichrome)

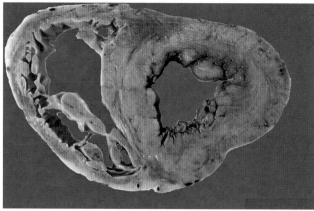

Fig. 14.43 The macroscopic transverse ventricle view of the case of Brugada syndrome showing some dilatation of the chambers but no histological clues. Bar marker 3 cm

the inflammatory cell density will allow confirmation of the diagnosis. However, many of the uncertainties in the diagnosis of myocarditis reflect a few common themes.

The tertiary center case reviews often include those cases with limited sampling and a few lymphoid cells being seen in the histology. Pragmatically, one should search for associated clinical history (recent viral-type illness, myocarditis symptoms/clinical evidence of cardiac failure) along with features of histological myocyte degeneration. Evidence of lymphoid attrition (in appropriate numbers) of myocytes is clearly supportive of myocarditis. However, a few lymphoid cells in an autopsy heart section without myocyte degeneration are a common finding, and these are readily seen in tissues of those dying of noncardiac disease. Nevertheless, there are also cases with scanty lymphocytes in association with patchy microscopic fibrosis (Fig. 14.42). These might reflect prior episodes of myocarditis (partially/ largely resolved), and these findings may also be the only clues for myocarditis-induced DCM. However, as has been described, some "recreational" drugs can cause patchy scarring in relation to focal ischemic phenomena, with these phenomena resulting in minor inflammatory consequences, that can be misinterpreted as resolving myocarditis. Thus, caution is needed before accepting any diagnosis of resolving myocarditis, and corroborative data also needs to be captured.

Channelopathies and the Long QT Syndrome (LQTS)

Sudden dysrhythmic deaths are well recognized. While many of these are reflective of underlying structural cardiac disease (e.g., valvular, ischemic heart disease), a percentage of these deaths have been identified within family kindreds. The initial realization that molecular disease was involved

grew from genetic/inheritance studies of some affected families with young age sudden deaths (Fig. 14.43). Those dying often had nonspecific findings or had an entirely normal study at autopsy (i.e., no structural, histological, ultrastructural lesion). These have been termed sudden adult dysrhythmic deaths (SADS) by some. The fact that some cases had altered antemortem ECG profiles (see Fig. 14.2), in particular prolonged QT intervals on the ECG, suggested problems in terms of cellular ion flux, and this allowed in the last 20 years the identification of a whole class of molecular pathologies [25–30].

Looking at the ventricular depolarization wave (see also chapter on cardiac physiology and electrophysiology) as a substrate for this disorder, it is clear that one can consider the depolarization potential and map it to different ion gate genes that have been identified [25, 26, 30]. The genes responsible relate to membrane-located ion gates, also known as pores or channels. These channels can allow high rate of electrolyte ions to transit and are responsible for the rapid changes in cell membrane potential with activation/ inactivation in a sequential fashion. It appears that the majority of LQTS cases are inherited in autosomal dominant fashion [25, 26, 30], but spontaneous mutations do occur and there are also some infrequent autosomal recessive inheritance patterns.

The sodium and calcium channels each comprise single large proteins. These are folded to span the cell membrane providing a central core through which the ions can variably flux. The opening and closing of the gate is controlled by the local electrical potential, explaining the opening (activation) and closing (inactivation) in a sequenced/timely manner. The potassium channels comprise multimer proteins which combine to make up a structurally similar ion channel. Consequently, more permutations of potassium channels are possible, compared with sodium channels. LQTS cases were seen initially to reflect a gain in function from sodium gates

Table 14.1 The channelopathies

Subtype	Gene	Ion current		Function change	Freq	Locus
LQT1	KCNQ1, KvLQT1	I	Ks	Loss	30–35%	11p15.5
LQT2	KCNH2, HERG	I	Kr	Loss	25–30%	7q35–36
LQT3	SCN5A	I	Na	Gain	5–10%	3p21–24
LQT4	ANKB, ANK2		Affects Na, K, Ca exchange	Loss	1–2%	4q25–27
LQT5	minK, IsK, KCNE1	I	Ks	Loss	1%	21q22.1–2
LQT6	MiRP1, KCNE2	I	Kr	Loss	Rare	21q22.1–2
LQT7	Kir2.1, KCNJ2	I	K1	Loss	Rare	17q23
LQT8	CACNA1C	I	Ca,L	Gain	Rare	12p13.3
LQT9	CAV3	I	Na	Gain	Rare	3p25
LQT10	SCBbeta4	I	Na	Gain	Rare	11q23

Summarized from Genet Med 2006:8;143–55 and http://www.geneticheartdisease.org/lqts_physician.htm

or a loss in function from potassium gates [27–29] although other effects have been described.

There are a variety of gene defects now recognized (Table 14.1) incorporating those with the deletions, frame shifts, etc. In addition, there are some specific familial syndromes associated with sensorineural deafness (Jervill and Lange-Nielsen syndromes) [27]. These tend to be autosomal dominant inherited. In addition, some appear to have multi-system functionality (Anderson's syndrome) [27] where there is a prolonged QT interval, periodic paralysis, and dysmorphogenetic events – the latter item indicating that these genes are involved in organ development. It has subsequently been realized that LQTS effect can also be potentiated/inhibited by drugs [31] and other factors that change the cardiac myocyte electrophysiological status. These other factors include background ischemic heart disease, hyperthermia, hypothyroidism, subarachnoid hemorrhage, exercise, emotional stress, and even auditory stimuli while asleep (especially in LQTS 3) to name but a few.

Approximately two thirds of LQTS cases have defects in LQTS genes 1–3 (see Table 14.1). There does overall appear to be some difference in the prevalence of these genetic lesions with some variation within racial groups – explaining the differing geographic densities across the globe. In addition, the functionality of the gene defects can vary with both age and sex, perhaps explaining the ages of presentation [27].

This chapter does not have time to consider in detail the stages of the ion gating sequences and associated genetic lesions, but being aware of where the genes interact with the cell depolarization potential explains how these genetic lesions prolong the plateau phase of the ventricular cell action potential and thereby introduce a risk of early after-depolarization. This electrical pathology ultimately can allow simultaneous depolarization and repolarization of focal areas of myocardium, promote a cyclical ineffective depolarization in the form of torsades de pointes (TdP) or ventricular fibrillation (VF).

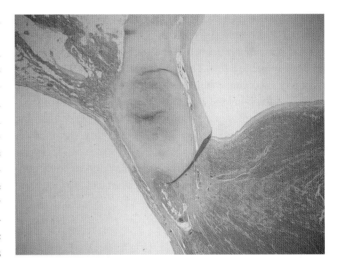

Fig. 14.44 The His bundle in this case of sudden death had a zone of chondroid tissue, although there was some moderate coronary disease also present. The significance of this finding is unclear, unless there is good antemortem clinical and ECG information pointing to nodal conduction problems

Other Diseases with Altered or Impaired Cardiac Conduction

Some cases of sudden death reflect common pathologies (infarction, amyloid, myocarditis, etc.), but a small number may be the consequence of abnormal tracts of tissue, usually of developmental origin [1, 2]. If one regularly samples the recognized common conduction pathways, then a variety of unusual pathologies may be found. Various metaplasias, such as fat, chondroid tissue, and infiltrates, may be found in the His bundle, for example (Fig. 14.44). They are potentially of significance but, to unequivocally include these items as the cause of death, there really needs to be antemortem ECG supportive data.

Structural abnormal cardiac conduction pathways may also be the cause of sudden death. They are subdivided according to the sites of aberrant muscle fascicles and are often defined antemortem along the lines of the ECG abnormalities that accompany the lesions. A good example would be Woolf-Parkinson-White syndrome (Fig. 14.45) with its delta wave ECG pattern. Rarely, such conduction pathways can be histologically sampled, particularly if electrophysiological mapping/consideration has taken place antemortem to ideally indicate the likely position of the lesion.

Thrombotic Thrombocytopenic Purpura

Thrombotic thrombocytopenic purpura [32] (also known as thrombotic microangiopathy) is characterized by small vessel occlusion by platelets and fibrin (Fig. 14.46). The precise trigger for this process is not clear, but the condition is recognized to complicate pregnancy, HIV infection, various neoplasms, some connective tissue disease, and sickle cell disease, to name a few. The coagulopathic process can affect a variety of organ/systems but characteristically affects the heart and explains the link to sudden death. The disorder is often only diagnosed at autopsy, but if recognized while the patient is alive, then there is the possibility for medical treatment.

Macroscopically at autopsy, there may appear to be generalized congestive features on the heart cut surface with

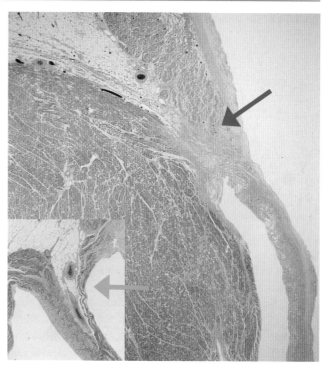

Fig. 14.45 Masson's trichrome composite image showing the normal separation (*blue arrow*) of the atrial and ventricular tissue on the lateral border of the heart. The *inset* (*low left*, hematoxylin and eosin) shows a wispy fiber connection running between the atrial and ventricular tissues in a case of Woolf-Parkinson-White syndrome (*green arrow*)

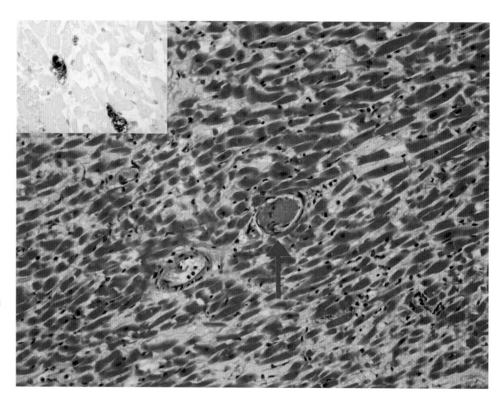

Fig. 14.46 Histological view (hematoxylin and eosin) in a case of thrombotic thrombocytopenic purpura showing small vessel occlusion by platelets (*arrowed*). The inset view (*top left*) demonstrates positive staining by CD61 platelet immunohistology

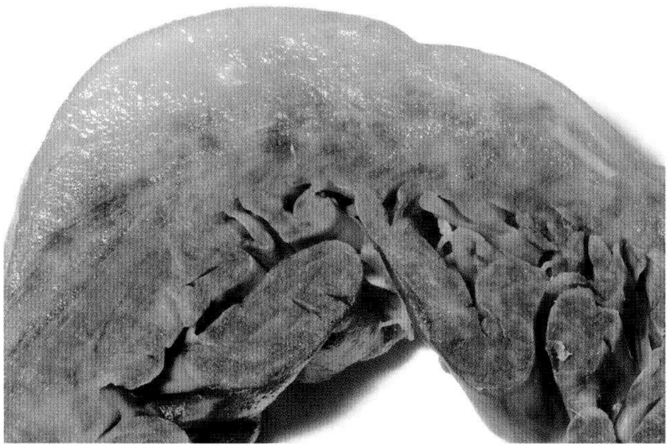

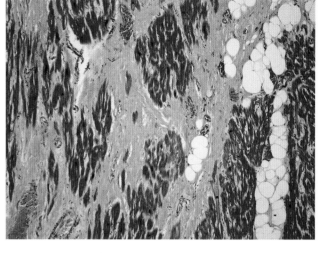

Fig. 14.47 A case of thrombotic thrombocytopenic purpura shows some variable hemorrhagic and congestive features macroscopically (Courtesy of Dr RD Start)

Fig. 14.48 Fibrous and fatty tissue replacement in a case of Duchenne's muscular dystrophy (Masson's trichrome)

petechial hemorrhages (Fig. 14.47). Histologically, the microthrombi are seen in the small blood vessels within the myocardial tissue. Other sites (brain, kidneys, etc.) can also be similarly affected. The histological thrombotic lesions can be highlighted with PAS histology but are best seen with platelet (CD61) immunohistochemistry (see Fig. 14.47). Given that the changes may be associated with local contraction band necrosis of myocytes, it appears reasonable to infer that microscopic infarction is taking place as part of this condition and that this process involves ischemia of the heart.

Obesity

The designation of clinically significant obesity, from a cardiac perspective specifically, is somewhat open to debate. However, individuals with a body mass index (BMI) in excess of 35–40 appear to have particular problems and may present with sudden cardiac death. Population statistics demonstrate that obesity is associated with an increased risk of early cardiovascular demise prompting some interest in the hearts of the obese [33, 34].

The reasons for this increased death rate are complicated but probably reflect a variety of different drivers. Firstly, the increased body mass will demand a higher workload from the heart per unit time – which may strain the heart. The cardiac mass of obese individuals also appears to be elevated, and this factor appears also to act independently, as a risk for sudden cardiac death.

Secondly, the heart in the obese is commonly diseased (usually with ischemic features). Certainly, the obese have an increased risk for ischemic heart disease probably as a consequence of their diabetes-like metabolic profile.

Thirdly, it is noted that there is some prolongation of QT interval within the obese population. It should not be forgotten that if the obese individual is undertaking a significant weight reduction diet, then fluctuations in some serum electrolytes and other biochemical factors may promote any dysrhythmic tendency for the patient. This metabolic status may be complicated by altered glucose handling, ketone production, and so on. Overall, these factors may adversely affect cardiac contractility and electrical conduction.

Finally, outside of the heart itself, the mass effect of the body itself may splint chest wall movement and limit oxygen delivery to the heart. There may also be other noncardiac compounding issues such as obstructive sleep apnea to be considered.

Muscular Dystrophies and Related Disorders

While many patients with a variety of muscular dystrophies [1, 2] die from noncardiac causes, such as terminal chest sepsis, there does appear to be a cohort within this broad group of patients who suffer sudden cardiac death at a relatively early age. A variety of histological changes have been reported in these conditions, including fibrous and fatty tissue replacement (Fig. 14.48) of muscular wall tissues for the ventricles and some similar changes within cardiac conduction. Classic disorders associated with sudden death include myotonic dystrophy (Steinert's disease) and Duchenne-type muscular dystrophy. It is not unreasonable to propose that the fibrous tissue with/or without fatty replacement of myocardial tissue produces problems for cardiac conduction and the risk for reentrant dysrhythmias. Some histological review of skeletal muscle is advised alongside autopsy cardiac tissue analysis in young adults with putative/proven muscular dystrophies.

Stress

Stress is a normal component of everyday life. It is appreciated as something that can vary cardiac work. Stress can be normal (i.e., physiological) or pathological. An example of physiological stress might be the regular exercise of a child, with this being maintained into adulthood as part of a healthy lifestyle. In general terms, if one has a normal coronary artery tree and myocardium, then the variable and routine stress should not adversely affect the individual. Indeed, it probably assists normal growth and development. By contrast, pathological stress is that which is capable of causing some degradation in cardiac status/function with adverse consequences for the individual concerned. This situation characteristically reflects an individual with a diseased heart.

In general terms (whether physiological/pathological), stress applied to the heart results in an increased rate of contraction and an increased force of contraction, thereby delivering more blood into the circulation per unit time (i.e., increased cardiac output). This reflects evolutionary realities whereby stress was necessarily linked to increased heart activity, as a reflex response to assist survival of the individual.

Stress can be acute or chronic in quality. Chronic stress is generally believed to be generally bad for cardiovascular health, presumably acting via hormonal and autonomic nervous system influences with mainly arterial/cardiovascular consequences. Chronic stress has been associated with arteriosclerosis, atheromatous disease, hypertension, and so on. Defining the impact of chronic stress on the heart and vascular system is fraught with difficulties. However, chronic stress is not usually invoked as part of the cause of death statement but rather features as the pathology consequences, namely, an acute coronary syndrome, cerebral bleed, etc.

By contrast, acute stress does appear to be associated with sudden death but is often a complex item to analyze as a component of the death of the individual [35–39]. Indeed, it is often difficult to prove this association as the chronological linkage may be complex, and the endpoint disease (e.g., acute myocardial infarction) is a natural event. However, the situation commonly encountered by pathologists is that of an individual with significant cardiac disease (e.g., unrecognized or medically controlled cardiomyopathy, ischemic heart disease, myocarditis, etc.) who has died suddenly, shortly after an acute stress.

When considering acute stress, one must appreciate that such stresses can be subdivided into endogenous and exogenous types. Endogenous stresses are generated from within the individual and may reflect a variety of situations – such as the emotional consequences after the death of a close relative. By contrast, exogenous stresses generally revolve around the "fright, flight, fight" reflex responses for the individual, caused by external factors. In simple terms, fright reflects an externally derived psychological stress to the individual, flight involves significant physical activity such as running, and fight involves the preparation/participation to an actual or perceived physical threat. All the fright, flight, and fight responses can interplay, with autonomic, neurohumoral, and higher cerebral processing of any perceived stress.

As stated, a fit and healthy person should cope adequately with normal daily stresses. However, for an individual with established cardiac disease, the cardiac reserve available to deliver an increased workload may be limited. Consequently, a sudden stress, requiring increased heart workload, may exceed the physiological tolerances for the heart and could result in acute cardiac decompensation and/or sudden death. The stressful situation can be compounded by changes in the individual's bloodstream with altered hormone levels and some variation in serum electrolytes even after the stress has receded [40–42]. These stressful events may also cause altered plaque stability with local thrombosis as a direct physical hemodynamic consequence.

It is therefore not surprising to find that an individual with cardiac disease, who has suddenly been required to deliver significant cardiac activity, dying suddenly. In this situation, one may not normally be concerned with the stressor event, as the disease can be regarded as natural in quality. For example, an elderly male with significant ischemic heart disease is found dead after struggling through a blizzard or after a period of shoveling snow [43]. This case will often simply be regarded as death due to ischemic heart disease.

By contrast, an alternative interpretation can be applied if the same elderly male (with ischemic heart disease) is suddenly confronted with an "unusual" stressful event. An example might be:

- Suddenly finding himself caught up in an armed robbery (fright)
- Attempting to run away from the robbery (flight)
- Becoming involved in a physical altercation with the robber (fight)

This elderly man with established heart disease may find that his cardiac reserve is rapidly exceeded and sudden death ensues. In this situation, the stress can be argued to be pathological. This consideration may be applied as armed robbery is deemed not part of a "normal" life and secondly, because it may be a pivotal (and criminal in this case) factor in the cause of death – interacting directly with the established ischemic heart disease. This scenario and similar situations commonly produce particular problems for pathologists, the police, and the legal profession. Each case is unique in quality and there is no easy way to control/test for the stressful event/s.

From a pragmatic perspective, when faced with such cases, it is perhaps best to commence by analyzing the individual and the underlying disease. Let us use the above ischemic heart disease example (although clearly similar arguments can apply to other cardiac disorders). This hypothetical example (designated case A) has a history of previous infarction and chronic angina of episodic quality. The individual has been able to live for many years in his own accommodation with some community supportive care. It can be argued that the ischemic heart disease here is stable, since the chronic ischemic heart disease reality has existed for some time before and since this individual was alive the day before the stressful event is applied, the week beforehand, and indeed many months before the stress. Indeed, the very stability of the ischemic heart disease is the key feature. While there is a chance of death on any day, this is seen as low – since the disease is apparently stable. Thus, it may be argued that the individual is no more likely to die on the day in question, as compared with any time in the recent past because his realities are not changing.

Next, we consider the sudden stress of the robbery. The introduction of this unexpected stressful event is now seen as changing the underlying cardiovascular dynamics (raised blood pressure, increased heart rate, altered oxygen requirements systemically). Thus, one moves from a low possibility of death, to that of a likelihood (heightened probability) of death – as cardiovascular tolerances are rapidly exceeded in the scenario given.

Conversely, let us now consider an individual with established ischemic heart disease with progressive cardiac failure (designated case B). This man has had increasingly severe angina attacks, progressively declining general debility and increasing care requirements. Now the argument will be applied that the death of the individual could be, as likely to reflect progressive cardiac disease realities, as that of the applied stress (i.e., the robbery).

Irrespective of whether the pathologist, the witnesses, and/or the relatives believe the stress is implicated in the death of cases A and B, the law courts have a different reality to consider. Indeed, it may well be that a court of law will be unable to prove that a (criminal/pathological) stress *can be proven* to be implicated in the death of case B but might accept linkage for case A. In short, the burden of proof for implicating a pathological stress clearly has to be seen as *having materially and substantially changed the individual's chances of surviving the day in question as a direct result/consequence of the stress*. To assist matters, the reverse consideration can be applied, wherein the following question is asked: *had the stress **not** been applied, would this individual have likely survived the day in question*? If one cannot unequivocally answer yes to this second question, then it is very unlikely that medicolegal proceedings will come to a conclusion that the stress has been proven as linked to the cause of death.

Finally, on this matter, the medicolegal realities of considering such stressful events as the cause of sudden cardiac death are complicated by aspects of law that vary across countries and continents, as well as the very unique scenarios and medical realities for the cases concerned.

Cardiac Surgery

It is inevitable that some degree of cardiac tissue reaction, or indeed damage, will occur as a consequence of all endovascular or open operation cardiac interventions. While such medical interventions are generally delivered with the aim, and indeed statistical probability, of improving the prognosis for the individual and curing symptoms, it has to be understood that no procedure is ever without risk of morbidity and/or mortality.

Given that the underlying heart is often constrained by some disease/pathology, it follows that a percentage of patients will not survive cardiac interventions. Some may die acutely during the intervention or in the immediate postoperative period. It is difficult to subdivide the effects of the surgery, the intervention, and other factors (changed electrolytes, stress hormones, altered clotting realities, etc.) in absolute terms. However, one should be aware that sudden death after cardiac surgery is not an uncommon endpoint for a percentage of patients. In most cases, this reflects the underlying cardiac disease, but a careful examination [44, 45] should be made to exclude surgical mishap or a specific pathology complication from the procedure (Fig. 14.49).

There is also another issue to be addressed in those patients with operated (grown-up) congenital heart disease (GUCH). Even with quality surgery nowadays being offered to children and adults with congenital heart disease, many individuals with apparently successful outcomes (in relation to their congenital lesion) appear to die suddenly between 30 and 50 years age (Fig. 14.50). Many have no overt provocation/etiology on the day in question – suggesting chronic heart disease-induced dysrhythmia.

Commotio Cordis

Direct, sudden, and significant blunt force applied to the chest can produce either chest compressive injury or simply a thoracic deformation that acts momentarily on the heart with cardiac standstill as a result. This process, often described as "commotio cordis," can really only be a diagnosis of exclusion – where all other cardiac, and other noncardiac, pathologies have been excluded [46]. It is difficult to introduce such a diagnosis when there is recognized cardiac disease. However, there are well-described cases where blunt force trauma to the chest, applied suddenly, has resulted in sudden death of a young, previously fit, and apparently healthy individual.

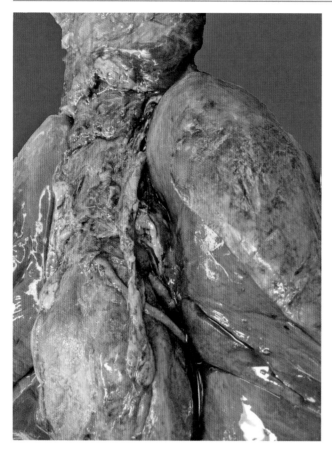

Fig. 14.49 Cases of death after cardiac bypass surgery need careful macroscopic and histological examination of vascular grafts. This case (*left oblique view*) shows the normal alignment of the left internal mammary graft and vein graft

An Approach to Assigning the Pathology to the Cause of Death

All of the above data demonstrates the complexity of considering cases of sudden death. This chapter author tries to balance the cardiac pathologies identified against a likelihood of the pathology, fully explaining the sudden death in the following schematic manner:

Very likely to have caused sudden cardiac death:

- Well-defined macroscopic/histological acute myocardial infarction
- Cardiac tamponade, due to infarct-related mural rupture or coronary artery dissection
- Root of the aorta dissection into pericardial sac/ mediastinum
- High-grade (tight) significant coronary artery stenosis (>95% stenosis)
- Tight aortic valve stenosis, often with left ventricle hypertrophy (+/−coronary artery disease)

Probably explaining the sudden death:

- High-grade atheromatous coronary disease (>70% stenosis) with, or sometimes without, myocardial ischemic changes
- Defined cardiomyopathy (e.g., HCM, ARVC, DCM)
- Muscular dystrophy (known history) with histological myocardial alterations
- Myocarditis (with myocyte degeneration)
- Known (or later confirmed) channelopathy
- Significant (i.e., widespread) amyloid deposition
- Widespread granulomatous inflammatory foci, in keeping with sarcoid

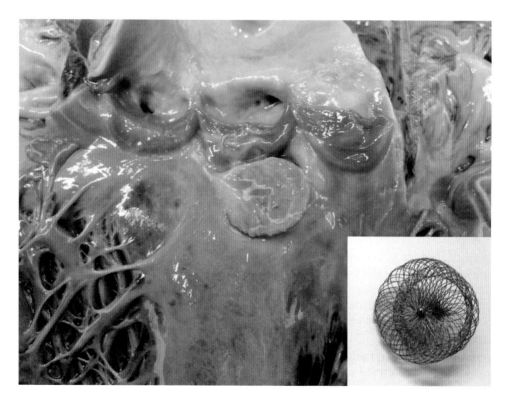

Fig. 14.50 The site of previous endovascular device closure of a ventricular septal defect (VSD) is seen in a young female. This case involved late diagnosis of the high-grade shunt across the VSD. There was significant pulmonary hypertension and despite the closure of the defect, the patient died suddenly a few years later

Possibly has caused the sudden death (*providing no significant other pathology*):

- Myocardial fibrosis, in keeping with prior infarction but without acute changes (this would require appreciable coronary atheroma to be present)
- Floppy mitral valve (supported by ballooning, atrial dilatation, jet lesions, etc.)
- Coronary artery anomaly (ideally with some myocardial ischemic evidence)
- Moderate coronary atheroma (40–60% stenosis) but would require need cardiac hypertrophy and/or old infarction scarring in the heart to substantiate

Having sorted this broad "batting order" of probability in one's mind, the converse question needs to be addressed: "what is inappropriate to list as a cardiac cause of sudden death?" This can conceivably cover virtually everything else, but problems that are regularly debated at autopsy include the following:

- Minor histological patchy fibrosis of the myocardium (i.e., without appreciable coronary disease or other antecedent ECG or clinical history, etc.)
- Minor cardiac hypertrophy alone (no more than 10% greater than the expected cardiac mass)
- Coronary calcification without significant narrowing (<40% stenosis)
- Serous pericardial effusion of less than 50 ml (unless there is antemortem evidence of tamponade/constrictive pericarditis)

This author does not recommend the above four pathological possibilities to be cited as the cause of sudden cardiac death, but as those practicing in this field are aware, each case must be considered and viewed on its own merits.

Final Comments

The pathology listing in this chapter is by no means total or exhaustive. There are many other lesions and pathologies, some infrequent and some very rare, which need to be considered on occasion. The case history and circumstances may guide one in this regard and focus investigations. However, all such investigations and considerations must be individually tailored to the case in question, where death is unexpected, sudden, or unusual.

References

1. Thiene G, Basso C, Corrado D. Cardiovascular causes of sudden death. In: Silver MD, Gotlieb AI, Schoen FJ, editors. Cardiovascular pathology. 3rd ed. New York: Churchill Livingstone; 2001. p. 326–74.
2. Virmani R, Burke A, Farb A, Atkinson JB. Sudden cardiac death. In: Cardiovascular pathology. 2nd ed. Philadelphia: WB Saunders; 2001. p. 340–85.
3. Soilleux EJ, Burke MM. Pathology and investigation of potentially hereditary sudden cardiac death syndrome in structurally normal hearts. Diagnostic Histopathology. 2009;15:1–26.
4. Basso C, Burke M, Fornes P, Gallagher PJ, de Gouveia Henriques R, Sheppard M, Thiene G, van der Wal A. Guidelines for autopsy investigation of sudden cardiac death. Vichow's Archiv. 2008; 452:11–8.
5. Kannel W, Thomas H. Sudden coronary death: the Framingham study. Ann N Y Acad Sci. 1982;382:3–21.
6. Basso C, Corrado D, Thiene G. Cardiovascular causes of sudden death in young individuals including athletes. Cardiol Rev. 1999;7: 127–35.
7. Bowker TJ, Wood DA, Davies MJ, Sheppard MN, Cary NR, Burton DJ, et al. Sudden, unexpected cardiac or unexplained death in England: a national survey. QJM. 2003;96(4):269–79.
8. 2005 Mortality statistics: cause (England and Wales) Health Stat Q 2007;89–92.
9. Maron BJ, Shirani J, Poliac LC. Sudden death in young competitive athletes. Clinical, demographic, and pathological profiles. JAMA. 1996;276:199–204.
10. Lucas S, Corbishley C, Leadbetter S, MacKenzie J, Moore I, Start R. The Royal College of Pathologists Working Party on the autopsy. Guidelines on autopsy practice- Scenario 1: Sudden death with likely cardiac disease. 2005. London: Royal College of Pathologists. www.rcpath.org/resources/pdf/AutopsyScenario1Jan05.pdf
11. Rutty GN, Burton JL. The hospital autopsy, 3rd edn. In: Burton JL, Rutty GN, editors. London: Arnold; 2010.
12. Davies MJ. Coronary artery remodelling and the assessment of stenosis by pathologists. Histopathology. 1998;33:497–500.
13. Davies MJ. Coronary disease – the pathophysiology of acute coronary syndromes. Heart. 2000;83:361–6.
14. Coroner's courts. A guide to law and practice (2nd edn). Dorries, CP. Oxford University Press; 2004.
15. Fletcher A, Ho SY, McCarthy KP. Sheppard MN. Spectrum of pathological changes in both ventricles of patients dying suddenly with arrhythmogenic right ventricular dysplasia. Relation of changes to age. Histopathology. 2006;48(4):445–52.
16. Tansey DK, Aly Z, Sheppard MN. Fat in the right ventricle of the normal heart. Histopathology. 2005;46:98–104.
17. Farrer-Brown G, Wolfe Medical Publications Ltd, 1982, p126, image 333.
18. Jefferies JL, Towbin JA. Dilated cardiomyopathy. Lancet. 2010;375(9716):752–62.
19. Fatkin D, MacRae C, Sasaki T, et al. Missense mutations in the rod domain of the lamin A/C gene as causes of dilated cardiomyopathy and conduction-system disease. N Engl J Med. 1999;341: 1715–24.
20. Kabbani SS, LeWinter MM. Diastolic heart failure. Constrictive, restrictive, and pericardial. Cardiol Clin. 2000;18(3):501–9; 18(3):501–9.
21. Angelini A, Calzolari V, Thiene G, Boffa GM, Valente M, Daliento L, et al. Morphologic spectrum of primary restrictive cardiomyopathy. Am J Cardiol. 1997;80(8):1046–50.
22. Mogensen J, Arbustini E. Restrictive cardiomyopathy. Curr Opin Cardiol. 2009;24:214–20.
23. Veinot JP, Johnston B. Cardiac sarcoidosis-an occult cause of sudden death: a case report and literature review. J Forensic Sci. 1998;43:715–7.
24. Ramaraj R, Sorrell VL. Peripartum cardiomyopathy: causes, diagnosis, and treatment. Cleve Clin J Med. 2009;76(5):289–96.
25. Schimpf R, Veltmann C, Wolpert C, Borggrefe M. Channelopathies: Brugada syndrome, long QT syndrome, short QT syndrome, and CPVT. Herz. 2009;34:281–8.
26. Kaufman ES. Mechanisms and clinical management of inherited channelopathies: long QT syndrome, Brugada syndrome, catecholaminergic polymorphic ventricular tachycardia, and short QT syndrome. Heart Rhythm. 2009;6:S51–5.

27. Modell SM, Lehmann MH. The long QT syndrome family of cardiac iron channelopathies: a HuGE review. Genet Med. 2006;8: 143–55.

28. Ackerman MJ. Cardiac channelopathies: it's in the genes. Nat Med. 2004;10:463–4.

29. Wang Q, Shen J, Splawski I, Atkinson D, Li Z, Robinson JL, et al. SCN5A mutations associated with an inherited cardiac arrhythmia, long QT syndrome. Cell. 1995;80:805–11.

30. Marban E. Cardiac channelopathies. Nature. 2002;415:213–8.

31. Postema PG, Wolpert C, Amin AS, Probst V, Borggrefe M, Roden DM, Priori SG, Tan HL, Hiraoka M, Brugada J, Wilde AA. Drugs and Brugada syndrome patients: review of the literature, recommendations and an up-to-date website (www.brugadadrugs.org). Heart Rhythm. 2009;6:1335–41.

32. Bell MD, Barnhart Jr JS, Martin JM. Thrombotic thrombocytopenic purpura causing sudden, unexpected death – a series of eight patients. J Forensic Sci. 1990;35:601–13.

33. Lucas SL. Derivation of new reference tables for human heart weights in light of increasing body mass index. J Clin Pathol. 2011;64:279–80.

34. Gaitskell K, Perera R, Soilleux EJ. Derivation of new reference tables for human heart weights in light of increasing body mass index. J Clin Pathol. 2011;64:358–62.

35. Meisel SR, Dayan KI, Pauzner H, Chetboun I, Arbel Y, David D. Kutz I Effect of Iraqi missile war on incidence of acute myocardial infarction and sudden death in Israeli civilians. Lancet. 1991;338: 660–1.

36. Cebelin MS, Hirsch CS. Human stress cardiomyopathy. Myocardial lesions in victims of homicidal assaults without internal injuries. Hum Pathol. 1980;11:123–32.

37. Lecomte D, Fornes P, Nicolas G. Stressful events as a trigger of sudden death. A study of 43 medico-legal autopsy cases. Forensic Sci Int. 1996;79:1–10.

38. Trichopoulos D, Katsouyanni K, Zavitsanos X, et al. Psychological stress and fatal heart attack: the Athens (1981) earthquake natural experiment. Lancet. 1983;26:441–3.

39. Sudden and rapid death during psychological stress. Engel GL. Ann Intern Med. 1971;74:771–83.

40. Young DB, et al. Potassium and catecholamine concentrations in the immediate post exercise period. Am J Med Sci. 1992;304:150–3.

41. Lindinger M. Potassium regulation during exercise and recovery in humans: Implications for skeletal and cardiac muscle. J Mol Cell Cardiol. 1995;27:1011–22.

42. Dimsdale JE, et al. Post exercise peril: plasma catecholamine and exercise. JAMA. 1984;252:630–2.

43. Glass RI, Zack Jr MM. Increase in deaths from ischaemic heart disease after blizzards. Lancet. 1979;1:485–7.

44. Lee AH, Gallagher PJ. Post-mortem examination after cardiac surgery. Histopathology. 1998;33:399–405.

45. Hickling MF, Pontefract DE, Gallagher PJ, Livesey AS. Post mortem examinations after cardiac surgery. Heart. 2007;93:761–5.

46. Madias C, Maron BJ, Weinstock J, Estes NA, Link MS. Commotio cordis – sudden cardiac death after chest wall impact. J Cardiovasc Electrophysiol. 2007;18:115–22.

Index

S.K. Suvarna (ed.), *Cardiac Pathology*,
DOI 10.1007/978-1-4471-2407-8, © Springer-Verlag London 2013